THE SEARCH FOR
NEW ANTICANCER DRUGS

CANCER BIOLOGY AND MEDICINE

Series Editors M. J. Waring and B. A. J. Ponder

THE SEARCH FOR NEW ANTICANCER DRUGS

Edited by

M. J. Waring

Reader in Chemotherapy,
University of Cambridge, UK

and

B. A. J. Ponder

Director, CRC Human Cancer Genetics Research Group,
Department of Pathology,
University of Cambridge, UK

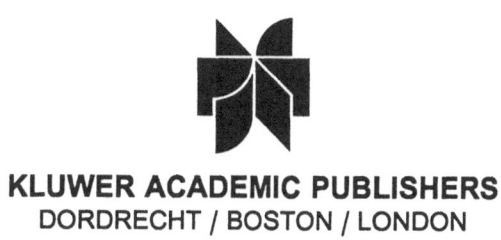

KLUWER ACADEMIC PUBLISHERS
DORDRECHT / BOSTON / LONDON

Distributors

for the United States and Canada: Kluwer Academic Publishers, PO Box 358,
Accord Station, Hingham, MA 02018-0358, USA
for all other countries: Kluwer Academic Publishers Group, Distribution
Center, PO Box 322, 3300 AH Dordrecht, The Netherlands

A catalogue record for this book is available from the British Library
ISBN-13: 978-94-010-6659-4   e-ISBN-13: 978-94-009-0385-2
DOI: 10.1007/978-94-009-0385-2

Library of Congress Cataloging in Publication Data

The Search for new anticancer drugs / edited by M. J. Waring and B. A. J. Ponder.
     p.   cm. — (Cancer biology and medicine; 3)
    Includes bibliographical references and index.

    1. Antineoplastic agents.   2. Cancer—Chemotherapy.   I. Waring, Michael J.
II. Ponder, B. A. J. (Bruce A. J.), 1944– .   III. Series.
    [DNLM: 1. Antineoplastic Agents—therapeutic use. 2. Neoplasms—drug therapy.
W1 CA673L v. 3 / QZ 267 S439]
RC271.C5S39 1992
616.99'4061— dc20
DNLM/DLC
for Library of Congress   92-49744
                                                    CIP

Copyright

Published in the United Kingdom by Kluwer Academic Publishers, PO Box 55,
Lancaster, UK.

Kluwer Academic Publishers BV incorporates the publishing programmes of D. Reidel,
Martinus Nijhoff, Dr W. Junk and MTP Press .

Typeset by Expo Holdings Sdn. Bhd., Malaysia.

Contents

List of Contributors

S. BREM
Division of Neurosurgery
Northwestern Memorial Hospital
233 E. Erie St, Suite 500
Chicago,
IL 60611-2906, USA

W. A. DENNY
Cancer Research Laboratory
University of Auckland
School of Medicine
Private Bag 92019
Auckland, New Zealand

T. -P. D. FAN
Department of Pharmacology
University of Cambridge
Tennis Court Road
Cambridge CB2 1QJ, UK

G. J. FINLAY
Cancer Research Laboratory
University of Auckland
School of Medicine
Private Bag 92019
Auckland, New Zealand

C. HÉLÈNE
Laboratoire de Biophysique
Muséum National d'Histoire Naturelle
43 rue Cuvier
75231 Paris Cedex 05, France

I. R. JUDSON
Drug Development Section
Institute of Cancer Research
Sutton
Surrey SM2 5NG, UK

H. P. KOEFFLER
Division of Hematology/Oncology
UCLA School of Medicine
11-934 Louis Factor, 10833 Le Conte
Los Angeles,
CA 90024-1678, USA

C. A. LAUGHTON
CRC Biomolecular Structure Unit
Institute of Cancer Research
Sutton
Surrey SM2 5NG, UK

J. G. McVIE
Scientific Department
Cancer Research Campaign
Cambridge House
6–10 Cambridge Terrace
Regent's Park
London NW1 4JL, UK

S. NEIDLE
CRC Biomolecular Structure Unit
Institute of Cancer Research
Sutton
Surrey SM2 5NG, UK

E. SAISON-BEHMOARAS
Laboratoire de Biophysique
Muséum National d'Histoire Naturelle
43 rue Cuvier
75231 Paris Cedex 05, France

M. F. G. STEVENS
Cancer Research Laboratories
Department of Pharmaceutical Sciences
University of Nottingham
University Park
Nottingham NG7 2RD, UK

A. TOBLER
Central Hematology Laboratory
University of Bern
Inselspital
CH-3010 Bern, Switzerland

W. R. WILSON
Oncology Section, Pathology Department
University of Auckland School of Medicine
Private Bag 92019
Auckland, New Zealand

Preface

Most of the anticancer drugs in use today were discovered by happy accident rather than design. Much the same might be said of antibiotics and drugs employed for antimicrobial chemotherapy, despite our good appreciation of differences between microbial and mammalian cells plus several decades' worth of scientific work to exploit those differences for clinical gain. Yet the rational design of better anticancer drugs remains a cherished goal, and one of the most important challenges facing medical science.

This book represents a compilation of views and progress reports which illustrate the diversity of the problem. Recent research has confirmed the belief that critical genetic changes are at work in cancer cells. The genome, then, (DNA in biological terms) surely represents a critical target for specific chemotherapy of cancer, and several chapters address the issue of attacking DNA, gene targeting, and the like. Others deal with principles of rational design, exploitation of novel modalities and targets, or the nuts and bolts of antitumour drug testing. While no attempt has been made to provide a comprehensive coverage of this wide-ranging and vitally important subject the editors hope the present volume in the series will provide further food for thought.

M. J. W.
B. A. J. P.
Cambridge, May 1992

1
Is there a future for the small molecule in developmental cancer chemotherapy?

M. F. G. STEVENS

INTRODUCTION

An objective observer tracking the literature relevant to the science of cancer treatment might conclude that all the important questions are now being engendered by advances in molecular biology. Whereas, in the last three decades, mathematicians, physicists and engineers led mankind in an exploration of the solar system, it will, so the molecular biologists argue, be a biology-driven space programme – one targeted at the innermost recesses of the cell itself – which will finally unravel the mysteries of the malignant state. However, even if the new biological revolution generates leaders with the vision of an Einstein or the imagination of an Arthur C. Clarke, it is unlikely that the power of molecular biology alone will give sufficient insights into how the disease might be *cured* even if it is fully understood.

For the foreseeable future, it will be necessary to administer to patients a 'therapeutic product' or, more likely, combination of products to attack the disease. The possibility that a chemist might synthesize, by chance, or extract from natural products, a molecule which cures cancer cannot be dismissed entirely. The history of chemotherapy in general is replete with examples of the serendipitous discovery of small molecules, often natural products, which subsequently acted as molecular probes to unravel biological processes. Penicillin, sulphonamides, chloramphenicol, methotrexate and bleomycin are examples of synthetic and natural product chemotherapeutic agents which were used clinically even before their (biological) modes of action were understood. "Interesting chemistry begets interesting biology", as the foregoing examples illustrate, is a proposition guaranteed to raise the hackles of biologists at any time, any place.

The great Swedish chemist Jöns Jakob Berzelius clearly expected chemistry to solve all ills:

> Of all the sciences contributing to medicine, chemistry is the primary one, and apart from the general light it throws on the entire art of healing, it will soon give some of its branches a perfection such as one could never have anticipated. (Lehrbuch der Chemie, 1808)

Nearly two centuries have elapsed and we still await a worthy claimant to the intellectual property of a cancer cure. What we have learned is that a determined onslaught on the cancer problem by mobilization of a single scientific discipline, however powerful, is unlikely to prevail over what can be achieved by a multidisciplinary effort. Thus, whereas advances in biology will identify the problems that need to be solved, it will be the rigorous techniques of the physico-organic chemist which will provide the breakthroughs in understanding the molecular events underlying aberrant cellular behaviour. At the end of the day, it is likely that the ingenuity of computational and synthetic chemists will be the key to the design and synthesis of small molecules capable of banishing the disease. That, at least, is the theme of this Chapter.

MOLECULAR WEIGHT AND ANTITUMOUR DRUGS

"Small is beautiful"

During the last decade, a diverse range of molecular structures has entered clinical trial: these moieties vary in complexity from tiny hydrazine sulphate containing just six atoms in the active base component with a molecular weight of 32 Da to the multikilobase gene coding for tumour necrosis factor (TNF).

Disciples of Schumacher would derive some comfort from the results of an analysis of the molecular weights of clinically active antitumour drugs conducted in 1988[1]. The data show that, of 44 drugs processed through the National Cancer Institute (NCI) and listed as having activity as single agents, no fewer than 33 were small molecules of less than 400 Da (Figure 1.1). It is

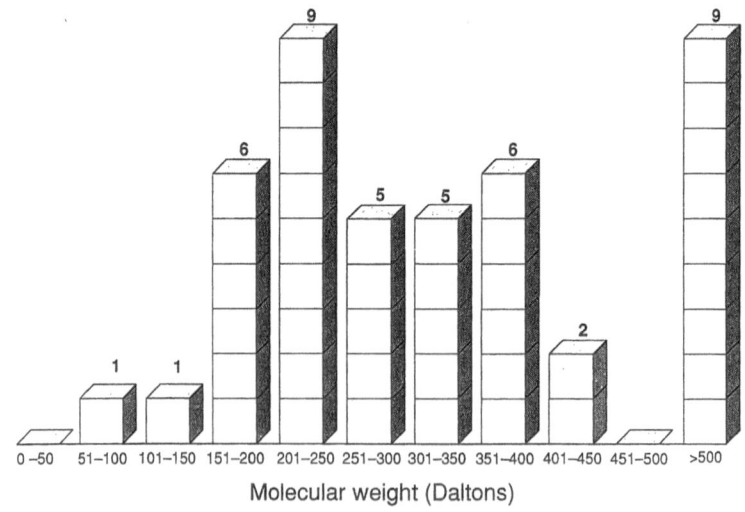

Figure 1.1 Molecular weights of 44 clinically active drugs (source of data, see reference 1)

intriguing to note that nearly one-third of the drugs have molecular weights in the range 200–299 Da. It was Paul Ehrlich in the 19th century who postulated that the ideal chemotherapeutic agent would have a molecular weight of about 250 Da. The larger the molecule, the more complex are likely to be the problems associated with large-scale synthesis, pharmaceutical formulation, and transport and distribution of the drug to its target site. The science and economics of drug development still dictate a strong preference for small molecules.

The highest ranking branded small synthetic drug – ICI's Nolvadex (tamoxifen) (Structure 1; Figure 1.2) is expected to achieve sales of $373 million in 1990 despite strong generic competition[2]. If impending trials on thousands of women at risk of contracting breast cancer identify a prophylactic indication for tamoxifen, the drug would be promoted to the 'block-busting' league. Moreover, prospects for the rational design of small-molecule inhibitors of enzymes involved in steroidogenesis pathways, with potential activity against breast and prostatic cancer, are particularly bright. Gene sequences coding for the enzyme structures have been cloned and expressed. Crystallographic and protein engineering studies will soon yield detailed insights into the structures of the target enzymes.

Small molecules have secured important roles in treating a range of cancer-associated diseases. The use of antibiotics and halogen-substituted nucleosides to treat bacterial and viral infections in immunocompromised patients is well established and life preserving. Infections caused by the opportunistic *Pneumocystis carinii* and Cytomegalovirus are routinely treated with pentamidine isethionate (Structure 2) and ganciclovir (Structure 3) respectively, and there are major research efforts worldwide directed to the discovery of novel agents with improved therapeutic efficacy.

Cancer cachexia, the wasting syndrome associated with the development of solid tumours in humans, has recently attracted attention as a novel biological target for drug intervention[3]. Studies have been facilitated by the identification of a relevant animal model of the syndrome – the MAC16 adenocarcinoma growing in mice[4]. Cachectic factors elaborated by this tumour, which are also present in the urine of cachectic patients bearing solid tumours, may tip the nutritional balance between tumour and host in favour of the tumour. Rational design of antagonists to these cachectic factors must await their structural elucidation but prototype small molecules, like eicosapentaenoic acid (EPA) (Structure 4), a constituent of fish oils, may be able both to reverse the cachexia and to inhibit solid tumour growth[5].

The uses of folinic acid to modulate methotrexate toxicity and mesna to counter the urothelial damage elicited by acrolein liberated in the metabolic activation of cyclophosphamide are well established in clinical practice. Chemoprotection is now an emerging discipline in cancer pharmacology. The thiol derivative, ethiofos (WR-2721) (Structure 5), was originally selected from a series of compounds screened for potential military use as radioprotectors. Preclinical studies[6] have indicated that ethiofos can reduce the mutagenic and carcinogenic action of radiotherapy and chemotherapy and ameliorate the nephro- and oto-toxicity of *cis*-platin. Whether or not this combination will bring greater clinical benefits than the use of the less toxic second-generation platinum agents is disputable even if dose-intensification in regimes including *cis*-platin is achievable.

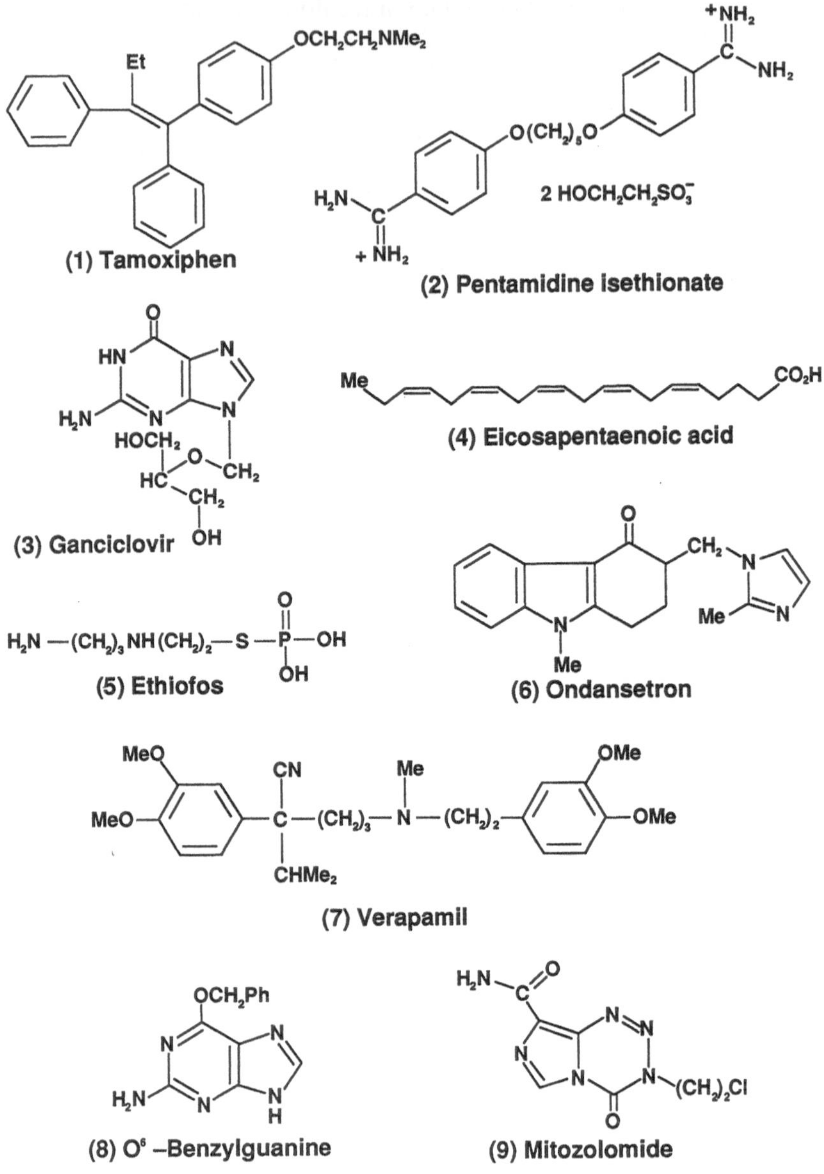

Figure 1.2 Structures (1–9) of small molecules with activity as anticancer agents, or activity in cancer-associated diseases

Nausea and vomiting are pernicious side-effects of many drugs, particularly *cis*-platin and electrophilic alkylating agents. The marketing of Glaxo's Zofran (ondansetron) (Structure 6) in 1990 marks a breakthrough in emesis control and a triumph for good old-fashioned receptor pharmacology and medicinal chemistry. Ondansetron, a simple carbazole derivative with molecular weight 293 Da, can discriminate between the currently identified eight functionally distinct 5-hydroxytryptamine (5-HT) receptors, antagonizing selectively the 5-HT_3 sub-type[7].

Considerable attention is now being devoted to the role of small molecules in modulating the development of resistance in those tumours which express the multi-drug resistance (MDR) phenotype[8]. This pleiotropic resistance is one of the most important and challenging topics in cancer treatment today[9]. Verapamil (Structure 7), a calcium channel blocker, has been used successfully to reduce resistance in B-cell neoplasms and other tumours that express the P-glycoprotein: however, cardiovascular side-effects can be severe[10]. Reports that tamoxifen[11], cyclosporin A[12], and new synthetic 1,4-dihydropyridine derivatives[13] can also modulate resistance in a range of tumour types expressing MDR suggests that a wide variety of molecular structures exhibit this property. A rational search for novel agents could uncover valuable new moieties with the potential to influence the outcome of cancer chemotherapy.

Mammalian O^6-alkylguanine-DNA alkyltransferase, a repair protein which stoichiometrically reacts with O^6-alkylguanine lesions in DNA[14] has a crucial effect on the outcome of therapy with alkylating agents of the nitrosourea and triazene classes. Tumours expressing the Mer[+] phenotype (repair-proficient) are inherently resistant to these drugs whereas Mer[-] tumours are relatively sensitive[15]. Clinical stratagems based on an initial depletion of the alkyltransferase (e.g. by a methylating agent) followed by treatment with a chloroethylnitrosourea[16] may allow nitrosoureas to realize the full potential they exhibited in preclinical screening. Of the small-molecule inactivators of the alkyltransferase, O^6-benzylguanine (Structure 8) is a useful lead structure amenable to further synthetic refinement[17].

On the evidence of the foregoing partial survey, small molecules are seen to be playing their part in a range of cancer treatment scenarios. However, the mid-1980s marked a watershed in drug discovery practices worldwide when the *in vivo* mouse tumour screening models hitherto used for selecting clinical candidates, in the main emanating from chemistry-driven (i.e. small molecule) synthetic projects or natural product sources, were discarded. Agents such as mitozolomide (Structure 9), which exhibited curative activity against a broad spectrum of mouse tumours[18] but performed disappointingly in the clinic[19], finally sealed the fate of the old screening procedures and accelerated their replacement by panels of human tumour cell lines cultured *in vitro*. The main goal of the new programme initiated by the NCI is to establish a *disease-orientated* drug screening strategy and its success will be monitored by the identification of novel agents with clinical activity against the major solid tumours in man[20]. In fact, the data presented in Figure 1.1 are open to an alternative conclusion to that presented so far – that is, since there are no really selective agents to treat the common solid tumours, then small-molecular-weight drugs have clearly failed. Nor is it likely that the efficacy of these agents could be dramatically improved by prodrug modification, conjugation with macromolecular carriers or antibodies, or by encapsulation in nanoparticles, erythrocytes, microspheres or liposomes. Other strategies to achieve site-directed delivery are unlikely to transform modest drugs into world-beaters.

'To cure a complicated disease requires a complicated molecule'

This intriguing proposition was advanced by Professor J. E. Baldwin of Oxford University in 1985 at the quinquennial site visit to an experimental chemotherapy group which concentrated on the development of small molecules! It makes a very taxing question on a finals examination paper for sure, but is there any fundamental scientific reason for believing that cancer is a more complicated disease than, say, stomach ulceration? The latter condition is readily treated with H_2-receptor antagonists with molecular weights in the 250–300 Da range. Twenty years ago, viral diseases appeared bafflingly complex and untreatable, until the discovery that acyclovir could be used for the chemotherapy of herpes infections offered a biochemical basis for the prospective downfall of other viral pathogens. Perhaps our collective failure as cancer scientists is that we have been unable to recognize that cancer may be a 'simple' disease.

Professor Baldwin's real point is that only a complex molecule presenting multiple binding possibilities to its 'receptor' is likely to be able to differentiate, selectively, between specific targets in multifunctional biological processes. There is no doubt that the large-molecular-weight products of the infant biotechnology industries have exquisite molecular selectivities that cannot be matched, as yet, by synthetic molecules. The high expectation of commercial rewards from biotechnology products explains the presence of 59 potential therapies for the treatment of cancer or cancer-related diseases amongst a total of 104 such products under development in the USA in 1990. Of these, monoclonal antibodies (MABs) account for 15 and include derivatives conjugated to drugs, toxins and radionuclides. The ADEPT technology (antibody directed enzyme prodrug therapy) developed by Bagshawe and his colleagues[21] is being progressed to clinical trial in the UK by the Cancer Research Campaign. In general, synthesis and pharmaceutical formulation of these large and fragile composites, and their inherent antigenicity, still present formidable problems, retarding the pace of clinical evaluation, but the development of truncated and/or humanized second-generation antibodies has rekindled optimism in the therapeutic potential of MABs[22].

The prospects for gene therapy were considered in gloomy terms in 1986[23] but, by 1990, more optimistic sentiments prevailed. It is timely to remind ourselves that genes are single molecules – albeit large ones – and many of the principles underlying development for the clinic are shared with their small-molecular-weight counterparts. It has been suggested that a suitable framework for conducting gene therapy trials should include the following elements[24]:

(1) The disease must have a severe and predictable phenotype;
(2) The inserted corrective gene should have been cloned;
(3) Expression of the gene product should not require too precise regulation nor particularly high levels of expression to overcome the defects;
(4) There must be a suitable delivery system for implantation of the genetically modified cells.

Both viral and physical methods for the insertion of cloned genes are continually being improved[25]. Whereas retroviral vectors have the potential to infect 100% of target cells, they are limited in that they can package only about

6

7 kb of inserted DNA; this capacity may not be sufficient to encode a complete gene and its promoter sequences. Also, retroviral vectors have the potential to combine with latent endogenous human viruses to generate infective virus in the patient: other vectors based on attenuated vaccinia, bovine papilloma and herpes viruses offer potentially safer alternatives.

Current physical methods of gene insertion involving, variously, co-precipitation of DNA with calcium phosphate, cell fusion techniques with protoplasts or erythrocyte ghosts, microinjection or electroporation, lead to low levels of integration. Recently, the successful insertion of genes into somatic mammalian cells has been achieved by coating the genes onto gold beads, accelerating the complex to high voltage and bombarding the genes through the cell membrane. Genes introduced by this aggressive technology have be successfully expressed in rodent liver, skin and muscle cells[26].

In early 1991, a pioneering clinical trial to exploit gene therapy to treat cancer was initiated at the National Cancer Institute under the direction of Dr Steven Rosenberg. Patients with advanced melanoma have been administered the gene encoding TNF spliced into tumour infiltrating lymphocytes. This is a 'high noon' for molecular biology with the very *raison d'être* of the science at stake.

In the case of the cytokines, just one molecule can trigger a cascade of events culminating in a cytotoxic or cytokinetic effect. Although cytokine therapy is still in its infancy, it is clear that the various interferon (INF) and interleukin (IL) products have only very modest activity against the major solid tumours as single agents[27]. Activity of IFN-α against hairy cell leukaemia and chronic myelogenous leukaemia, and of IL-2 against melanoma and renal cell carcinoma are unlikely to bring sufficient commercial rewards to banish the biotech blues. Signs of stiffening regulatory resistance to the approval of new IFNs and ILs reflect these clinical setbacks.

In defence of cytokines, it is possible to argue that clinical scientists are still learning how to tune the dosage and timing schedules of these novel high-molecular-weight compounds effectively and their role in combination regimes with cytotoxic agents remains to be explored thoroughly. For example, a recent comprehensive survey[28] on the use of combinations of IFN and small-molecular-weight drugs has highlighted the complexities of the interactions involved and the vagaries of translating preclinical studies to clinical investigations.

Two eagerly awaited biotechnology products which received their first regulatory approvals in 1991 were Amgen's granulocyte colony stimulating factor (G-CSF) and Immunex-Behringwerke's granulocyte macrophage colony stimulating factor (GM-CSF). These haemopoietic growth factors have the potential to stimulate the recovery of bone marrow and may significantly reduce the severity of neutropenia associated with chemotherapy using myelo-suppressive cytotoxic agents.

In concluding this section, the point has to be made that the clinician still awaits one really effective drug, irrespective of size, for treatment of the major common tumours. Speculative experimental juggling of cytokines and cytotoxic agents in combination does not make a scientifically edifying spectacle. Shakespeare found words which precisely and appositely describe the predicament confronting cancer scientists:

7

Diseases desperate grown
By desperate appliance are reliev'd,
Or not at all.   (Hamlet, Act IV, Scene III)

PROSPECTS FOR CHEMOTHERAPY BEYOND THE BIOTECHNOLOGY REVOLUTION

Convergence of immunotherapy and chemotherapy

The growth of tumours and the development of metastases are highly complex processes, the outcome of which hinges on an interplay between the intrinsic characteristics of tumours and host factors, many of which are uncharacterized chemically. The immune status of the host clearly has a bearing on tumour initiation and progression. Notwithstanding their disappointing clinical activity so far, the cytokines as a class are potent and specific biological probes which may allow for a detailed evaluation of immunological intervention as a means of recruiting the antitumour potential of the immune system.

Efforts to treat cancer with crude bacterial broths date back to the 1890s[29]. Evidence of clinical efficacy is, at best, anecdotal: only the Japanese, apparently, are prepared to believe in the efficacy of these products. The term 'biological response modifier' (BRM) was coined to describe agents whose putative mode of action may involve priming of the host immune response. Although the designation BRM adds scientific respectability to what is now a burgeoning discipline, it is also a convenient catch-all term, which has been used to embrace all biologically active compounds which have an unexplained mode of action!

Many BRMs operate by provoking the intracellular release of cytokines. For example ImuVert, a sterile suspension of ribosomes and membrane vesicles fractionated from *Serratia marcescens,* is claimed to stimulate the release of IL-1, GM-CSF, IFN-α, IFN-β, IFN-γ and TNF in cultures of fresh human mononuclear peripheral blood cells[30], and OK-432 (picibanil), a streptococcal preparation popular in Japan, induces TNF production in mice and humans[31]. Muramyl dipeptide, a structural fragment of enteric bacteria, can also prime induction of endogenous TNF when administered orally to mice[32].

Certain familiar molecules,such as uracil mustard (Structure 10, Figure 1.3), cyclophosphamide (Structure 11) and DTIC (Structure 12), can exert immuno-enhancing activity which may be a component of their antitumour properties, although such agents are conventionally used in a high-dose cytotoxic mode. It is now clear that the intriguing synthetic flavanoid, flavone acetic acid (FAA) (Structure 13), originally selected for clinical trial on the basis of its activity against the murine colon adenocarcinoma 38, has an indirect effect which may be mediated by augmentation of systemic natural killer (NK) activity. Antitumour activity of the drug in mice is strongly influenced by the immune status of the host[33]. Interestingly, systemic alkalinization inhibits the ability of the drug to augment NK activity, induce cytokine gene expression, and synergize with IL-2 for the treatment of murine renal cancer[34]. FAA has been shown to augment NK activity in the peripheral blood of some cancer patients[35], but it is unlikely that high-dosage cytotoxic schedules, employed in conjunction

8

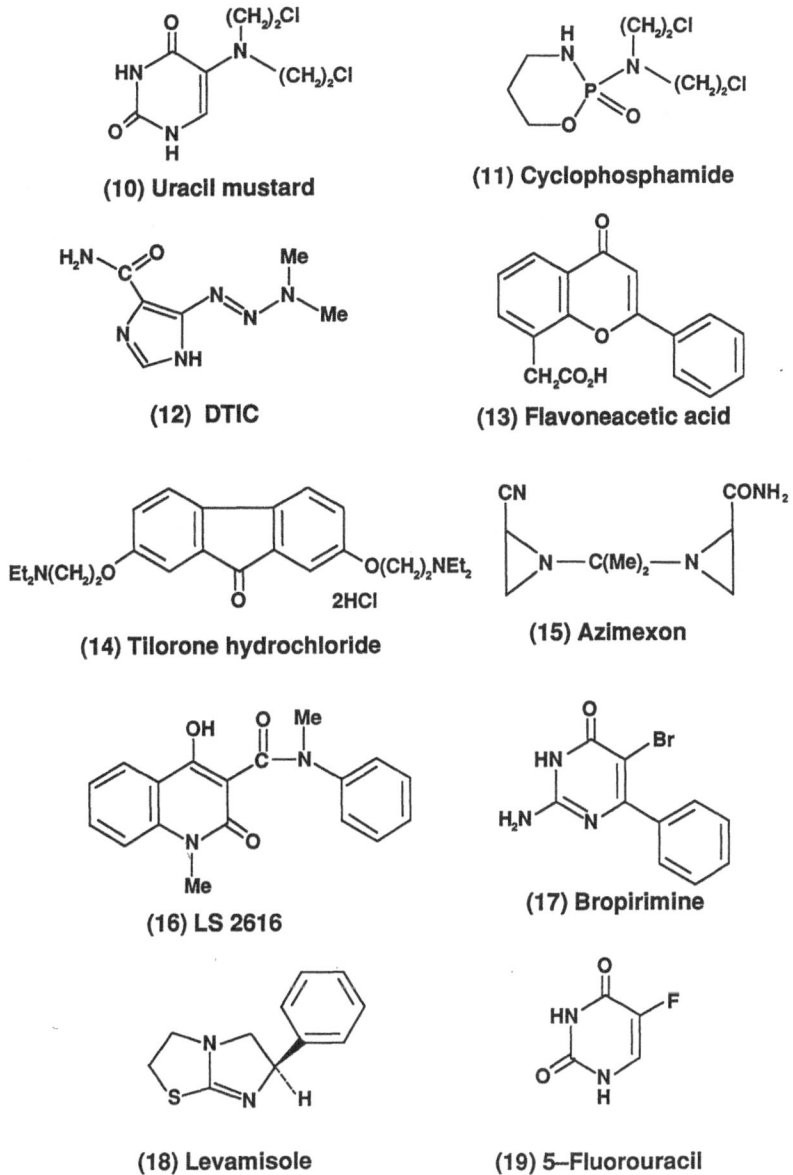

Figure 1.3 Structures (10–19) of small molecules with immunomodulatory activity

with urine alkalinization[36], would allow the more subtle immuno-enhancement component of the activity of the drug to be discerned.

A group of structurally disparate compounds, including the fluorenone derivative, tilorone hydrochloride (Structure 14), and polyamines and polyanions, have been shown to induce the endogenous production of IFNs[37]. In addition, a series of carboxamides and cyclic carboxamides has been shown recently to have immunomodulatory activity. The carbamoyl aziridine, azimexon (Structure 15),[38] has already progressed to clinical trial and the quinoline-3-carboxamide, LS2616 (Structure 16), has been shown to exert an immunostimulatory effect on T cell responses[39] and NK activity[40] in mice. Bropirimine (Structure 17) is the lead compound in a new class of pyrimidinone BRMs which induce IFNs[41] and may act partially through the endogenous liberation of TNF[42].

There is a clear picture emerging of a significant role for small-molecule immunomodulatory agents as clinical partners with 'conventional' cytotoxic agents (Figure 1.4). As with all experimental combinations, the timing and dosages of administration of the separate agents may be critical and fundamental questions on whether the immunotherapeutic component should be administered prior to, or after, debulking therapy with the cytotoxic component have yet to be answered[43].

A key paper published by Moertel and his colleagues in 1990 proposed that a combination of levamisole (Structure 18) and 5-fluorouracil (5-FU) (Structure 19) – both very small molecules – should be standard adjuvant treatment for Stage C colon carcinoma[44]. The combination is better than 5-FU alone and treatment with levamisole alone had no effect. Levamisole is an immuno-

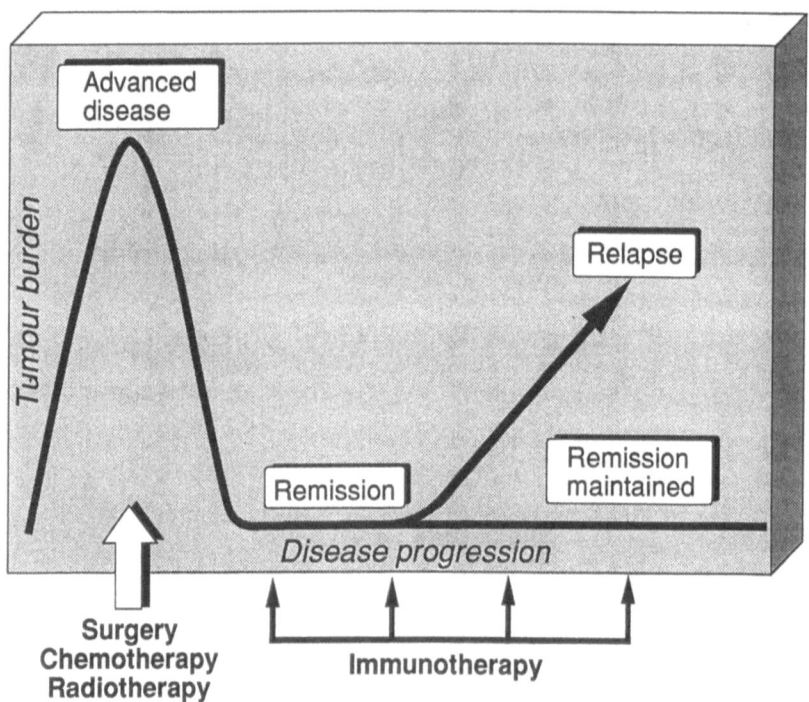

Figure 1.4 Remission maintenance by combination of treatment modalities

suppressant in high doses, and an immunostimulant in low doses. Although the clinical results obtained by adding levamisole to 5-FU may, conceivably, be an example of biochemical modulation completely independent of an immune effect, the possibility that levamisole may act by stimulating depressed cell-mediated immunity is exciting. Colonic cells are naturally chemoresistant: low doses of levamisole might trigger the intracellular release of natural cytokines which lower the dosage threshold at which 5-FU initiates programmed cell death in colon carcinoma cells.

There is now an opportunity to develop new and specific small-molecule BRMs which might be used in new combinations with existing cytotoxic agents – in fact, such discoveries could completely transform our appreciation of the value of conventional cytotoxic agents.

To date, all small-molecule BRMs have emerged quite by accident. If a rational search for new agents were to be mounted, a suitable high-throughput *in vitro* screen incorporating human tumour cells and endogenous infiltrating

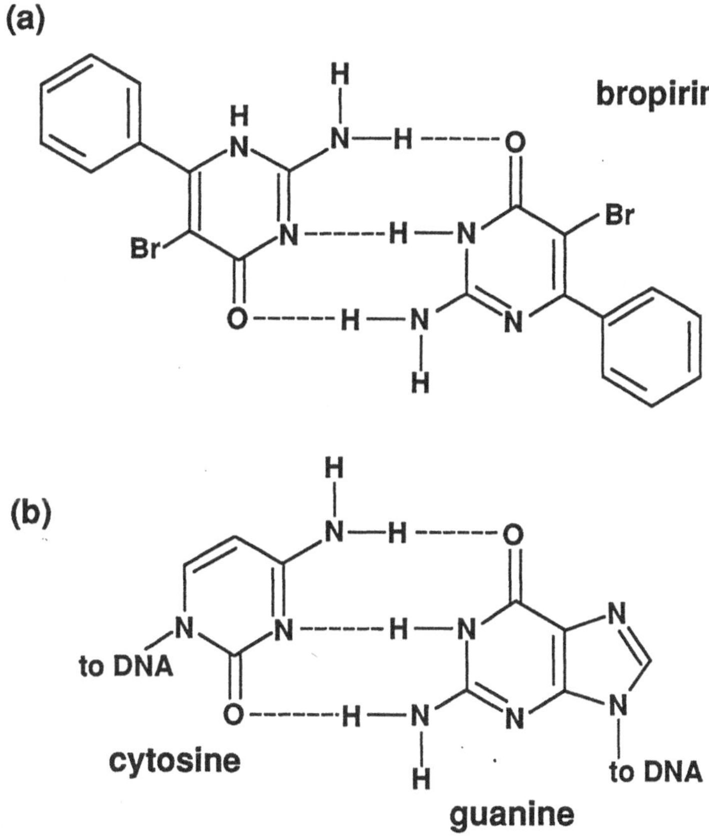

Figure 1.5 Intermolecular hydrogen bonding between (a) the 1H- and 3H-tautomers of bropirimine and (b) a Watson–Crick cytosine–guanine base pair

effector cells would be required; also, some BRMs display antitumour activity *in vivo* in the growth and metastasis models of the B16 melanoma growing in mice[45]. In this new research area, dealing with agents whose molecular mechanism of action is not understood, there are few chemical leads upon which to base a rational synthetic chemistry programme. However, the X-ray crystal structure of bropirimine displays an interesting feature (Schwalbe, C.H. and Stevens, M.F.G., unpublished). Two equally populated tautomers, one with the pyrimidin(1H)-one structure, the other in the pyrimidin(3H)-one arrangement, are hydrogen bonded in the manner of a Watson-Crick cytosine:guanine base pair in DNA (Figure 1.5). Thus, bropirimine has the potential to hydrogen bond to either cytosine or guanine residues in single-stranded DNA, or to double-stranded DNA in a Hoogsteen base pairing arrangement. This raises the possibility that bropirimine could be acting by influencing the transcription of genes coding for the peptide sequences of cytokines or other regulatory proteins. In addition, the structural resemblance between the bropirimine 'base-pair' and poly I:poly C, a known immunomodulatory double-stranded DNA molecule, is very striking.

Reductionism in drug design

In a prophetic article in 1984, Vane and Cuatrecasas discussed the future of drug design beyond the biotechnology revolution[46]. Recombinant DNA technology, it was argued, now provides the means of large-scale synthesis of proteins with therapeutic potential and, in the future, genetic engineering will engender exquisite probes for the study of the molecular basis of cellular control. Given the exhilarating pace of scientific advance, scientists might reasonably expect to understand, by the end of this decade even, the key molecular event(s) switching a cell from normality to malignancy.

But what then? The focus of excitement in the drive to develop new cancer treatments will switch from cell and molecular biology to physical and organic chemistry (Figure 1.6). The techniques of the X-ray crystallographer will be used to determine the structures of controlling proteins, and ever-increasing high-field NMR spectroscopy will give insights into the conformations and dynamics of these proteins in the physiologically relevant solution state[47]. It is a sign of the times that many of the articles in recent issues of the journal *Biochemistry* are devoted to NMR studies. In the future, it should be possible to predict protein structures from amino acid sequences alone by employing computational methods[48]. Protein engineering can then provide information on close encounters of the molecular kind between these proteins and their targets. These encounters involve only transient contacts: the bulk of a protein structure is required only to bring relatively few atoms into functioning juxtaposition at its combining region, or active site. Thus, it is entirely realistic to predict that new generations of designer drugs[49], probably small heterocyclic moieties with correctly positioned functionalities – a carbonyl group here, an N–H bond there, a hydrophobic or hydrophilic domain elsewhere – will be able to supplant or antagonize regulatory proteins. One might speculate that the prototype differentiating agents *N*-methylformamide (Structure 20; Figure 1.7) and hexa-

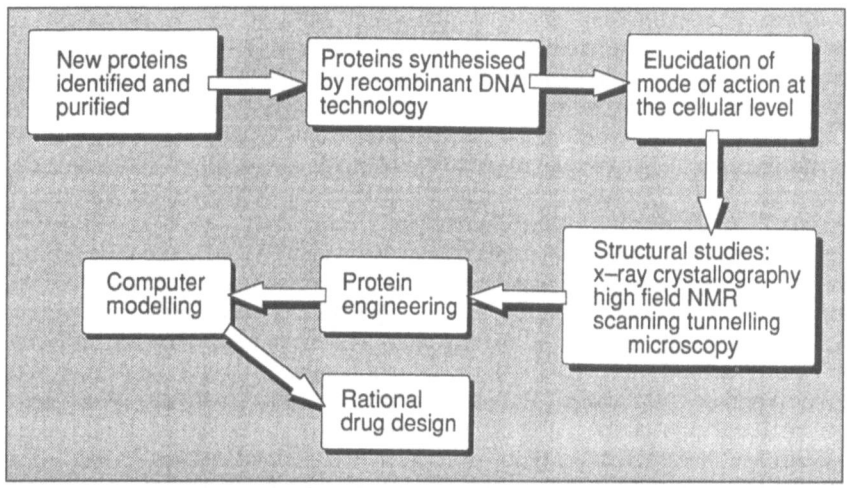

Figure 1.6 Structured rational drug design beyond the biotechnology revolution

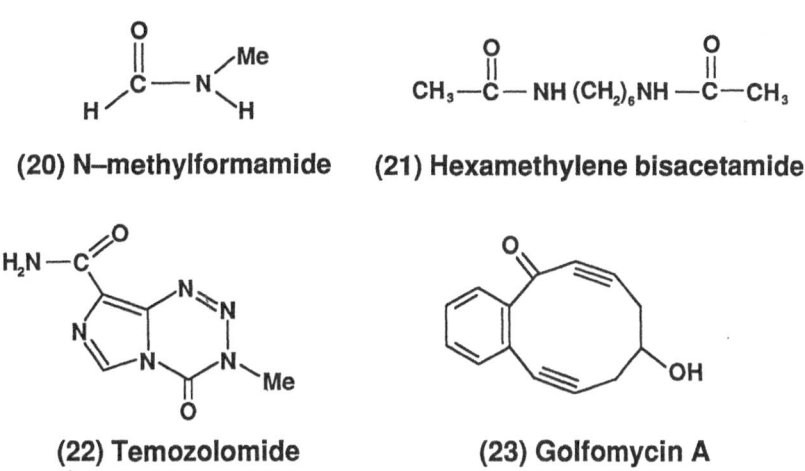

(20) N–methylformamide   **(21) Hexamethylene bisacetamide**

(22) Temozolomide   **(23) Golfomycin A**

Figure 1.7 Small molecular probes with novel biological properties (Structures 20–23)

methylene bisacetamide (Structure 21) might act by mimicking such regulatory molecules.

Finally, if cancer is a disease which results from aberrant gene expression and if we are to develop cures for the major malignancies, then we must develop molecular strategies to control gene expression. This may involve developing novel agents to switch *on*, or up-regulate, expression of tumour-suppressor genes, or switch *off*, or down-regulate, malignancy-associated oncogenes. There has been much thoughtful speculation recently that this might be achieved by developing new drugs directed to cell membrane targets[50,51]. However, nature controls gene expression with proteins which bind in the major groove of DNA[52] employing structural motifs such as helix-turn-helix units to recognize their operators. It is logical that the search for agents to modulate gene expression should start with DNA as the prime target.

Gene-specific recognition has been achieved in experimental systems by synthetic oligonucleotides homing in on, and binding to, unique DNA sequences by triple helix formation through Hoogsteen base pairing in the major groove[53-55]. Delivering intact oligonucleotides to target genes may, however, engender insurmountable pharmaceutical problems[56,57] and tumour cells may yet activate a range of mechanisms to develop resistance to such agents. An alternative approach would be to synthesize small-molecular-weight heterocyclic compounds (e.g. 'lexitropsins') which can read DNA sequences as a blind person can read Braille[58]. Encouragingly, a small molecule, like temozolomide (Structure 22) molecular weight 194 Da, with ideal pharmaceutical properties to achieve high drug levels in the brain, can achieve a measure of sequence selectivity in its covalent interactions within the major groove of DNA[59]. Possibly, such an agent can be attached to an appropriate helix-turn-helix peptide motif to attain gene-specific recognition.

The recent total synthesis of the mighty molecule, palytoxin ($C_{129}H_{223}N_3O_{54}$), a natural product from the coral *Palythoa toxica*[60], and the small DNA-cleaving cyclodecadiynone, golfomycin A (Structure 23), a mimic of the esperamicin and calicheamicin DNA-cutting antibiotics[61], demonstrates that the power of modern organic chemistry is boundless and its future role can be much more than solely that of handmaiden to biology and medicine. Confidence remains high that the answer to the question posed in the title to this Chapter will be affirmative.

References

1. Lomax, N. R. and Narayanan, V. L. (1988). *Chemical Structures of Interest to the Division of Cancer Treatment*, Vol. VI. (Bethesda: Drug Synthesis and Chemistry Branch, Developmental Therapeutics Program, National Cancer Institute)
2. De Pass, J. and Wood-Gush, G. (1990). In *Pharmaceutical Industry Perspectives*. (London: Barclays de Zoete Wedd)
3. Tisdale, M. J. (1991). Cancer cachexia. *Br. J. Cancer*, **63**, 337–342
4. Bibby, M. C., Double, J. A., Ali, S. A., Fearon, K. C. H., Brennan, R. A. and Tisdale M. J. (1987). Characterisation of a transplantable adenocarcinoma of the mouse producing cachexia in recipient animals. *J. Natl. Cancer Inst.*, **78**, 539–544
5. Tisdale, M. J. and Beck, S. A. (1991). Inhibition of tumour-induced lipolysis *in vitro* and cachexia and tumour growth *in vivo* by eicosapentaenoic acid. *Biochem. Pharmacol.*, **41**, 103–107
6. Smoluk, G. D., Fahey, R. C., Calabro-Jones, P. M., Aguilera, J. A. and Ward, J. F. (1988). Radioprotection of cells in culture by WR-2721 and derivatives: form of the drug responsible for protection. *Cancer Res.*, **48**, 3641–3647
7. Barnes, J. M., Barnes, N. M., Costall, B. and Naylor, R. J. (1991). Development of $5HT_3$ receptor antagonists as anti-emetics. *Pharm. J.*, 112–114
8. Brown, R. and Kaye, S. B. (1990). Drug resistance and the problem of treatment failure. In Ponder, B. A. J. and Waring, M. J. (eds.) *The Science of Cancer Treatment*, pp. 55–82. (Lancaster: Kluwer Academic Publishers)
9. Marx, J. L. (1986). Drug resistance of cancer cells probed. *Science*, **234**, 818–820
10. Pennock, G. D., Dalton, W. S., Roeske, W. R., Appleton, C. P., Mosley, K., Plezia, P., Miller, T. P. and Salmon, S. E. (1991). Systemic toxic effects associated with high-dose verapamil infusion and chemotherapy administration. *J. Natl. Cancer Inst.*, **83**, 105–110

11. Foster, B. J., Grotzinger, K. R., McKoy, W. M., Rubinstein, L. V. and Hamilton, T. C. (1988). Modulation of induced resistance to adriamycin in two human breast cancer cell lines with tamoxifen or perhexilene maleate. *Cancer Chemother. Pharmacol.*, **22**, 147–152

12. Twentyman, P. R., Fox, N. E. and White, D. J. G. (1987). Cyclosporin A and its analogues as modifiers of adriamycin and vincristine resistance in a multi-drug resistant human lung cancer cell line. *Br. J. Cancer*, **56**, 55–57

13. Watanabe, Y., Takano, H., Kiue, A., Kohno, K. and Kuwano, M. (1991). Potentiation of etoposide and vincristine by two synthetic 1,4-dihydropyridine derivatives in multidrug-resistant and atypical multidrug-resistant human cancer cells. *Anti-cancer Drug Design*, **6**, 47–58

14. Pegg, A. E. (1990). Mammalian O^6-alkylguanine-DNA alkyltransferase: regulation and importance in response to alkylating carcinogenic and therapeutic agents. *Cancer Res.*, **50**, 6119–6129

15. Yarosh, D. B., Barnes, D. and Erickson, L. C. (1986). Transfection of DNA from a chloroethylnitrosourea-resistant tumour cell line (Mer^+) to a sensitive tumour cell line (Mer^-) results in a tumour cell line resistant to MNNG and CNU that has increased O^6-methylguanine-DNA methyltransferease levels and reduced levels of DNA interstrand crosslinking. *Carcinogenesis* (London), **7**, 1603–1606

16. Lee, S. M., Thatcher, N. and Margison, G. P. (1991). O^6-Alkylguanine-DNA alkyltransferase depletion and regeneration in human peripheral lymphocytes following dacarbazine and fotemustine. *Cancer Res.*, **51**, 619–623

17. Dolan, M. E., Moschel, R. C. and Pegg, A. E. (1990). Depletion of mammalian O^6-alkylguanine-DNA alkyltransferase activity by O^6-benzylguanine provides a means to evaluate the role of this protein in protection against carcinogenic and therapeutic alkylating agents. *Proc. Natl. Acad. Sci. USA*, 5368–5372

18. Hickman, J. A., Stevens, M. F. G., Gibson, N. W., Langdon, S. P., Fizames, C., Lavelle, F., Atassi, G., Lunt, E. and Tilson, R. M. (1985). Experimental antitumour activity against murine tumor model systems of 8-carbamoyl-3-(2-chloroethyl)imidazo[5,1-d]-1,2,3,5-tetrazin-4(3H)-one (Mitozolomide), a novel broad spectrum agent. *Cancer Res.*, **45**, 3008–3013

19. Newlands, E. S., Blackledge, G., Slack, J. A., Goddard, C., Brindley, C. J., Holden, L. and Stevens, M. F. G. (1985). Phase I clinical trial of mitozolomide. *Cancer Treatment Rep.* **69**, 801–805

20. Boyd, M. R. (1989). Status of the NCI preclinical antitumor drug discovery screen. *Principles Pract. Oncol.*, **3**, 1–12

21. Bagshawe, K. D. (1987). Antibody directed enzymes revive anticancer prodrugs concept. *Br. J. Cancer*, **56**, 531–532

22. Coghlan, A. (1991). A second chance for antibodies. *New Scientist*, 9th February, 34–39

23. Robertson, M. (1986). Gene therapy: desperate appliances. *Nature (London)*, **320**, 213–214

24. Kinnon, C. and Levinsky, R. J. (1990). Gene therapy for cancer. *Eur. J. Cancer*, **26**, 638–640

25. Wang, C. Y. and Huang, L. (1989). Highly efficient DNA delivery mediated by pH-sensitive immunoliposomes. *Biochemistry*, **28**, 9508–9514

26. Yang, N.-S., Burkholder, J., Roberts, B., Martinell, B. and McCabe, D. (1990). *In vivo* and *in vitro* gene transfer to mammalian somatic cells by particle bombardment. *Proc. Natl. Acad. Sci. USA*, **87**, 9568–9572

27. Kelly, S. A., Malik, S. and Balkwill, F. R. (1990). Cytokine therapy. In Ponder, B. A. J. and Waring, M. J. (eds.) *The Science of Cancer Treatment*, pp. 127–159. (Lancaster: Kluwer Academic Publishers)

28. Wadler, S. and Schwartz, E. L. (1990). Antineoplastic activity of the combination of interferon and cytotoxic agents against experimental human malignancies: A review. *Cancer Res.*, **50**, 3473–3486

29. Coley, W. B. (1893). The treatment of malignant tumors by repeated innoculations of erysipelas with a report of ten original cases. *Am. J. Med. Sci.*, **105**, 487–511

30. Weisenthal, L. M., Dill, P. L. and Pearson, F. C. (1991). Effect of prior cancer chemotherapy on human tumor-specific cytotoxicity *in vitro* in response to immunopotentiating biologic response modifiers. *J. Natl. Cancer Inst.*, **83**, 37–42

31. Satoh, M., Inagawa, H., Shimada, Y., Soma, G.-I., Oshima, H. and Mizuno, D. (1987). Endogenous production of tumor necrosis factor in normal mice and human cancer patients by interferons and other cytokines combined with biological response modifiers of bacterial origin. *J. Biol. Response Modifiers*, **6**, 512–514

32. Okutomi, T., Inagawa, H., Nishizawa, T., Oshima, H., Soma, G.-I. and Mizuno, D. (1990). Priming effect of orally administered muramyl dipeptide on induction of endogenous tumor necrosis factor. *J. Biol. Response Modifiers*, **9**, 564–569

33. Bibby, M.C., Phillips, R.M., Double, J.A. and Pratesi, G. (1991). Anti-tumour activity of flavone acetic acid (NSC-347512) in mice – influence of immune status. *Br. J. Cancer*, **63**, 57–62

34. Futami, H., Hornung, R. L., Back, T. T., Bull, R., Gruys, E. and Wiltrout, R. H. (1990). Systemic alkanization inhibits the ability of flavone acetic acid to augment natural killer activity, induce cytokine gene expression, and synergize with interleukin-2 for the treatment of murine renal cancer. *Cancer Res.*, **50**, 7926–7931

35. Urba, W., Longo, D. L., Lombardo, F. A., and Weiss, R. B. (1988). Enhancement of natural killer activity in human peripheral blood by flavone acetic acid. *J. Natl. Cancer Inst.*, **80**, 521–525

36. Kerr, D. J., Kaye, S. B., Cassidy, J., Bradley, C., Rankin, E. M., Adams, L., Setanoians, A., Young, T., Forrest, G., Soukop, M. and Clavel, M. (1987). Phase I and pharmacokinetic study of flavone acetic acid. *Cancer Res.*, **47**, 6776–6781

37. Mayer, G. D., Krueger, R. F., Betts, R. F., Douglas, R. G., Breinig, M. C. and Morahan, P. S. (1980). In Stringfellow, D. A. (ed.) *Interferon and Interferon Inducers: Clinical Applications.* (New York: Marcel Dekker, Inc.)

38. Srikishnan, T. (1990). Structural studies of immunomodulators. Part 2. Crystal structure and conformation of azimexon (BM 12.531) an immunostimulant and an anti-tumor drug. *Anti-Cancer Drug Design*, **5**, 213–220

39. Larsson, E.-L., Joki, A. and Stålhandski, T. (1987). Mechanism of action of the new immunomodulator LS 2616 on T cell responses. *Int. J. Immunopharmacol.*, **9**, 425–431

40. Kalland, T., Alm, G. and Stålhandski, T. (1985). Augmentation of mouse natural killer cell activity by LS 2616, a new immunomodulator. *J. Immunol.*, **134**, 3956–3961

41. Li, L. H., Wallace, T. L., Wierenga, W., Stulnick, H. I. and DeKoning, T. F. (1987). Antitumour activity of pyrimidinones, a class of small molecule biological response modifiers. *J. Biol. Response Modifiers*, **6**, 44–55

42. Scherina, M., Ijzermans, J. N. M., Jeekel, J. and Marquet, R. L. (1990). The antitumour activity of the interferon inducer bropirimine is partially mediated by endogenous tumour necrosis factor α. *Cancer Immunol. Immunother.*, **32**, 251–255

43. Weistenthal, L. M., Dill, P. L. and Pearson, F. C. (1991). Effect of prior cancer chemotherapy on human tumor-specific cytotoxicity *in vitro* in response to immunopotentiating biologic response modifiers. *J. Natl. Cancer Inst.*, **83**, 37–42

44. Moertel, C. G., Fleming, T. R., MacDonald, J. S., Haller, D. G., Laurie, J. A., Goodman P. J., Ungerleider, J. S., Emerson, W. A., Tormey, D. C., Glick, J. H., Veeder, M. H. and Mailliard, J. A. (1990). Levamisole and fluorouracil for adjuvant therapy of resected colon carcinoma. *N. Eng. J. Med.*, **322**, 352–358

45. Kalland, T. (1986). Effects of immunomodulator LS 2616 on growth and metastasis of the murine B16-F10 melanoma. *Cancer Res.*, **46**, 3018–3022

46. Vane, J. and Cuatrecasas, P. (1984). Genetic engineering and pharmaceuticals. *Nature (London)*, **312**, 303–305

47. Wüthrich, K. (1989) Protein structure determination in solution by nuclear magnetic resonance spectroscopy. *Science*, **243**, 45–50

48. Sternberg, M. J. E. and Zvelebil, M. J. J. M. (1990). Prediction of protein structure from sequence. *Eur. J. Cancer*, **26**, 1163–1166

49. Blundell, T.(1990). Designer drugs head for the market place. *New Scientist*, 9th June, 61–64

50. Workman, P. (1990). The cell membrane and cell signals: New targets for novel anticancer agents. *Ann. Oncol.*, **1**, 100–111

51. Powis, G., Hickman, J. A., Workman, P., Tritton, T. R., Abita, J. P., Berdel, W. E., Gescher, A., Moses, H. L. and Nicolson, G. L. (1990). The cell membrane and cell signals as targets in cancer chemotherapy. *Cancer Res.*, **50**, 2203–2211

52. Ptashne, M. (1986). Gene regulation by proteins acting nearby and at a distance. *Nature (London)*, **322**, 697–701

53. Maher, L. J., Wold, B. and Dervan, P. B. (1989). Inhibition of DNA binding proteins by oligonucleotide-directed triple helix formation. *Science*, **245**, 725–730

54. Strobel, S. A. and Dervan, P. B. (1991). Single-site enzymatic cleavage of yeast genomic DNA mediated by triple helix formation. *Nature (London)*, **350**, 172–174

55. Hélène, C. and Toulmé, J.-J. (1990). Specific regulation of gene expression by antisense, sense and antigene nucleic acids. *Biochim. Biophys. Acta*, **1049**, 99–125

56. Stein, C. A. and Cohen, J. S. (1988). Oligonucleotides as inhibitors of gene expression: a review. *Cancer Res.*, **48**, 2659–2668

57. Rothenberg, M., Johnson, G., Laughlin, C., Green, I., Cradock, J., Sarver, N. and Cohen, J. S. (1989). Oligonucleotides as anti-sense inhibitors of gene expression: therapeutic implications. *J. Natl. Cancer Inst.*, **81**, 1539–1544

58. Thurston, D. E. and Thompson, A. S. (1990). The molecular recognition of DNA. *Chem. Britain*, **26**, 767–772

59. Clark, A. S., Stevens, M. F. G., Sansom, C. E. and Schwalbe, C. H. (1990). Anti-tumour imidazotetrazines. Part XXI. Mitozolomide and temozolomide: probes for the major groove of DNA. *Anti-Cancer Drug Design*, **5**, 63–68

60. Armstrong, R. W., Beau, J. N., Cheon, S. H., Christ, W. J., Fujioka, H., Ham, W. H., Hawkins, L. D., Jin H., Kang, S. H., Kishi, Y., Martinelli, M. J., McWhorter, W. W., Mizuno, M., Nakata, M., Stutz, A. E., Talamas, F. X., Taniguchi, M., Tino, J. A., Ueda, K., Uerishi, J., White, J. B. and Yonaga, M. (1989). Total synthesis of palytoxin carboxylic acid and palytoxin amide. *J. Am. Chem. Soc.*, **111**, 7530–7533, and references quoted therein

61. Nicolaou, K. C., Skokotas, G., Furuya, S., Suemune, H. and Nicolaou, D. C. (1990). Golfomycin A, a novel designed molecule with DNA-cleaving properties and antitumour activity. *Angew. Chem. Int. Ed. Engl.*, **29**, 1064–1068

2

The role of medicinal chemistry in the discovery of DNA-active anticancer drugs: from random searching, through lead development, to *de novo* design

W. A. DENNY

THE CHANGING PHILOSOPHY OF ANTICANCER DRUG DISCOVERY

Systematic attempts to use chemotherapy as a primary method of cancer treatment began in the late 1940s, with the use of nitrogen mustard to treat leukaemias and lymphomas[1], and, from that time, the search for effective small-molecule anticancer drugs has been one of the significant goals of medicinal chemistry. The history of this endeavour has an important theme running through it: the changing relative importance of different scientific disciplines and how they have influenced the philosophy behind the medicinal chemistry of anticancer drug discovery.

Random searching

Initially, with very little knowledge upon which to base rational design, most effort focused on the random screening of compounds, using simple high-throughput screening systems (primarily mouse leukaemia models). Many of today's useful drugs were derived *directly* in this way. The cutting-edge disciplines were synthetic and structural chemistry, required to elucidate the often complex structures, whereas the biological testing was predominantly phenomenological. Drugs were advanced to clinical trial largely on the basis of screening results, and most of the drugs which reached the clinic did so long before their mechanism of action was understood.

The largest single such effort has been the US National Cancer Institute screening programme[2] where, over thirty years from the mid-1950s to the mid-1980s, approximately 600 000 materials (both pure compounds and crude extracts from synthetic and natural sources) were screened, primarily against mouse leukaemia cell lines both *in vitro* and *in vivo*. From this work, about 300 different compounds eventually proceeded to some level of evaluation in humans, resulting in a total of 42 drugs being approved by the US Federal Drug Administration as available medicines[2].

While this process of drug discovery is of very low productivity at all steps, and is now less important for direct procurement of clinical agents, it remains an important source of *new leads*, since it is still not possible to predict the usefulness of the compounds of diverse structure now in use as clinical anticancer drugs by modelling or computational methods. The sophistication of the procedure has improved, as the critical importance of the screening systems to be used has been recognized. Biochemical screens (enzyme assay, receptor binding, specially characterized and even constructed cell lines) give information on the effectiveness of the compound at the critical site of action, and early insights into its mode of action. However, they do not delineate the likely ability of the drug to reach the active site with a suitable concentration/time profile, or its toxic side-effects (see Chapter 3, this volume).

Lead development

In recent years, emphasis in the search for anticancer drugs has moved away from structural chemistry, with studies of the mechanism of action, pharmacology and toxic side-effects of drugs becoming a more important part of drug development. In fact, the elucidation (in broad terms at least) of the mechanisms of both the therapeutic action and the limiting toxicities of the major classes of anticancer drugs has probably been the most important achievement of the field in the last 20 years. This knowledge has influenced clinical practice, with drugs now being used in more mechanistically appropriate combinations. It has also powerfully influenced drug design by providing both starting points (existing drugs of known mechanism) and clear goals to aim for (improvements in specific properties) in the process of drug optimization for a particular purpose.

During the same period, the techniques available for such optimization (from a known lead compound) have improved greatly. Small molecules can now be defined quite accurately in terms of patterns of forces, determined by both the nature of their constituent atoms and their spatial arrangement. The critical physicochemical properties which result can be increasingly accurately described by quantifiable parameters: molecular charge distribution, energies of molecular orbitals, and both local (substituent) and global (whole-molecule) electronic, steric and hydrophobic effects[3]. Statistical methods have been developed for relating drug structure (defined in terms of the above quantifiable properties) to measures of biological activity, to provide relationships of predictive value[4].

De novo design

The ultimate goal of medicinal chemistry is the design of useful new drugs for a particular disease directly from knowledge of that disease. The basic premise behind *de novo* drug design is that specific drug–receptor interactions exist, mediated through a set of specific forces, which themselves result from the properties of the drug molecules and their receptors (see Chapter 5, this volume). Much has been achieved towards the goals of describing these forces and properties quantitatively, and in learning how to put together a group of atoms in such a way that the basic force patterns that result provide a desired and defined set of physicochemical properties. Computer modelling of macromolecule–ligand interactions is now an important technique in medicinal chemistry.

Recent work in molecular and cell biology has also revolutionized our knowledge about the nature of cancer, and indicated real differences between cancer and normal cells which are potentially exploitable as drug targets. These differences are often very subtle, and the new discoveries are placing medicinal chemistry in the uncomfortable position of having a plethora of potential targets that it does not yet have the ability to fully exploit. Thus, the philosophy behind small-molecule anticancer drug design is changing again, with the cutting-edge disciplines becoming structural and computational chemistry, and with medicinal chemistry as a whole struggling to exploit, via *de novo* drug design, the opportunities opened up by molecular and cell biology.

'SMALL' VERSUS 'LARGE' MOLECULES AS ANTICANCER DRUGS

This chapter is focused on the development of 'small-molecule' anticancer drugs which act directly on DNA. These are defined less by molecular weight (although usually below 1500 Da) than by concept (small-molecule 'drugs' versus large-molecule 'biological factors'). Despite enormous efforts, there has been little success in the last 15 years in the development of broad-spectrum small-molecule anticancer agents (whether through 'searching' or 'design'). This failure has fuelled much debate about the value of the continued development of small molecules as anticancer drugs[5] (see also Chapter 1, this volume), with a particular criticism being the presumed inherent inability of such compounds to exert sufficient selectivity for cancer cells.

Thus, much work is being invested in new approaches using 'large molecules'. A major concept is the targeting of various cytotoxins and radio-isotopes to tumour cells by attachment to monoclonal antibodies raised against tumour antigens[6,7]. The T-cell proliferation factor, IL-2, is being used more specifically to expand certain immune cell populations (lymphokine-activated killer cells and tumour-infiltrating lymphocytes) to bolster the host immune response[8]. IL-2[9] and other cellular cytokines, such as interferons[10,11], are also being explored as drugs in their own right. However, while specificity can be shown to tumour cell populations both *in vitro* and *in vivo* by these approaches, major disadvantages remain. The two most critical are the availability on human tumours of suitable antigenic determinants to provide consistent targets[12], and the difficulties of achieving effective distribution of such large molecules *in vivo*[13].

A concept which seeks to combine the favourable selectivity of 'large-molecule' entities with the distributive properties of 'small-molecule' drugs is the ADEPT (antibody-directed enzyme prodrug therapy) approach[14]. Specific enzymes (preferably non-mammalian) are conjugated to suitable tumour-specific antibodies, allowing them to localize at tumour sites. A prodrug which is a substrate only for the attached enzyme is then administered at a later time, when there has been localization of the antibody complex at tumour sites, so that the prodrug is preferentially metabolized to a cytotoxic species at these sites. Incomplete tumour coverage by the antibody (due to poor distribution or limited antigen expression) is less important than with other immunotoxins, since the (small-molecule) drug can subsequently diffuse to adjacent tissues. The process is also catalytic with respect to the conjugate, since one enzyme molecule can activate many molecules of prodrug. As noted by Bagshawe[14], the challenge to medicinal chemistry is to provide the enzyme and prodrug pairs to exploit fully this ingenious concept. The most well-studied approach to date has been the use of a carboxypeptidase enzyme[15].

However, it is the thesis of this chapter that small-molecule anticancer therapy also has a promising future in its own right. While the age of *direct* drug discovery by random screening is probably largely over, such methods will still provide new *lead compounds* for design. Improved statistical methods for determining structure–activity relationships will allow more efficient optimization of present drugs, exploiting existing knowledge to design out toxic side-effects as well as maximizing desired pharmacological effects (both of which will improve therapeutic ratios). However, the future lies with *de novo* design. Improving computational and modelling techniques will allow the determination of the 'essential pharmacophores' of larger biomolecules[5]. A deeper understanding of the chemistry of drug–receptor interactions and an increasing ability to predict molecular properties from structure will enable the precise tailoring of molecules for highly defined roles. A recent commentary about drug design in general, headlined "The reign of trial and error draws to a close"[16], is no less true for anticancer drug design.

CENTRAL PROBLEMS IN ANTICANCER DRUG DEVELOPMENT

There are three general phenomena which limit the effectiveness of small-molecule cytotoxic compounds as anticancer drugs: poor intrinsic selectivity for cancer cells, the limited distributive ability of many drugs, and the dynamics of the target cancer cell populations (which result in the rapid development of resistance in initially sensitive populations). Much has been learned about these concepts in the last few years. They *should* dominate thinking about the *de novo* design of small-molecule anticancer drugs, but probably have not been kept enough in mind by medicinal chemists involved in anticancer drug development.

Drug selectivity

Achieving selectivity for tumour cells has always been the limiting factor in the development of cytotoxic substances as anticancer drugs. In theory, this can be achieved at any one of three different levels[17].

Primary (subcellular)

Cell division controlled by small molecules (growth factors) which initiate the process by binding to transmembrane receptors. These pass on the signal through a complex multi-step 'growth signal transduction pathway' to the nucleus[18]. Many of the oncogenes (genes which, when activated, convert a normal cell into a cancer cell) which have now been identified code for components of the growth signal transduction pathway, leading in some cases to altered proteins[19,20]. Such differences between cancer and normal cells are real and important, and drugs which can target them successfully may provide the long-sought 'tumour-selective chemotherapy'. Two broad classes of potential targets can be identified at this subcellular level of tumour cell biochemistry and genetics: (a) oncogenes and their nucleic acid products (e.g. mRNAs), and (b) their protein products. Drugs targeted at the nucleic acid level include antisense oligonucleotides[21,22] and DNA minor groove binding drugs[17,23]. Drugs targeted at the protein level include those aimed at selective inhibition of protein function in the growth signal transduction pathway[24,25].

Secondary (cellular)

The great majority of clinically used anticancer drugs exert their therapeutic effects by being selective at this level, being most successful against cancers with a high rate of cell proliferation (leukaemias, lymphomas). The fact that most drugs are antiproliferative is not surprising, since nearly all of them came out of the large random screening programmes which used rapidly dividing animal tumours as the primary screens[26]. While much remains to be done in refining the profiles of action and toxicity of antiproliferative drugs (see below), the fundamental problem of their poor selectivity for slowly-dividing tumour cells compared with rapidly-dividing host cell populations will remain.

Tertiary (supracellular)

Recent research in tumour biology has shown that solid tumours are structurally very complex. As well as being biochemically heterogeneous, cells in solid tumours exist in a number of distinct microenvironments, which can be defined largely by the accessibility of the cells to oxygen. In most solid tumours, this is dictated by the limitation of tumour vascular networks, which, although stimulated to develop by angiogenesis factors secreted by tumour cells[27], remain growth-limiting on the tumour[28]. This microenvironmental heterogeneity provides a third level at which to seek tumour cell selectivity. Unique and potentially exploitable microenvironmental factors which cells in solid tumours experience include poor venous drainage, low intracellular pH due to increased glycolysis, a primitive vasculature, and chronic hypoxia[17,29].

Drug distribution

While anticancer agents share with many other types of drugs the necessity to have good vascular distribution (in order to reach remote tumour sites), they also have the additional requirement for efficient extravascular penetration to reach cells distant from the vasculature within solid tumours[29]. Recent experimental[30] and theoretical[31,32] work has shown that the ability of agents to penetrate into cell masses by extravascular diffusion depends critically on their DNA-binding properties, with the rate of penetration being inversely proportional to the tightness of DNA binding.

Drug resistance

The development of drug-resistant cells (either by the expansion of pre-existing resistant clones or as the direct result of drug-induced selection pressure) is one of the major causes of treatment failure. Resistance to particular drugs takes many different forms, and several extensive reviews exist[33,34]. The development of analogues of existing clinical agents is often motivated by the need to find compounds which will not be susceptible to the particular form of resistance shown towards the parent drug. However, the most important form of resistance is multi-drug resistance (MDR), where exposure to one particular drug gives rise to cell sublines which are then colaterally resistant to a wide variety of other drugs in addition to the inducing compound.

The most widely studied and clinically important[35] form of MDR, particularly evident with DNA-binding agents, arises from increased production of a family of membrane-spanning glycoproteins termed P-glycoproteins, which act as an energy-dependent 'pump' to accelerate the removal of intracellular drugs[36,37]. The apparently low structural specificity of this enzyme family has made it difficult to design out the property, although a recent quantitative structure–activity relationship study[38] has suggested that lipophilic compounds[39] of either very high or very low molecular weight are least subject to this phenomenon. This form of MDR may be at least partially reversed by treatment with second agents[37], which probably work by competing for enzyme sites[40]. Again, the structural requirements for this activity appear wide, although some conclusions have been drawn[41].

CURRENT TRENDS IN THE CHEMISTRY OF ANTICANCER DRUG DEVELOPMENT

Rather than discussing the chemistry of particular compounds in detail, this section attempts to summarize what appear to be the current medicinal chemistry concepts and design trends in the major classes of small-molecule DNA-active anticancer drugs. Classification of the drugs is (as far as possible) according to the chemistry of their biological action, rather than the chemistry of their structures. Although the former approach poses some difficulties, since the mechanisms of action of some compounds are not yet known (and may be multiple), it is the more logical. It is also a reminder that drug design is the science of putting together a group of atoms so that they have *a defined and desired set of physicochemical properties*. The exact atom arrangement is not critical, since it is the set of physicochemical properties which is important. We cannot always exactly predict the set of physicochemical properties we will get from a given atom configuration, and even less often do we know exactly what that set should be. Nevertheless, this is the ultimate goal of medicinal chemistry.

DNA adduct-forming agents (alkylators)

Introduction

As noted above, these were the earliest type of synthetic anticancer drugs. A variety of different alkylating moieties were explored, but the only ones still widely used clinically in combination protocols are the nitrogen mustards (particularly chlorambucil (1), melphalan (2) and cyclophosphamide (3)) and the platinum complexes (which are not covered here). This section will concentrate only on recent aspects of the chemistry and design of the covalent alkylating agents, since a number of excellent historical reviews exist[42].

1 : chlorambucil   2 : melphalan   3 : cyclophosphamide

Chemistry of cross-linking

The nitrogen mustard alkylating agents exert their antiproliferative cytotoxic effects by interstrand cross-linking of DNA[43], although there is recent evidence[44] that they also cause termination of transcription. Early work on the isolation of cross-linked fragments from digested alkylator-treated DNA showed that these cross-links were predominantly between the C7 positions on guanines[45]. The residues in DNA most likely to be attacked are guanines in runs of contiguous guanines[46], which have the lowest molecular electrostatic potentials[47]. Although it has been widely assumed that these cross-links were between adjacent guanines, recent work shows that the simple nitrogen mustard, mechlorethamine (4), preferentially cross-links between non-adjacent guanines[48]. Studies on the kinetics of cross-linking have shown that the second alkylation event, to form the cross-link, can be very slow[49], and recent work[50] on the sequence-specificity of cross-linking by mitomycin C (5) suggests that a critical factor is the correct spatial placement of the second substrate site.

4 : mechlorethamine   5 : mitomycin C

DNA-targeting of cross-linking agents

Simple alkylating agents suffer from a number of drawbacks. Although their site of action is DNA, they have no particular affinity for it. Thus, due to their necessarily high chemical reactivity, a large proportion of the drug may be completely inactivated by hydrolysis, or lost by interactions with other cellular macromolecules, before reaching the DNA. When reaction does occur, the majority of events (ca. 95%) are mono-alkylations, due to the slow kinetics of the second alkylation step (see above), allowing *in situ* hydrolysis to compete with cross-linking. Such monoadducts are considered to be genotoxic rather than cytotoxic[51]. Simple alkylators have little ability to recognize sequences larger than a single nucleotide[52]. Finally, resistance to such reactive electrophiles is easily developed by an increase in the cellular level of low-molecular-weight thiols (particularly glutathione)[53].

Many of these drawbacks could, in principle, be ameliorated by attaching the mustard to a carrier molecule having some affinity for DNA. Such targeting to DNA (in a general sense) should result in less diversion of active drug by reaction with other cell components, and the use of sequence-specific carriers should direct the pattern of alkylation sites on DNA, ultimately allowing targeting to particular genes. An improvement in the proportion of lethal cross-links with respect to more genotoxic monoalkylation events might limit the known[54] carcinogenicity of alkylators. Finally, the development of resistance to such compounds by elevated cellular thiol levels is likely to be less effective.

Thus, the most well-defined new approach in this class of drugs is the development of 'DNA-targeted alkylators'. Results for compounds based on a number of different carrier molecules show that some of these goals can be met. Nitrogen mustards targeted by intercalating carriers such as acridines (6) and

6 : acridine-linked mustards
(n = 2-5)

7

anthraquinones (**7**) can achieve 10–100-fold improvements in potency and improved antileukaemic activity compared with the corresponding untargeted mustards of similar reactivity[55-58], and show altered patterns of DNA alkylation[52]. Similar results have been shown for intercalator-targeted Pt complexes[59,60].

DNA minor groove alkylators

Much greater scope exists for using minor groove binders as carriers, since these have a larger binding site size, with some showing specific reversible binding to DNA sequences as large as 4–5 base pairs[61,62]. The most susceptible alkylation sites in the minor groove are the N3 of adenine and the exocyclic 2-amino group of guanine. A nitrogen mustard derivative (**8**) based on the well-known class of polybenzamide minor groove binders[63] was shown to be a very potent cytotoxin, and to alkylate exclusively at adenine in runs of adenines[64]. Although a less potent cytotoxin, a bromoacetyl analogue (**9**) of the minor groove binding polypyrrole antibiotic distamycin was reported to have very high sequence-specificity of DNA alkylation[65], while a mustard analogue (**10**) showed good activity against solid tumours *in vivo*[66,67]. In contrast, mustard analogues (**11**) based on the anilinoquinoline carboxamide minor groove binder[62] were less effective[68], although apparently binding in the minor groove[69].

However, most of the recent work with DNA minor groove alkylators has not been concerned with synthetic mustard compounds, but with the natural products CC-1065 (**12**)[70] and anthramycin (**13**)[71] and their analogues. These compounds are monoalkylating agents, reacting in the minor groove respectively at the N3 of adenine at the 5'-end of runs of adenines, and at the exocyclic amino group of guanine. Despite forming only monoadducts, they are extraordinarily potent cytotoxins, possibly because they do not readily induce

DNA repair enzymes[72]. A great deal of work has been carried out on CC-1065 analogues. The stereochemistry of the reaction is known in detail[70,73], and the delayed toxicity, which is a feature of the parent compound, has been successfully designed out to provide a derivative (**14**) which is now in clinical trial[74].

12 : CC-1065

13 : anthramycin

14 : U73975

A resurgence of interest?

Although DNA-alkylating agents are among the oldest type of anticancer drugs, and the clinical agents now in use were all introduced before 1965, there have recently been sufficient new insights and techniques to suggest a resurgence of interest. Certainly this is an area where enough information is now available for medicinal chemists to attempt the *de novo* design of specific inhibitors of gene expression. In addition, the primary goal of new concepts, such as the ADEPT approach, many immunotoxins (see above), and hypoxia-selective cytotoxins (see below), is to deliver DNA-alkylating agents selectively to chosen tumour cell populations.

DNA-binding agents (topoisomerase II inhibitors)

Introduction

These are a very important class of clinical anticancer drugs. The first examples were all natural products, found by random screening programmes, e.g. actinomycin D (**15**)[75], daunomycin (**16**)[76], doxorubicin (**17**)[77] and 9-methoxyellipticine (**18**)[78]. Since these are all structurally complex molecules with multiple biological effects, it was not obvious for some time whether they collectively constituted a particular class. As methods were developed for determining how ligands bind to DNA, it was clear that one thing they had in common was their ability to bind to DNA by intercalation. This is the favoured mode of binding of all molecules which possess a flat aromatic chromophore, with the driving force for the interaction being stacking interactions between the drug and the base pairs, and also the increase in entropy by the release of structured water from both the DNA minor groove and the ligand. Because this binding mode distorts DNA structure, and because these compounds all inhibit nucleic acid synthesis, the latter was originally thought to be the mechanism by which their cytotoxicity and anticancer activity was expressed (the distortion being assumed to prevent template or polymerase binding).

The class was soon expanded by a variety of synthetic DNA-intercalating ligands, which were, in the main, deliberately designed as DNA-intercalators. The first of these synthetic compounds to reach clinical use was the 9-anilinoacridine derivative, amsacrine (19)[79], to be followed by a large number of other synthetic compounds, including bisantrene (20)[80], mitoxantrone (21)[81], celipticinium acetate (22)[82], oxantrazole (23)[83], amonafide (24)[84] and crisnatol (25)[85].

29

Early trends: targeting to DNA

Detailed structure–activity relationship studies with several classes of DNA-intercalating agents suggested that the *mode* of binding was important. Intercalative binding appeared to be a necessary but not sufficient condition for antitumour activity. While several studies showed that altering the structure of active compounds to prevent them binding by intercalation abolishes activity[86,87], there are also many examples of ligands which do bind by intercalation but which have no antitumour activity.

Many studies with different classes of DNA-intercalating compounds showed that their potency (both as cell culture cytotoxins and as antitumour drugs) often correlated positively with their *strength* of binding to DNA[88–91], although this is not always true[92]. The perceived relationship between high DNA-binding and efficacy led to much work developing ever more tightly binding compounds. One obvious approach was to use compounds (e.g. **26–28**) containing more than one DNA-intercalating ligand[93–96], since theoretical studies[97] showed that these (subject to certain restrictions) should bind very much more tightly than the corresponding monomers. Although some of these bis- and tris-intercalating ligands bind to DNA nearly as tightly as do regulatory proteins[96,98], there is in fact no clear relationship between binding level and even cytotoxicity *in vitro*, let alone activity *in vivo*, and no clinically useful drugs have resulted from this work. The only bis-intercalating drugs to receive clinical trials have been the antibiotic, echinomycin[99], and the pyridocarbazole derivative, ditercalinium (**29**) (quoted in reference 100). Although the latter has a unique mechanism of action, involving rapid degradation of mitochondrial DNA triggered by "futile repair"[101], it has not shown clinical efficacy.

26 : diphenanthridinium

27 : pyrazole diacridine

28 : triacridine

29 : ditercalinium

More recently, it has become clear that tight DNA-binding, far from being a positive factor, in fact severely limits the extravascular distributive properties of drugs[30]. Consideration of this has led to the concept of 'minimal' DNA-intercalating ligands, and work delineating the minimum chromophore necessary for intercalative binding has provided several new series of active DNA-intercalating drugs (e.g. **30–34**) based on the acridine, phenazine, 2-phenylquinoline, 2-phenylbenzimidazole and dibenzodioxin chromophores)[87,102–106].

There has also been interest in the relationship between biological activity and the *kinetics* of binding to DNA, especially the average residence time of the drug at any particular binding site. An NMR study of a wide variety of DNA-intercalating agents[107] concluded that there was some correlation between biological activity and long drug/DNA residence times, an observation generally supported by detailed stopped-flow spectrophotometric studies of the dissociation of analogues of actinomycin D[108], 9-aminoacridine carboxamides[109], anthraquinones[110,111], bisantrene analogues[112,113] and diacridines[95]. One strategy for attaining such long residence times is use of 'DNA-threading agents', compounds in which a DNA-intercalating chromophore is flanked by two bulky groove-residing side chains, one of which has to disengage through the helix to achieve dissociation. The natural product nogalamycin (**35**), which has very slow dissociation kinetics[114], has been shown by both NMR[115] and X-ray[116] studies to bind in such a fashion. A subclass of amsacrine-4-carboxamides (e.g. **36**) with slow dissociation kinetics has also been suggested to be DNA-threading agents[117]. These relationships provided a useful set of constraints on the design of DNA-intercalating agents, but no satisfactory overall picture relating drug structure and DNA interactions to activity (even cytotoxicity *in vitro*) could be deduced.

Later trends: targeting to enzyme

The observation[118] that the antitumour activity of many DNA-intercalating agents was due primarily to their production of DNA double-strand breaks by interfering with the normal functioning of the DNA enzyme topoisomerase II[119] explained the failure of DNA-binding studies to predict fully the activities of DNA-intercalating agents. It also accounted for the fact that these compounds show marked selectivity for cycling cells, since topoisomerase II was shown to

31

35 : nogalamycin

36 : amsacrine-4-carboxamide

be cell cycle dependent, and also to occur at higher levels in malignant and transformed cells[120]. Thus, plateau-phase AA8 cells are many-fold more resistant than log-phase cells to amsacrine, although drug accumulation and metabolism are similar in both cases[121]. Finally, it explained why compounds such as the epipodophyllotoxin etoposide (37), which is structurally related to tubulin inhibitors[122] and which has very little DNA-binding ability[123], possess very similar patterns of activity and resistance to those of the DNA-intercalators, by showing that these compounds also act via topoisomerase II inhibition. There is now good evidence[124] that the critical event is formation of a ternary complex between drug, DNA and enzyme. Thus, an ability to bind to DNA alone is less important than the ability to form a stable ternary complex.

37 : etoposide

Clearly, a full understanding of structure–activity relationships among the so-called 'DNA-binding topoisomerase II agents' will have to consider both DNA-binding and protein-binding properties. An important aspect of this is to delineate if possible, in each class of compounds, the DNA-binding and protein-binding domains. At the present time, this is most clearly defined for the 9-anilinoacridine class of compounds to which amsacrine belongs. The crystal structure of amsacrine shows that the plane of the anilino side chain is oriented almost orthogonally (about 70°) to the plane of the acridine chromophore[125], such that, when the acridine binds parallel to the base pair long axis, the side chain must protrude into one of the DNA grooves, probably the minor groove[126], from which it could make contacts with the enzyme.

Recently, the topoisomerase II enzyme was shown to consist of multiple isozymes arising from two separate genes[127]. The IIα form is the one regulated during the cell cycle, with the IIβ form becoming predominant in both non-cycling cells and cells resistant to 'classical' topo II-inhibiting agents[127,128]. The cell lines used to date in the development of DNA-intercalating agents possess the isozyme topoisomerase IIα. This identification of a second topoisomerase II isozyme has provided a new potential target for drug therapy of tumours, and studies with analogues of amsacrine[129,130] have already shown that redesign of the protein-binding domain can provide analogues (e.g. 38) which have greatly improved activity both *in vitro* and *in vivo* against 'drug-resistant' cell lines expressing topoisomerase IIβ.

Current design goals

As noted above, a major problem associated with DNA-intercalating agents is their susceptibility to P-glycoprotein-mediated multiple drug resistance (MDR). Thus, a major goal is to identify compounds not subject to this phenomenon. Studies with amsacrine analogues have shown that changes in the DNA-binding domain can provide the requisite property, with compounds such as CI-921 (39) lacking susceptibility to this form of MDR[131] (although still highly susceptible to MDR caused by changes in topoisomerase isozymes). Anthracycline 3'-cyanomorpholide analogues, such as MRA-CN (40) are also not cross-resistant. Reasons advanced for this are: their high lipophilicity which facilitates cell entry; the lack of basicity which may limit binding to the efflux pump; and the low levels of these very potent drugs which are required for activity[132].

Many classes of topoisomerase II inhibitors (anthracyclines, 9-anilino-acridines, anthraquinones, ellipticines, epipodophyllotoxins) are also redox-active compounds, via quinone-like structures which are present in either the parent molecule or in rapidly formed oxidative metabolites[133–137]. Although this is now not considered to be their primary mechanism of action, it may well be a factor contributing to their therapeutic effects (it appears to be a mandatory property for activity of the epipodophyllotoxins)[137]. However, the concomitant cardiotoxicity which the more active redox-cycling agents (particularly many anthracyclines) engender, through free radical damage of cardiac lipids[138], probably outweighs these beneficial effects. Another constraint on future design

39 : CI-921

40 : MRA-CN

is therefore to avoid structures with redox-cycling capability. Finally, there have been reports that some lipophilic DNA-intercalators particularly anthracyclines[139] and the arylmethylaminopropanediol class of compounds (e.g. crisnatol, 25)[140], also have cell-membrane-directed activity.

Thus, the development of this class of compounds, which had its origins in the random screening of complex natural products, now largely proceeds by lead development, within a large number of constraints imposed by the studies described above. It is debatable whether we yet know enough about these compounds to undertake the *de novo* design of completely novel and 'better' topoisomerase II inhibitors.

DNA-cutting agents (free radical generators)

Introduction

There is nothing inherently remarkable about breaking DNA by radical chemistry, and in fact many metal complexes and redox-active compounds are known to nick DNA under oxidative conditions. However, useful antitumour activity via such a mechanism appears to be limited to compounds which can target the radicals to DNA in such a way as to generate double-strand breaks. The compounds which do this most successfully are complex natural products, which are now providing starting points for synthesizing new classes of synthetic compounds with the same ability.

Oxygen free radical generators

The only compound of this type in clinical use is the glycopeptide, bleomycin A2 (41), the principal component of a complex mixture isolated from the micro-organism *Streptomyces verticillus*[141]. Bleomycin is a very useful drug clinically. Its mode of selectivity is unique, resulting from a combination of selective tissue distribution (concentrating particularly in lung and skin tissue) and selective deactivation by an enzyme called bleomycin hydrolase, a cysteine protease in which lung and skin tissue are particularly deficient[142].

41 : bleomycin A2

The molecule consists of two functional domains. The DNA-targeting domain consists of the charged dimethylsulphonium ion (providing long-range targeting to DNA), the bithiazole ring (providing local positioning by intercalation), and possibly some of the carbohydrate elements, which contribute to DNA targeting in undefined ways. The radical-generating domain consists of five seemingly unconnected nitrogens which actually make up a 5-point metal co-ordination site. There has been much speculation concerning the activated species (produced in the presence of oxygen and thiols), which is now thought to be an Fe(III)OOH compound, produced by reduction of the initially formed Fe(III)O$_2$ complex[143].

The activated antibiotic molecule, due to its specific binding, is able to abstract a hydrogen atom from DNA in a very specific fashion, from the 4'-position of the deoxyribose. This initiates a complex reaction which results in a one-base gap in the DNA strand[144]. The cutting is sequence selective, occurring most often at Cs and Ts 3' to G (i.e. at GC and GT sequences). The high cytotoxicity of bleomycin is due to the fact that this is a catalytic reaction, with a single drug molecule initiating formation of several radicals in the same place, leading to a high frequency of double-strand breaks (a ratio of ca. 9:1 over single-strand breaks)[144].

There has been relatively little work on the deliberate design of oxygen radical generators as antitumour drugs[145]. Research on close analogues of bleomycin showed that changes in the radical-generating domain usually abolish activity[145]. Changes in the bithiazole part of the DNA-targeting domain are permitted and may even be positively beneficial[146], but synthesis has been limited because of its difficulty. No synthetic compounds have been evaluated clinically.

35

Carbon free radical generators

The antitumour antibiotic, neocarzinostatin (NCS), shows good experimental activity against both leukaemia and solid tumours, and has been used for the treatment of pancreatic and gastric cancer and leukaemia in humans (quoted in reference 147). Although it was first isolated in 1965 from *Streptomyces carzinostaticus*, the structure (**42**) of the unstable non-protein chromophore (which contains all the biological activity) was not deduced until twenty years later[148]. The molecule contains a DNA-targeting domain (the methoxy-naphthalene and amino sugar moieties) which locates the drug in the minor groove[149], and a unique enediyne grouping which is the radical-generating domain[150].

The primary DNA damage caused by NCS (again in the presence of oxygen and thiols) consists of DNA single- and double-strand breaks (under some conditions, up to 25% double-strand breaks), initiated by free radical attack on the C-5' of deoxyribose[151]. The mechanism of this process is considered to proceed via radical attack by thiol at C12, which results in opening of the epoxide ring and formation of a cumulene structure which rapidly undergoes a spontaneous electrocyclic reaction to the indene diradical[152]. This *simultaneously* abstracts protons from the C5' positions of two spatially close deoxyribose sugars on the DNA, leading to a double-strand break.

42 : neocarzinostatin chromophore

43 : esperamicins : R_1, R_2 = polyglycosides
44 : calichemicins : R_1=H, R_2 = polyglycosides

More recently, two other classes of extremely potent enediyne cytotoxins, esperamicins (e.g. **43**) and calicheamicins (e.g. **44**) were isolated from soil bacteria[153,154]. Some of these compounds are effective against a variety of mouse tumours *in vivo* at around 0.1 μg/kg, making them the most potent anticancer agents known (ca. 5000-fold more potent than doxorubicin). The DNA-targeting domains of these compounds, and the way in which they orient the molecules on DNA, have not been fully delineated. Computer modelling suggests that the thiobenzoate of calicheamicin acts as a sequence non-specific locator in the minor groove, with the ethylamino and rhamnose sugars also being involved[155]. The radical-generating domain of these compounds is a 3-ene-1,5-diyne moiety, held in a rigid tricyclic framework. Activation is by thiol-induced reduction of the trisulphide group to the sulphide anion, which then undergoes a rapid internal addition reaction, a process which significantly alters the geometry of the enediyne moiety, bringing the conjugated multiple bonds closer together[156]. This permits an electrocyclic cyclization reaction[157] to form the transient benzene 1,4-diradical, the driving force for this reaction being a relief of about 12 kcal/mol of strain energy.

The end result is very efficient generation of the extremely reactive benzene 1,4-diradical in the minor groove of DNA, with each radical centre able efficiently to abstract a ribose C-5' hydrogen atom at two spatially close sites on opposite DNA strands. As with neocarzinostatin, an oxygen-dependent cleavage process then follows, resulting in a DNA double-strand break. The potency of these compounds *in vitro* is again due to very efficient generation of highly lethal double-strand breaks. Calicheamicin causes site-specific double-stranded DNA cleavage at *very* low concentrations (down to 7 nmol/L), with very few single-strand breaks observed.

Other enediyne antibiotics have since been described[158]. The details of their activation chemistry are different, but the concept (creation of a diradical in close proximity to the DNA via an electrocyclic process) is the same. Several synthetic enediynes which possess the radical-generating domain, and which cause DNA double-strand breaks on reductive activation, have been prepared[159,160].

Future prospects

The radical generators are a novel class of cytotoxin, acting by delivery of highly reductive oxygen- or carbon-centred diradicals to specific regions of DNA. The singular advantage of bleomycin (the only compound of the type in clinical use) is its novel toxicity profile, particularly its lack of myelo-suppression. It would also appear difficult for cells to develop resistance to the actual toxic event, and the potency of the compounds (at least the carbon radical generators) militates against the development of transport-based resistance. However, resistance might be developed by the cells via the obligative bioreductive step. A possible use for these compounds (because of their extraordinary potency) is as the toxin component in monoclonal antibody-targeted drugs. Most work to date has been at the random screening level, but enough has been discovered about the mechanism of radical generation to have stimulated work on *de novo* synthesis.

Hypoxia-selective cytotoxins

Introduction: The phenomenon of tumour hypoxia

For a solid tumour to reach a diameter greater than a few millimetres, it must develop its own vascular network[27]. This neoplastic vasculature is not efficient[28], and results in many cells existing in a state of chronic hypoxia because of their relatively long distance from the nearest blood vessel; such cells have been termed 'diffusion-limited'[161]. Another type of hypoxia, acute or transient hypoxia, caused by the spasmodic closing off of a blood vessel due to compression by the growing tumour, has also been demonstrated in animal tumours[162] and has been termed 'perfusion hypoxia'[161]. Such hypoxic cells have been shown to exist in human solid tumours[28,163], and have been shown to be resistant to chemotherapy[164] by virtue of their inaccessibility to drugs[29,30], their low extracellular pH[165] and their non-cycling status[166]. Despite these difficulties, the hypoxic microenvironment is an attractive target since nearly all normal tissue is well perfused, and drugs which could be activated only in hypoxic regions offer the possibility of being truly specific for solid tumours[167] (see also Chapter 4 of this volume).

Early trends: hypoxia selectivity as a side-effect

Most nitroaromatic compounds which have sufficiently high redox potentials to undergo efficient cellular reduction give products which are not markedly cytotoxic, and therefore show little hypoxia-selective cytotoxicity. However, compounds which fragment on reduction to especially reactive species do display this property. The most well-studied class are the 2-nitroimidazoles, which were developed as radiosensitizers, but which also show significant hypoxic-selective cytotoxicity[168]. The parent 2-nitroimidazole compound (azomycin: **45**) is itself a hypoxia-selective cytotoxin, but the best-known example is the *N*-substituted derivative, misonidazole (**46**)[169]. *N*-Alkyl-2-nitroimidazoles have a complex reduction chemistry, with the key intermediates appearing to be dihydroxyimidazolium adducts formed from the hydroxylamine. These eventually yield glyoxal and guanidinium ions, or react with nucleophiles[170]. Studies with radiolabelled misonidazole have shown that the cytotoxic event is formation of DNA adducts[171,172]. The 2-nitroimidazoles show about a 10-fold selectivity for hypoxic cells *in vitro*, but are not sufficiently potent for clinical use as hypoxia-selective cytotoxins. They have little DNA affinity[173], and the small monoadducts formed represent a class of relatively non-toxic (although mutagenic) and easily repaired DNA lesions[51].

45 : R=H : azomycin

46 : R=CH$_2$CH(OH)CH$_2$OMe : misonidazole

Parameters for hypoxia selectivity

The requirements of efficient vascular distribution and extravascular diffusion to reach hypoxic regions in solid tumours, followed by rapid and selective activation there to very cytotoxic species, place severe constraints on the *de novo* design of hypoxia-selective cytotoxins.

Selective activation is normally sought by utilizing reductive mechanisms which are, at some early point, reversible by molecular oxygen in oxygenated cells, rather than mechanisms which are exclusive to hypoxic cells. Thus, nitroaromatic compounds, such as the 2-nitroimidazoles, are reduced in cells by a number of flavoprotein enzymes[174] which effect stepwise addition of up to six electrons. The key process is addition of the first electron to form the nitro radical anion, an electron transfer process whose rate is related to the difference in the reduction potentials of the nitroaromatic compound and the cellular enzyme[175]. To be reduced sufficiently rapidly by cellular enzymes, drugs appear to need a redox potential above about $-450\,mV$[167]. In oxygenated tissues, the initially formed radical anion can be scavenged by molecular oxygen in another electron-transfer process, to re-form the nitro compound with the concomitant production of superoxide (futile metabolism). This back-reaction slows as the nitro group redox potential increases, and the useful upper limit of the nitro group redox potential appears to be ca. $-300\,mV$[167,175].

Mechanisms for enhanced cytotoxicity following reduction

Several specific concepts have also been explored to provide very cytotoxic species following such (hypoxia-selective) reduction. As noted above, some nitroaromatics, such as the 2-nitroimidazoles, spontaneously fragment on reduction, to form cytotoxic DNA-alkylating agents. In attempts to improve the intrinsic cytotoxicity of the 2-nitroimidazoles, while preserving their selectivity, they have been attached to various types of reversible DNA-binding carriers. Thus, the phenanthridinium analogue, NLP-1 (**47**) shows 10–100-fold greater potency than misonidazole as a hypoxia-selective cytotoxin, even though the compound does not bind particularly strongly to DNA[173,176]. The related acridine-borne analogue, NLA-1 (**48**), is also a highly potent hypoxia-selective cytotoxin *in vitro*, but is not active *in vivo*[177]. Thus, while the concept of DNA-targeting has been successful in terms of improving potency, the carriers used to date appear to bind too strongly to DNA; and it remains to be seen whether a suitable compromise can be reached.

47 : NLP-1   48 : NLA-1

A related approach involves the use of compounds which exhibit both hypoxia selectivity and DNA affinity in the same chromophore. The best-known examples are 1-nitroacridines, such as nitracrine (**49**). This compound shows very potent hypoxia-selective cytotoxicity against tumour cells in culture[178], but is not active against hypoxic cells in solid tumours *in vivo*, due probably to a combination of a high reduction potential ($-303\,mV$), resulting in rapid metabolism even in well-oxygenated tissues, and a relatively high DNA-binding constant, resulting in slow extravascular diffusion[179]. 4-Substituted analogues with lower redox potentials had improved metabolic stability[180], with the 4-methoxy derivative (50) showing some activity against hypoxic cells *in vivo*. Analogous but less tightly DNA-binding 5-nitroquinolines, such as 51, show both improved extravascular penetration properties and greater hypoxia selectivity than nitracrine[179]. However, even 51 shows no *in vivo* hypoxia-selective activity, suggesting that it still binds too tightly to DNA[181]. Providing appropriate rates of extravascular diffusion thus seems likely to be the critical determinant for this class of compound.

49 : R=H : nitracrine
50 : R=OMe

52

The 4-nitropyrazoloacridines (e.g. 52), developed primarily for their solid-tumour activity, are another group of DNA-binding nitroaromatic compounds which show hypoxia selectivity[182] *in vitro*, but no data on their hypoxia selectivity *in vivo* has been reported.

An alternative strategy for providing very cytotoxic species on reduction, which has been discussed by several authors in varying detail[165,183,184], is the use of nitroaromatic compounds as prodrugs. In these compounds, a DNA-alkylating moiety is activated by cellular reduction of the nitro group. Since the stability and alkylating reactivity of aromatic nitrogen mustards is determined almost entirely by the electron density on the nitrogen[185], conversion of the powerfully electron-withdrawing nitro group (Hammett σ value 0.78) to the electron-donating hydroxylamine (σ −0.32) or amino (σ −0.66) metabolites activates the mustard considerably[165,186]. The first such compound demonstrated to have hypoxic selectivity was the dinitroaziridine CB1954 (53)[187]. A recent report on the synthesis and cell culture evaluation of a series of substituted aniline chloromustards showed that the simplest such prodrug, *N,N*-bis(2-chloroethyl)-4-nitroaniline (54), also has modest but significant hypoxic selectivity[186]. This is despite a very low nitro group reduction potential of about −510 mV, which implies very slow metabolic reduction, even under hypoxic conditions, and provides encouraging evidence that the concept is viable if compounds with the correct combination of physicochemical properties can be constructed.

53 : CB1954   54

The other well-known class of compounds, apart from nitroaromatics, that can undergo 1-electron reduction (in two 1-electron steps, first to the semiquinone radical and then to the hydroquinone) are quinones. The semiquinone radical is capable of being scavenged by oxygen in oxygenated normal tissues, resulting in hypoxia-selective metabolism, although direct oxygen-irreversible two-electron reduction pathways (e.g. by DT diaphorase) are also possible. The aziridoquinone mitomycin C (**5**), which has been used as an adjunct to radiotherapy in head and neck cancer[188,189], has been claimed to be a hypoxia-selective cytotoxin, although its level of cytotoxicity *in vitro* is modest and cell line dependent (presumably depending on the enzyme present)[190]. The lethal event is DNA cross-linking via the 2-amino group of guanine[191], which occurs following a complex activation process[192].

The benzotriazine-N-oxides, originally developed as antimalarials, have recently been identified[193] as hypoxia-selective cytotoxins with a novel mode of action. The most well studied is 3-amino-1,2,4-benzotriazine-1,4-dioxide (SR4233) (**55**) which is metabolized by sequential reduction of first the 4- and then the 1-oxide groups in two 2-electron steps. The mechanism of hypoxia selectivity is considered to be an initial one-electron reduction to the C3-centred radical anion, which can be back-scavenged by oxygen. In the absence of oxygen, this radical anion abstracts hydrogen atoms from cellular targets (including DNA deoxyribose) to form the mono-oxide, which reacts (at a much lower rate due to a lower redox potential) in another 2-electron step[194]. A dose-dependent hypoxia-selective formation of both single- and double-strand DNA breaks is seen, and these correlate with cytotoxicity.

55 : SR4233

Various metals form substitutionally-inert co-ordination complexes with nitrogen ligands; for example $Co(NH_3)_6^{3+}$ has a displacement halflife[195] of

6×10^9 sec. One-electron reduction to a Co(II) complex results in enormous labilization of such ligands[196]. Hypoxia-selective metabolism is therefore possible, with ligand displacement by water to form the very stable hexa-aquo Co(II) cation competing (in oxygenated cells) with reoxidation of the Co(II) complex by molecular oxygen (futile metabolism). Such compounds are capable of hypoxia-selective cytotoxicity provided that the free ligands are much more cytotoxic than when metal bound. Recent studies[197] show this to be the case, since complexes of aziridine with Co(III) (e.g. **56**) are greatly stabilized with respect to hydrolysis. Such complexes are not hypoxia selective, probably because the reduced Co(II) forms are too labile, but related complexes employing chelating alkylating agents as ligands (e.g. **57**) do show limited hypoxia-selective cytotoxicity *in vitro*[198].

Future de novo design

Of all the areas of anticancer drug development discussed here, the hypoxia-selective cytotoxins are among the most suited to *de novo* design at the current time. Although dependent on reductase enzymes for activation, the target is primarily a physical condition (lack of oxygen). Strategies to maximize their extravascular diffusion, selectivity of activation, and toxicity of the reduced species depend primarily on a knowledge of chemistry, and this class should be an attractive goal for medicinal chemists.

Radiosensitizers

Introduction

The hypoxic cells in solid tumours have long been known to have a limiting effect on the efficacy of clinical radiotherapy[199]. Thus there have been many efforts to develop 'oxygen-mimetic' radiosensitizers; electron-affinic compounds which will take the place of oxygen by transferring an electron to the initially formed DNA radicals, but will not be actively metabolized, so that they can reach the hypoxic interior of solid tumours. The 'sensitization efficiency' of nitroaromatic radiosensitizers is governed largely by their reduction potentials[200], increasing with higher redox potentials since the rate of electron transfer between nitroaromatic substance and DNA radical depends on the difference in the redox potentials[175]. However, the dose-limiting cytotoxicity of these compounds (caused by the products of enzymic nitro group reduction) is similarly dependent on redox potential[201]. This parallel between the electronic requirements for both sensitization and cytotoxicity remains a fundamental problem in the development of nitroaryl radiosensitizers.

Early trends: optimization of nitroimidazole pharmacology

The first clinically useful radiosensitizer was the 2-nitroimidazole derivative, misonidazole (**46**)[202]. However, this compound has such limited potency that it is very difficult to achieve sufficiently high concentrations in tumours to obtain useful sensitization. The limiting clinical toxicity of misonidazole is peripheral neuropathy due to its uptake into the brain at these high doses. Most of the early work on developing 'second-generation' analogues has focused on improving the pharmacology of misonidazole[203], to improve cell uptake (and thus potency) while lowering the relative uptake into the brain. It was found that tumour/brain ratios increased as the drugs became more hydrophilic, and there appeared to be an optimum value of drug lipophilicity (log P about -1.35), which resulted in a maximal '*in vivo* therapeutic index'. The compound with the closest value to the ideal was an analogue of misonidazole known as etanidazole (**58**)[204]. Other studies focused on cationic compounds with rapid renal clearance (sensitization depends largely on peak drug concentration at the time of irradiation, while toxicity relates more to the plasma concentration $\times$ time integral)[205]. From these studies, a relatively lipophilic piperidine analogue (pimonidazole, **59**) was selected. Both of these compounds are now in clinical trial.

58 : etanidazole   59 : pimonidazole

Recent trends: DNA-targeting

One strategy for improving the radiosensitization efficiency of the 2-nitroimidazoles was to attach to the molecule an alkylating agent which would purportedly locate the drug on DNA. The most well-studied such compound is the aziridine analogue, RSU-1069 (**60**)[206], which does show greater radiosensitization efficiency. However, clinical trials showed it to cause unacceptable gastrointestinal toxicity[207]. More recently, the use of reversible DNA-binding carriers has been explored. Both the acridine- and phenanthridium-targeted 2-

nitroimidazoles, NPL-1 and NLA-1 (**47** and **48**), mentioned above as hypoxia-selective cytotoxins, also show increased radiosensitization efficiency *in vitro*[173,177]. The nitroacridines discussed above are also very potent radio-sensitizers *in vitro*. However, most of the improvement in potency (compared with neutral compounds, such as misonidazole) is due to high cell uptake factors driven by the DNA-binding of the compounds[208].

60 : RSU-1069

Future trends

Despite much work, nitroaryl compounds have not yet proved clinically useful as oxygen-mimetic radiosensitizers. The similar dependence of both radiosensitizing potency and reductively mediated cytotoxicity on nitro group redox potential is a fundamental problem in the development of nitroaryl radiosensitizers. It remains to be seen whether non-nitro compounds (for example, metal complexes[209]), which might not be subject to this limitation, can be successfully developed as radiosensitizers.

SUMMARY AND CONCLUSIONS

No area of drug development is homogeneous, so that generalizations are difficult to draw. Nevertheless, anticancer drug development has undoubtedly undergone greater changes in philosophy over the last 15–20 years than is the case for almost any other class of drugs. From a field dominated by structural chemistry, random screening and simplistic biological models, it has developed to the point where it is today on the brink of being dominated by biotechnology. However, it is the thesis of this chapter that small molecules should remain a major concept in anticancer drug design. Slow progress to date lies more perhaps with the inadequacy of the screening systems[26] than with any inherent lack of selectivity of such compounds. Medicinal chemistry still has much to do in new drug development in this area.

Random testing against more sophisticated screens, coupled with a greatly increased ability to delineate modes of action, will continue to produce novel compounds. Increased capabilities in organic synthesis mean that such compounds serve increasingly as new leads for design rather than as drugs in their own right: the enediyne compounds[153–160] are a good example. Computer-based methods (both statistical and graphical) which permit more efficient optimization of the biological profiles of known classes of drugs, and delineation of the essential pharmacophores of more complex biological molecules, are drastically changing drug design methods.

Finally, the recent explosion of knowledge about the nature of cancer, and the identification of numerous (if subtle) differences between cancer and normal cells at the genetic and tumour microenviroment levels, have provided many potential targets for new drug design. It will take all of the new tools of medicinal chemistry to exploit these opportunities fully.

References

1. Goodman, L. S., Wintrobe, M. M., Damesheck, W., Goodman, M. J., Gilman, A. and McLennan, M. T. (1946). Nitrogen mustard therapy. Use of methyl-bis(β-chloroethyl)amine hydrochloride and tris-(β-chloroethyl)amine hydrochloride for Hodgkin's disease, lymphosarcoma, leukemia and certain allied and miscellaneous disorders. *J. Am. Med. Assoc.*, **132**, 126–132
2. Zee-Cheng, R. K.-Y. and Cheng, C. C. (1988). Screening and evaluation of anticancer agents. *Methods Finding Exptl. Clin. Pharmacol.*, **10**, 67–101
3. Hansch, C. and Leo, A. J. (1979). *Substituent Constants for Correlation Analysis in Chemistry and Biology*. N Y: Wiley-Interscience
4. Martin, Y. C. (1978). *Quantitative Drug Design: A Critical Introduction*. In Marcel Dekker, NY: Magee, P. S., Henry, D. R. and Block, J. H. (eds.) (1990) *Probing Bioactive Mechanisms*, ACS Symposium Series 413. NY: ACS
5. Vane, J. and Cuatrecasas, P. (1984). Genetic engineering and pharmaceuticals. *Nature (London)*, **312**, 303–305
6. Upeslacis, J. and Hinman, L. (1988). Chemical modification of antibodies for cancer chemotherapy. *Ann. Rep. Med. Chem.*, **23**, 151–160
7. Blattler, W. A., Lambert, J. M. and Goldmacher, V. S. (1989) Realising the full potential of immunotoxins. *Cancer Cells*, **1**, 50–55
8. Rosenberg, S (1985) Lymphokine-activated killer cells: a new approach to the immunotherapy of cancer. *J. Natl. Cancer Inst.*, **75**, 595–603
9. Lotze, M. T., Frana, L. W., Sharrow, S. O., Robb, R. J. and Rosenberg, S. A. (1985). *In vivo* administration of purified human interleukin 2. *J. Immunol.*, **134**, 157–166
10. Thompson, J. A., Brady, J., Kidd, P. and Feter, A. (1985). Recombinant α-2-interferon in the treatment of hairy cell leukemia. *Cancer Treatment Rep.*, **69**, 791–793
11. Blick, M., Sherwin, S. A., Rosenblum, M. and Gutterman, J. (1987). Phase I study of recombinant tumor necrosis factor in cancer patients. *Cancer Res.*, **47**, 2986–2989
12. Cillo, C., Mach, J.-P., Schreyer, M. and Carrel, S. (1984). Antigenic heterogeneity of clones and subclones from human melanoma sublines demonstrated by a panel of monoclonal antibodies and microfluorometric analysis. *Int. J. Cancer*, **34**, 11–21
13. Sutherland, R., Buchegger, F., Schreyer, M., Vacca, A. and Mach, J.-P. (1987). Penetration and binding of radiolabelled anti-carcinoembryonic antigen monoclonal antibodies and their antigen binding fragments in human colon multicellular tumor spheroids. *Cancer Res.*, **47**, 1627–1633
14. Bagshawe, K. D. (1990). Antibody directed enzyme prodrug therapy. *Anal. Proc.*, **27**, 5.
15. Springer, C. J., Antoniw, P., Bagshawe, K. D., Searle, F., Bisset, G. M. F. and Jarman, M. (1990). Novel prodrugs which are activated to cytotoxic alkylating agents by carboxypeptidase G2. *J. Med. Chem.*, **33**, 677–681
16. Waldrop, M. M. (1990). The reign of trial and error draws to a close. *Science*, **247**, 28–29
17. Denny, W. A. (1988). New directions in the design and evaluation of anticancer drugs. *Drug Design Deliv.*, **3**, 99–124
18. Bishop, J. M. (1987) The molecular genetics of cancer. *Science*, **235**, 305–310
19. Weinberg, R. A. (1987). The action of oncogenes in the cytoplasm and nucleus. *Science*, **230**, 770–776
20. Weinstein, I. B. (1987). Growth factors, oncogenes and multi-stage carcinogenesis. *J. Cell. Biochem.*, **33**, 312–324
21. Stein, C. A. and Cohen, J. S. (1988). Oligodeoxynucleotides as inhibitors of gene expression: a review. *Cancer Res.*, **48**, 2659–2668

22. Rothenburg, M., Johnson, G., Laughlin, C., Green, I., Cradock, J., Sarver, N. and Cohen, J. S. (1989). Oligodeoxynucleotides as inhibitors of gene expression: therapeutic implications. *J. Natl. Cancer Inst.*, **81**, 1539–1544

23. Lown, J. W. (1988). Lexitropsins: rational design of DNA sequence reading agents as novel anti-cancer drugs and potential cellular probes. *Anti-Cancer Drug Design*, **3**, 25–40

24. Shiraishi, T., Owada, M. K., Tatsuka, M., Yamashita, T., Wanatabe, K. and Kakunaga, T. (1989). Specific inhibitors of tyrosine-specific tyrosine kinases: properties of 4-hydroxycinnamamide *in vitro*. *Cancer Res.*, **49**, 2374–2378

25. Gescher, A. and Dale, L. L. (1989). Protein kinase C: a novel target for rational anti-cancer drug design? *Anti-Cancer Drug Design*, **4**, 93–105

26. Grindey, G. B. (1990). Current status of cancer drug development: failure or limited success? *Cancer Cells*, **2**, 163–171

27. Folkman, J., Watson, K., Ingber, D. and Hanahan, D. (1988). Induction of angiogenesis during the transition from hyperplasia to neoplasia. *Nature* (*London*), **339**, 58–61.

28. Vaupel, P., Kallinowski, F. and Okunieff, P. (1989). Blood flow, oxygen and nutrient supply, and metabolic microenvironment of human tumors: a review. *Cancer Res.*, **49**, 6449–6465

29. Jain, R. K. (1989). Delivery of novel therapeutic agents in tumors: physiological barriers and strategies. *J. Natl. Cancer Inst.*, **81**, 570–576

30. Durand, R. E. (1989). Distribution of and activity of antineoplastic drugs in a tumor model. *J. Natl. Cancer Inst.*, **81**, 146–152

31. Casciari, J. J., Sotirchos, S. V. and Sutherland,R. M. (1988). Glucose diffusivity in multicellular tumor spheroids. *Cancer Res.*, **48**, 3905–3909

32. McFadden, R. and Kwok, C. C. (1988). Mathematical model of simultaneous diffusion and binding of antitumor antibodies in multicellular human tumor spheroids. *Cancer Res.*, **48**, 4032–4037

33. Curt, G. A., Clendeninn, N. J. and Chabner, B. A. (1984). Drug resistance in cancer. *Cancer Treatment Rep.*, **68**, 87–99

34. Harris, A .L. and Hickson, I. D. (1989). Drug resistance, DNA repair and growth factors. In Kessel, D. (ed.) *Resistance to Antineoplastic Drugs*. (Boca Raton: CRC Press)

35. Park, J.-G., Kramer, B. X., Lai, S.-L., Goldstein, L. J. and Gazdar, A. F. (1990). Chemosensitivity patterns and expression of human multidrug resistance-associated MDR1 gene by human gastric and colorectal carcinoma cell lines. *J. Natl. Cancer Inst.*, **82**, 193–198

36. Georges, E., Bradley, G., Gariepy, J. and Ling, V. (1990). Detection of P-glycoprotein isoforms by gene-specific monoclonal antibodies. *Proc. Natl. Acad. Sci. (USA)*, **87**, 152–156

37. Endicott, J. A. and Ling, V. (1989). The biochemistry of P-glycoprotein-mediated multidrug resistance. *Ann. Rev. Biochem.*, **58**, 351–375

38. Selassie, C. D., Hansch, C. and Khwaja, T. A. (1990) Structure–activity relationships of antineoplastic agents in multidrug resistance. *J. Med. Chem.*, **33**, 1914–1919

39. Hofsli, E. and Nissen-Meyer, J. (1990). Reversal of multidrug resistance by lipophilic drugs. *Cancer Res.*, **50**, 3997–4002

40. Zamora, J. M., Pearce, H. L. and Beck, W. T. (1988). Physicochemical properties shared by compounds that modulate multidrug resistance in human leukemic cells. *Mol. Pharmacol.*, **33**, 454–462

41. Pearce, H. L., Winter, M. A. and Beck, W. T. (1990). Structural characteristics of compounds that modulate P-glycoprotein-associated multidrug resistance. *Adv. Enzyme Regul.*, **30**, 357–373

42. Wilman, D. E. V. and Connors, T. A. (1983). In Neidle S. and Waring, M. J. (eds.) *Molecular Aspects of Anticancer Drug Action*, p. 234. (London: MacMillan)

43. Hansson, J., Lewensohn R., Ringborg. U. and Nilsson, B. (1987). Formation and removal of DNA cross-links induced by melphalan and nitrogen mustard in relation to drug-induced cytotoxicity in human melanoma cells. *Cancer Res.*, **47**, 2631–2637

44. Peiper, R. O., Futscher, B. W., and Erickson, L. C. (1989). Transcription-terminating lesions induced by bifunctional alkylating agents *in vivo*. *Carcinogenesis*, **10**, 1307–1314

45. Singer, B. (1975). The chemical effects of nucleic acid alkylation, and their relationship to mutagenesis and carcinogenesis. *Prog. Nucl. Acids Res. Mol. Biol.*, **15**, 219–284

46. Kohn, K. W., Hartley, J. A. and Mattes, W. B. (1987). Mechanisms of DNA sequence-selective alkylation of guanine N7 positions by nitrogen mustards. *Nucleic Acids Res.*, **15**, 10531–10549

47. Perehia, D. and Pullman, A. (1979). The molecular electrostatic potential of the B-DNA helix. II. The region of the adenine–thymine base pair. *Theor. Chim. Acta*, **50**, 351–354

48. Millard, J. T., Raucher, S. and Hopkins, P. B. (1990). Mechlorethamine crosslinks deoxyguanosine residues at 5'-GNC sequences in duplex DNA fragments. *J. Am. Chem. Soc.,* **112**, 2459–2460

49. Butour, J. L. and Johnson, N. P. (1986). Chemical reactivity of monofunctional platinum-DNA adducts. *Biochemistry,* **25**, 4534–4539

50. Teng, S. P., Woodson, S. A. and Crothers, D. M. (1989). DNA sequence specificity of mitomycin C cross-linking. *Biochemistry,* **28**, 3901–3907

51. Brendel, M. and Ruhland, A. (1984). Relationship between functionality and genetic toxicology of selected DNA-damaging agents. *Mutat. Res.,* **133**, 51–85

52. Prakash, A. S., Denny, W. A., Gourdie, T. A., Valu, K. K., Woodgate, P. D. and Wakelin, L. P. G. (1990). DNA-directed alkylating ligands as potential antitumor agents: sequence specificity of alkylation by DNA-intercalating acridine-linked aniline mustards. *Biochemistry,* **29**, 9799–9807

53. Suzukake, K., Vistica, B. P. and Vistica, D. T. (1983). Dechlorination of L-phenylalanine mustard by sensitive and resistant tumor cells and its relationship to intracellular glutathione content. *Biochem. Pharmacol.,* **32**, 165–167

54. Schmahl, D. (1986). Carcinogenicity of anticancer drugs and especially alkylating agents. In Schmahl, D. and Kaldor, J. M. (eds.) *Carcinogenicity of Alkylating Cytostatic Drugs,* pp. 143–146. IARC Sci. Publ. No. 78. (Lyon: IARC)

55. Creech, H. J., Preston, R. K., Peck, R. M., O'Connell, A. S. and Ames, B. N. (1972). Antitumor and mutagenesis properties of a variety of heterocyclic nitrogen and sulfur mustards. *J. Med. Chem.,* **15**, 739–746

56. Koyama, M., Takahashi, K., Chou, T.-C., Darzynkiewicz, Z., Kapuscinski, J., Kelly, T. T. and Wanatabe, K. A. (1989). Intercalating agents with covalent bond forming capability. A novel type of potential anticancer agents. 2. Derivatives of chrysophanol and emodin. *J. Med. Chem.,* **32**, 1594–1599

57. Gourdie, T. A., Valu, K. K., Gravatt, G. L., Boritzki, T. J., Baguley, B. C., Wilson, W. R., Woodgate, P. D. and Denny, W. A. (1990). DNA-directed alkylating agents. 1. Structure–activity relationships for acridine-linked aniline mustards: consequences of varying the reactivity of the mustard. *J. Med. Chem.,* **33**, 1177–1186

58. Valu, K. K., Gourdie, T. A., Gravatt, G. L., Boritzki, T. J., Woodgate, P. D., Baguley, B. C. and Denny, W. A. (1990). DNA-directed alkylating agents. 3. Structure–activity relationships for acridine-linked aniline mustards: consequences of varying the length of the linker chain. *J. Med. Chem.,* **33**, 3014–3019

59. Sundquist, W. I., Bancroft, D. P. and Lippard, S. J. (1990). Synthesis, characterization and biological activity of *cis*-diammineplatinum (II) complexes of the DNA intercalators 9-aminoacridine and chloroquine. *J. Am. Chem. Soc.,* **112**, 1590–1596

60. Palmer, B. D., Lee, H. H., Johnson, P., Baguley, B. C., Wickham, G., Wakelin, L. P. G., McFadyen, W. D. and Denny, W. A. (1990). DNA-directed alkylating agents. 2. Synthesis and biological activity of platinum complexes linked to 9-anilinoacridine. *J. Med. Chem.,* **33**, 3008–3014

61. Kopka, M., Yoon, C., Goodsell, D., Pjura, P. and Dickerson, R. E. (1985). The molecular origin of DNA-drug specificity in netropsin and distamycin. *Proc. Natl. Acad. Sci. (USA),* **82**, 1376–1380

62. Leupin, W., Chazin, W., Hyberts, S., Denny, W. A., Stewart, G. M. and Wuthrich, K. (1986). 1D and 2D NMR study of the complex between the decadeoxyribonucleotide d(GCATTAATGC)$_2$ and a minor groove binding drug. *Biochemistry,* **25**, 5902–5910

63. Denny, W. A., Atwell, G. J., Baguley, B. C. and Cain, B. F. (1979). Potential antitumor agents. Part 29. QSAR for the antileukemic bisquaternary ammonium heterocycles. *J. Med. Chem.,* **22**, 134–151

64. Prakash, A. S., Valu, K. K., Wakelin, L. P. G. and Denny, W. A. (1991). Synthesis and antitumour activity of the spatially-separated mustard bis-N,N'-[3-(N-(2–chloroethyl)-N-ethyl)amino-5-((N,N-dimethylamino)methyl)aminophenyl]-1,4-benzenedicarboxamide, which alkylates DNA exclusively at adenines in the minor groove. *Anticancer Drug Design,* **6**, 195–206

65. Baker, B. F. and Dervan, P. B. (1989). Sequence-specific cleavage of DNA by N-bromoacetyldistamycin. Product and kinetic analyses. *J. Am. Chem. Soc.,* **111**, 2700–2712

66. Arcamone, F. M., Animati, F., Barbieri, B., Configliacchi, E., D'Alessio, R., Geroni, C., Giuliani, F. C., Lazzari, E., Menozzi, M., Mongelli, N., Penco, S. and Verini, M.A. (1989).

Synthesis, DNA-binding properties and antitumor activity of novel distamycin derivatives. *J. Med. Chem.*, **32**, 774–778

67. Krowicki, K., Balzarini, J., De Clercq, E., Newman, R. A. and Lown, J. W. (1988). Novel DNA minor groove binding alkylators: design, synthesis and biological activity. *J. Med. Chem.*, **31**, 341–345

68. Gravatt, G. L., Baguley, B. C., Wilson, W. R. and Denny, W. A. (1991). DNA-directed alkylating agents. 4. 4-Anilinoquinoline-based minor groove-directed aniline mustards. *J. Med. Chem.*, **34**, 1552–1560

69. O'Connor, C. J., Denny, W. A. and Fan, J.-Y. (1991). Alkylation of nucleic acids by DNA-targeted 4-anilinoquinolinium aniline mustards: kinetic studies. *Chem. Biol. Int.*, **77**, 223–241

70. Hurley, L. H., Lee, C.-S., McGovren, J. P., Warpehoski, M. A., Mitchell, M. A., Kelly, R. C. and Aristoff, P .A. (1988). Molelcular basis for sequence-specific DNA alkylation by CC-1065. *Biochemistry*, **27**, 3886–3892

71. Hurley, L. H. and Needham-vanDevanter, D. R. (1986). Covalent binding of antitumor antibiotics in the minor groove of DNA. Mechanism of action of CC-1065 and the pyrrolo(1,4)benzodiazepines. *Acc. Chem. Res.*, **19**, 230–237

72. Tang, M. S., Lee, C.-S., Doisy, R., Ross, L., Needham-vanDevanter, D. R. and Hurley, L. H. (1988). Recognition and repair of the CC-1065-(N3-adenine)-DNA adduct by the UVR-ABC nucleases. *Biochemistry*, **27**, 893–901

73. Warpehoski, M. A. and Hurley, L. H. (1988). Sequence selectivity of DNA covalent modification. *Chem. Res. Tox.*, **1**, 315–333

74. Li, L. H., Kelly, R. C., Warpehoski, M. A., McGovren, I. P., Gebhard, I. and Dekoning, T. F. (1991). Adozelesin, a selected lead among cyclopropylpyrroloindole analogues of the DNA binding antibiotic CC-1065. *Invest. New Drugs*, **9**, 137–148

75. Farber, S., D'Angio, G., Evans, A. and Mitus, A. (1960). Clinical studies of actinomycin D with special reference to Wilms' tumor in children. *Ann. N.Y. Acad. Sci.*, **89**, 421–425

76. Weiss, R. B., Sarosy, G., Clagett-Carr, K., Russo, M. and Leyland-Jones, B. (1986). Anthracycline analogues: past, present and future. *Cancer Chemother. Pharmacol.*, **18**, 185–197

77. Ghione, M. (1975). Development of adriamycin (NSC 123127). *Cancer Chemother. Rep.*, **58**, 83–89

78. Mathe, G., Hayat, M. and de Vassal, F. (1970). Methoxy-9-ellipticine lactate. III. Clinical screening: its action in acute myeloid leukemia. *Eur. J. Clin. Biol. Res.*, **15**, 541–547

79. Denny, W. A., Baguley, B. C., Cain, B. F. and Waring, M. J. (1983). Antitumour acridines. In *Molecular Aspects of Anticancer Drug Action*, pp. 1–34. Neidle, S. and Waring, M. J. (eds.) (London: MacMillan)

80. Von Hoff, D. D., Myers, W., Kuhn, J., Sandbach, J. F., Pocelinko, R., Clark, G. and Coltman, C. A. (1981). Phase I clinical investigation of 9,10-anthracenedicarboxaldehyde bis[(4,5-dihydro-1H-imidazol-2-yl)hydrazone] dihydrochloride (CL 216942). *Cancer Res.*, **41**, 3118–3121

81. Cornbleet, M. A., Stuart-Harris, R. C., Smith, I. E., Coleman, R. E., Rubens, R. D., McDonald, M., Mouridsen, H. T., Rainer, H., van Oosterom, A. T. and Smyth, J. F. (1984). Mitoxantrone in the treatment of advanced breast cancer. *Eur. J. Cancer Clin. Oncol.*, **20**, 1141–1147

82. Clarysse, A., Brugarolas, A., Siegenthaler, P., Abele, R., Cavalli, F., de Jager, R., Renard, G., Rozencweig, M. and Hansemn, H. H. (1984). Phase II study of 9-hydroxy-2N-methylellipticinium acetate. *Eur. J. Cancer Clin. Oncol.*, **20**, 243–247

83. Ames, M. M. and Loprizini, C. L. (1988). Preliminary pharmacologic and toxicologic data from a Phase I clinical trial of oxantrazole incorporating a pharmacologically-guided dose escalation. *Proc. Am. Assoc. Cancer Res.*, **29**, 196

84. Kris, M. G., Gralla, R. J., Berger, M. Z., Marks, L. A., Potanovich, L. M., DiMaggio, J. J. and Heelan, R. T. (1989). Phase II trial of amonafide in patients with advanced non-small-cell lung cancer. *Proc. Am. Assoc. Cancer Res.*, **30**, 270

85. Harman, G. S., Craig, J. B., Kuhn, J. C., Luther, J. S., Turner, J. N., Weiss, G. R., Tweedy, D. A., Koeller, J., Tuttle, R.C., Lucas, S. V., Wargin, W. Whisnant, J. K. and von Hoff, D. D. (1988). Phase I and clinical pharmacology trial of crisnatol (BW A770U mesylate) using a monthly single-dose schedule. *Cancer Res.*, **48**, 4706–4710

86. Denny, W. A., Twigden, S. J. and Baguley, B. C. (1986). Steric constraints for DNA binding and biological activity in the amsacrine series. *Anti-Cancer Drug Design*, **1**, 125–132

87. Atwell, G. J., Bos, C. D., Baguley, B. C. and Denny, W. A. (1988). Potential antitumor agents. 56. 'Minimal' DNA-intercalating ligands as antitumor drugs: phenylquinoline-8-carboxamides. *J. Med. Chem.*, **31**, 1048–1052

88. Baguley, B. C., Denny, W. A., Atwell, G. J. and Cain, B. F. (1981). Potential antitumor agents. Part 35. Quantitative relationships between antitumor (L1210) potency and DNA binding for 4'-(9-acridinylamino)methanesulfon-m-anisidide analogues. *J. Med. Chem.*, **24**, 520–525

89. Le Pecq, J-B., Dat-Xuong, N., Gosse, C. and Paoletti, C. (1974). A new antitumoral agent; 9-hydroxyellipticine. Possibility of a rational design of anticancerous drugs in the series of DNA intercalating drugs. *Proc. Natl. Acad. Sci. USA*, **71**, 5078–5084

90. Hartley, J. A., Reszko, K., Zuo, E. T., Wilson, W. D., Morgan, A. R. and Lown, J. W. (1988). Characteristics of the interaction of anthrapyrazole anticancer agents with deoxyribonucleic acids; structural requirements for DNA binding, intercalation and photosensitisation. *Mol. Pharmacol.*, **33**, 265–271

91. Valentini, L., Nicolella, V., Vannini, E., Menuzzi, M., Penco, S. and Arcamone, F.M. (1985). Association of anthracycline derivatives with DNA: a fluorescence study. *Il Farmaco Ed. Sci.*, **40**, 376–382

92. Bair, K.W., Tuttle, R. L., Knick, V. C., Cory, M. and McKee, D. D. (1990). (1-Pyrenylmethyl)amino alcohols, a new class of antitumor DNA intercalators. Discovery and initial sidechain structure–activity studies. *J. Med. Chem.*, **33**, 2385–2393

93. Esnault, C., Roques, B. P., Jacquemin-Sablon, A. and Le Pecq, J.-B. (1984). Effects of new antitumor bifunctional intercalators derived from 7H-pyridocarbazole on sensitive and resistant L1210 cells. *Cancer Res.*, **44**, 4355–4360

94. Cory, M., McKee, D. D., Kagan, J., Henry, D. W. and Miller, J. A. (1985). Design, synthesis and DNA binding properties of bifunctional intercalators. Comparison of polymethylene and diphenylether chains connecting phenanthridines. *J. Am. Chem. Soc.*, **107**, 2528–2536

95. Denny, W.A., Atwell, G. J., Baguley, B. C. and Wakelin, L. P. G. (1985). Potential antitumor agents. 44. Synthesis and antitumor activity of new classes of diacridines: importance of linker chain rigidity for DNA binding kinetics and biological activity. *J. Med. Chem.*, **28**, 1568–1574

96. Wakelin, L. P. G. (1986). Polyfunctional DNA intercalators. *Med. Res. Rev.*, **6**, 275–340

97. Capelle, N., Barbet, J., Dessen, P., Blanquet, S., Roques, P. B. and Le Pecq, J.-B. (1979). Deoxyribonucleic acid bifunctional intercalators: kinetic investigation of the binding of several acridine dimers to deoxyribonucleic acid. *Biochemistry*, **18**, 3354–3362

98. Becker, M. M. and Dervan, P. B. V. (1979). Molecular recognition of nucleic acids by small molecules. Binding affinity and structural specificity of bis(methidium)spermine. *J. Am. Chem. Soc.*, **101**, 3664–3666

99. Kuhn, J. G., von Hoff, D. D., Hersch, M., Melink, T., Clark, G. M., Weiss, G. R. and Coltman, C. A. (1989). Phase I trial of echinomycin (NSC 526417), a bifunctional intercalating agent, administered by 24-hour continuous infusion. *Eur. J. Cancer Clin. Oncol.*, **25**, 797–803

100 Segal-Bendirjian, E., Coulaud, D., Roques, B. P. and Le Pecq, J.-B. (1988). Selective loss of mitochondrial DNA after treatment of cells with ditercalinium (NSC 335153), an antitumor bis-intercalating agent. *Cancer Res.*, **48**, 4982–4992

101. Esnault, C., Brown, S. C., Segal-Bendirjian, E., Coulaud, D., Mishal, Z., Roques, B. P. and Le Pecq, J-B. (1990). Selective alteration of mitochondrial function by ditercalinium (NSC 335153), a DNA bisintercalating agent. *Biochem. Pharmacol.*, **39**, 109–122

102. Atwell, G. J., Rewcastle, G. W., Baguley, B. C. and Denny, W. A. (1987). Potential antitumor agents. 50. *In vivo* solid tumor activity of derivatives of N-[2-(dimethylamino)ethyl]acridine-4-carboxamide. *J. Med. Chem.*, **30**, 664–669

103. Rewcastle, G. W., Denny, W. A. and Baguley, B. C. (1987). Potential antitumor agents. 51. Synthesis and antitumor activity of phenazine-1-carboxamides. *J. Med. Chem.*, **30**, 843–851

104. Atwell, G. J., Baguley, B. C. and Denny, W. A. (1989). Potential antitumor agents. 57. 2-Phenylquinoline-8-carboxamides as 'minimal' DNA-intercalating antitumor agents with *in vivo* solid tumor activity. *J. Med. Chem.*, **32**, 396–401

105. Denny, W. A ., Baguley, B. C. and Rewcastle, G. W. (1990). Potential antitumor agents. 59. Structure–activity relationships for 2-phenylbenzimidazole-4-carboxamides, a new class of 'minimal' DNA-intercalating agent which may not act via topoisomerase II. *J. Med. Chem.*, **33**, 814–819

106. Palmer, B. D., Lee, H. H., Baguley, B. C. and Denny, W. A. (1992). Potential antitumor agents. 64. Synthesis and antitumor evaluation of dibenzo[1,4]dioxin-1-carboxamides, a new class of weakly-binding DNA-intercalating agents. *J. Med. Chem.* **35**, 258–266

107. Feigon, J., Denny, W. A., Leupin, W. and Kearns, D. R. (1984). The interactions of antitumor drugs with natural DNA: a ^{1}H NMR study of binding mode and kinetics. *J. Med. Chem.*, **27**, 450–465

108. Muller, W.. and Crothers, D. M. (1968). Studies of the binding of actinomycin D and related compounds to DNA. *J. Mol. Biol.*, **35**, 251–290

109. Wakelin, L. P. G., Atwell, G. J., Rewcastle, G. W. and Denny, W. A. (1987). Relationships between DNA binding kinetics and biological activity for the 9-aminoacridine-4-carboxamide class of antitumor agents. *J. Med. Chem.*, **30**, 855–862

110. Krishnamoorthy, C. R., Yen, S.-F., Smith, J. C., Lown, J. W. and Wilson, W. D. (1986). Stopped-flow kinetic analysis of the interaction of anthraquinone anticancer drugs with calf thymus DNA, poly[d(G-C)].poly[d(G-C)] and poly[d(A-T).poly[d(A-T)]. *Biochemistry*, **25**, 5933–5940

111. Denny, W. A. and Wakelin, L. P. G. (1990). Kinetics of the binding of mitoxantrone and analogues to DNA: relationship to binding mode and antitumour activity. *Anti-Cancer Drug Design*, **5**, 189–200

112. Denny, W. A. and Wakelin, L. P. G. (1987). Mode and kinetics of binding of the antitumour agent bisantrene. *Anti-Cancer Drug Design*, **2**, 71–77

113. Elliott, J. A., Wilson,W. D., Shea, R. G., Hartley, J. A., Reszka, K. and Lown, J. W. (1989). Interaction of bisantrene anti-cancer agents with DNA: footprinting, structural requirements for DNA unwinding, kinetics and mechanism of binding and correlation of structural and kinetic parameters with anti-cancer activity. *Anti-Cancer Drug Design*, **3**, 271–282

114. Fox, K. R., Brasset, C. and Waring, M. J. (1985). Kinetics of dissociation of nogalamycin from DNA: comparison with other anthracycline antibiotics. *Biochim. Biophys. Acta*, **840**, 383–392

115. Searle, M. S., Hall, J. G., Denny, W. A. and Wakelin, L. P. G. (1988). NMR studies of the interaction of the antibiotic nogalamycin with the hexadeoxyribonucleotide duplex d(5'-GCATGC)$_2$. *Biochemistry*, **27**, 4340–4349

116. Gao, Y-G., Liaw, Y.-C., Robinson, H. and Wang, H.-J. (1990). Binding of the antitumor drug nogalamycin and its derivatives to DNA: structural comparison. *Biochemistry*, **29**, 10307–10316

117. Wakelin, L. P. G., Chetcuti, P. and Denny, W. A. (1990). Kinetic and equilibrium studies of amsacrine-4-carboxamides: a class of asymmetric DNA-intercalating agents which must bind by threading through the DNA helix. *J. Med. Chem.*, **33**, 2039–2044

118. Zwelling, L. A., Michaels, S., Erickson, L. C., Ungerleider, R. S., Nichols, M. and Kohn, K. W. (1981). Protein-associated deoxyribonucleic acid strand breaks in L1210 cells treated with the deoxyribonucleic acid intercalating agents 4'-(9-acridinylamino)methanesulfon-*m*-anisidide and adriamycin. *Biochemistry*, **20**, 6553–6563

119. Drlica, K. and Franko, R. J. (1988). Inhibitors of DNA topoisomerases. *Biochemistry*, **27**, 2253–2259

120. Heck, M. M. S., Hittelman, W. N. and Earnshaw, W. C. (1988). Differential expression of DNA topoisomerases I and II during the eukaryotic cell cycle. *Proc. Natl. Acad. Sci. USA*, **85**, 1086–1090

121. Robbie, M. A., Baguley, B. C., Denny, W. A., Gavin, J. G., and Wilson, W. R. (1988). Mechanism of resistance of non-cycling mammalian cells to 4'-(9-acridinyl-amino)methanesulfon-*m*-anisidide (m-AMSA): comparison of uptake, metabolism and DNA breakage in log- and plateau-phase Chinese hamster fibroblast cell cultures. *Cancer Res.*, **48**, 310–319

122. Stahelin, H. and von Wartburg, A. (1989). From podophyllin glucoside to etoposide. *Prog. Drugs Res.*, **33**, 169–266

123. van Maanen, J. M. S., Retel, J., de Vries, J. and Pinedo, H. M. (1988). Mechanism of action of antitumor drug etoposide: a review. *J. Natl. Cancer Inst.*, **80**, 1526–1533

124. Huff, A. C. and Kreuzer, K. N. (1990). Evidence for a common mechanism of action for antitumor and antibacterial agents that inhibit type II topoisomerases. *J. Biol. Chem.*, **265**, 20496–20505

125. Abraham, Z. H. L., Cutbush, S. D., Kuroda, R., Neidle, N., Acheson, R. M. and Taylor, G. N. (1985). Nucleic acid binding drugs. Part 12. X-ray crystallographic and conformational studies on the anticancer drug *m*-AMSA and its mesyl derivative. *J. Chem. Soc. (Perkin II)*, 461–466

126. Chen, K. X., Gresh, N. and Pullman, B. (1988). Groove selectivity in the interaction of 9-aminoacridine-4-carboxamide antitumor agents with DNA. *Nucleic Acids Res.*, **16**, 3061–3074

127. Chung, T. D. Y., Drake, F. H., Tan, S. R., Per, M., Crooke, S. T. and Mirabelli, C. K. (1989). Characterization and immunological identification of cDNA clones encoding two human DNA topoisomerase isozymes. *Proc. Natl. Acad. Sci. USA*, **86**, 9431–9435

128. Drake, F. H., Hofmann, G. A., Bartus, H. F., Mattern, M. R., Crooke, S. T. and Mirabelli, C. K. (1989). Biochemical and pharmacological properties of p170 and p180 forms of topoisomerase II. *Biochemistry*, **28**, 8154–8160

129. Rewcastle, G. W., Baguley, B. C., Atwell, G. J. and Baguley, B. C. (1987). Potential antitumor agents. 52. Carbamate analogues of amascrine with *in vivo* activity against multidrug-resistant P388 leukemia. *J. Med. Chem.*, **30**, 1576–1581

130. Baguley, B. C., Holdaway, K. M. and Fray, L. M. (1990). Design of DNA intercalators to overcome topoisomerase II-mediated multidrug-resistance. *J. Natl. Cancer Inst.*, **82**, 398–402

131. Baguley, B. C. and Finlay, G. J. (1988). Derivatives of amsacrine: determinants required for high activity against the Lewis lung carcinoma. *J. Natl. Cancer Inst.*, **80**, 195–199

132. Scudder, S. A., Brown, J. M. and Sikic, I. B. (1988). DNA crosslinking and cytotoxicity of the alkylating cyanomorpholide derivative of doxorubicin in multidrug-resistant cells. *J. Natl. Cancer Inst.*, **80**, 1294–1298

133. Mukherjee, T., Land, E. J., Swallow, A. J. and Bruce, J. M. (1989). One-electron reduction of adriamycin and daunomycin: short-term stability of the semiquinones. *Arch. Biochem. Biophys.* **272**, 450–458

134. Jurlina, J. L., Lindsay, A., Baguley, B. C. and Denny, W. A. (1987). Redox chemistry of the 9-anilinoacridine class of antitumor agents. *J. Med. Chem.*, **30**, 473–480

135. Kolodziejczyk, P., Reszka, K. and Lown, J. W. (1988). Enzymatic oxidative activation and transformation of the antitumor agent mitoxantrone. *Free Radical Biol. Med.*, **5**, 13–25

136. Bernadou, J., Meunier, G., Paoletti, C. and Meunier, B. (1983). *o*-Quinone formation in the biochemical oxidation of the antitumor drug N(2)-methyl-9-hydroxyellipticinium acetate. *J. Med. Chem.*, **26**, 574–579

137. Long, B. H., Musial, S. T. and Brattain, M. G. (1984). Comparison of cytotoxicity and DNA breakage activity of congeners of podophyllotoxin including VP16-213 and VM26: a quantitative structure–activity relationship. *Biochemistry*, **23**, 1183–1188

138. Schwartz, H. S. (1983). Mechanisms of selective toxicity of adriamycin, daunomycin and related anthracyclines. In Neidle, S. and Waring, M. J. (eds) *Molecular Mechanisms of Anticancer Drug Action*, p. 93. (London: MacMillan)

139. Ferrer-Mantiel, A. V., Ferraught, J. A. and Gonzalez-Ros, J. M. (1990). Role of membrane lipids in the interaction of daunomycin with plasma membranes of tumor cells. Implications in drug resistance phenomena. *Biochemistry*, **29**, 7275–7282

140. Adams, D. J., Watkins, P. J., Knick, V. C., Tuttle, R. L. and Bair, K. W. (1990). Evaluation of arylmethylaminopropanediols by a novel *in vitro* pharmacodynamic assay: correlation with antitumor activity *in vivo*. *Cancer Res.*, **50**, 3663–3669

141. Umezawa, H., Maeda, K., Takeuchi, T. and Okami, Y. (1966). New antibiotics, bleomycin A and B *J. Antibiot. Ser. A.*, **19**, 200–209

142. Umezawa, H. (1987). Studies on antibiotics and enzyme inhibitors. *Rev. Infect. Dis.*, **9**, 147–164

143. Hecht, S. M. (1990). The chemistry of activated bleomycin. In: Wilman, D. E. V. (ed.) *The Chemistry of Antitumour Agents* (London: Blackie) p. 395

144. Rabow, L. E., Stubbe, J. and Kozarich, J. W. (1990). Identification and quantitation of the lesion accompanying base release in bleomycin-mediated DNA degradation. *J. Am. Chem. Soc.*, **112**, 3196–3203

145. Stubbe, J. and Kozarich, J. W. (1987). Mechanism of bleomycin-induced DNA degradation. *Chem. Rev.*, **87**, 1107–1136

146. Vloon, W. J. Kruk, C., Pandit, U., Hofs, H. and McVie, J. (1987). Synthesis and properties of side-chain modified bleomycins. *J. Med. Chem.*, **30**, 20–24

147. Wender, P. A., McKinney, J. A. and Mukai, C. (1990). General methodology for the synthesis of neocarzinostatin chromophore analogues: intramolecular chromium-mediated closures for strained-ring synthesis. *J. Am. Chem. Soc.*, **112**, 5369–5370

148. Edo, K., Mitzukagi, M., Koido, Y., Seto, H., Furihata, K., Otake, N. and Ishida, N. (1985). The structure of neocarzinostatin chromophore possessing a novel bicyclo[7,3,0]dodecadiyne system. *Tet. Lett.*, **26**, 331–334

149. Lee, S. H. and Goldberg, I. H. (1989). Sequence-selective, strand-selective and directional binding of neocarzinostatin chromophore to oligodeoxyribonucleotides. *Biochemistry*, **28**, 1019–1026

150. Chin, D.-H., Zeng, C.-H., Costello, C. E. and Goldberg, I. H. (1988). Sites in the diyne-ene bicyclic chromophore of neocarzinostatin chromophore responsible for hydrogen abstraction from DNA. *Biochemistry*, **27**, 8106–8114

151. Povirk, L. F. and Goldberg, I. H. (1985). Detection of neocarzinostatin chromophoredeoxyribose adducts as exonuclease-resistant sites in defined-sequence DNA. *Biochemistry*, **24**, 4035–4040

152. Myers, A. G., Proteau, P. J. and Handel, T. M. (1988). Stereochemical assignment of neocarzinostatin chromophore. Structures of neocarzinostatin chromophore-methyl thioglycolate adducts. *J. Am. Chem. Soc.*, **110**, 7212–7214

153. Lee, M. D., Dunne, T. S., Siegel, M. M., Chang, C. C., Morton, G. O. and Borders, D. B. (1987). Calicheamicins, a novel family of antitumour antibiotics. 1. Chemistry and partial structure of calicheamicin γ_1^I. *J. Am. Chem. Soc.*, **109**, 3464–3466

154. Golik, J., Clardy, J., Dubay, G., Groenewold, G., Kawaguchi, H., Konishi, M., Krishnan, B., Ohkuma, H., Saitoh, K. and Doyle, T.W. (1987). Esperamicins, a novel class of potent antitumour antibiotics. Structure of esperamicin X. *J. Am. Chem. Soc.*, **109**, 3461–3462

155. Zein, N., Poncin, M., Nilakatan, R. and Ellestad, G. A. (1989). Calicheamicin γ_1^I and DNA: Molecular recognition process responsible for site specificity. *Science*, **244**, 697–699

156. Nicolaou, K. C., Zuccarello, G., Ogawa, Y., Schweiger, E. J. and Kumazawa, T. (1988). Cyclic conjugated enediynes related to calicheamicins and esperamicins: calculations, synthesis and properties. *J. Am. Chem. Soc.*, **110**, 4866–4868

157. Bergman, R. G. (1973). Reactive 1,4-dehydroaromatics. *Acc. Chem. Res.*, **6**, 25–31

158. Snyder, J. P. and Tipsword, G. E. (1990). Proposal for blending classical and biradical mechanisms in antitumor antibiotics: dynemicin A. *J. Am. Chem. Soc.*, **112**, 4040–4042

159. Nicolaou, K. C., Maligres, P., Shin, J., de Leon, E. and Rideout, D. (1990). DNA cleavage and antitumor properties of designed molecules with conjugated phosphine oxide-allene-ene-yne functions. *J. Am. Chem. Soc.*, **112**, 7825–7826

160. Nicolaou, K. C., Skokotas, G., Furuya, S., Suemume, H. and Nicolaou, D. C. (1990). Golfomycin, a novel designed molecule with DNA-cleaving properties and antitumor activity. *J. Angew. Chem. Intl. Ed. Engl.*, **29**, 1064–1067

161. Coleman, C. N. (1988). Hypoxia in tumors: a paradigm for the approach to biochemical and physiologic heterogeneity. *J. Natl. Cancer Inst.*, **80**, 310–317

162. Chaplin, D. J., Olive, P. L. and Durand, R. E. (1987). Intermittent blood flow in a murine tumor: radiobiological effects. *Cancer Res.*, **47**, 597–601

163. Urtasun, R. C., Chapman, J. D., Raleigh, J. A., Franko, A. J. and Koch, C. J. (1986). Binding of 3H-misonidazole to solid human tumors as a measure of tumor hypoxia. *Int. J. Radiat. Oncol. Biol. Phys.*, **12**, 1263–1267

164. Teicher, B. A., Holden, S. A., Al-Achi, A. and Herman, T. S. (1990). Classification of antineoplastic treatments by their differential toxicity towards putative oxygenated and hypoxic tumor subpopulations *in vivo* in the FSaIIC murine fibrosarcoma. *Cancer Res.*, **50**, 3339–3344

165. Tannock, I. F. and Rotin, D. (1989). Acid pH in tumors and its potential for therapeutic use. *Cancer Res.*, **49**, 4373–4384

166. Tannock, I. F. (1968). The relation between cell proliferation and the vascular system in a transplanted mouse mammary tumour. *Br. J. Cancer*, **22**, 258–272

167. Denny, W. A. and Wilson, W. R. (1986). Considerations for the design of nitrophenyl mustards as drugs selectively toxic for hypoxic mammalian cells *J. Med. Chem.*, **29**, 879–887

168. Adams, G. E. and Stratford, I. J. (1986). Hypoxia-mediated nitroheterocyclic drugs in the radio- and chemotherapy of cancer. *Biochem. Pharmacol.*, **35**, 71–76

169. Brown, J. M. (1982). The mechanisms of cytotoxicity and chemosensitization by misonidazole and other nitroimidazoles. *Int. J. Rad. Oncol. Biol. Phys.*, **8**, 675–682

170. McClelland, R. A., Panicucci, R. and Rauth, A. M. (1987). Products of the reductions of 2-nitroimidazoles. *J. Am. Chem. Soc.*, **109**, 4308–4314

171. Raleigh, J. A. (1985). Binding of misonidazole to hypoxic cells in monolayer and spheroid culture: evidence that a sidechain label is bound as efficiently as a ring label. *Br. J. Cancer*, **51**, 229–235

172. Franko, A. J., Raleigh, J. A., Sutherland, R. G. and Soderlind, K. J. (1989). Metabolic binding of misonidazole to mouse tissues: comparison between labels on the ring and side chain, and the production of tritiated water. *Biochem. Pharmacol.*, **38**, 665–670

173. Panicucci, R., Heal, R., Laderoute, K., Cowan, D. M. S., McClelland, R. A. and Rauth, A. M. (1989). NLP-1, a DNA-intercalating hypoxic cell radiosensitiser and cytotoxin *Int. J. Radiat. Oncol. Biol. Phys.*, **16**, 1039–1043

174. Kedderis, G. L. and Miwa, G. T. (1988). The metabolic activation of nitroheterocyclic therapeutic agents. *Drug Met. Rev.*, **19**, 33–62

175. Wardman, P. A. (1984). Radiation chemistry in the clinic: hypoxic cell radiosensitisers for radiotherapy. *Radiat. Phys. Chem.*, **24**, 293–305

176. Cowan, D. M. S., Panicucci, R., McClelland, R. A. and Rauth, A. M. (1991). Targeting radiosensitisers to DNA by attachment of an intercalating group: nitroimidazole-linked phenanthridines. *Radiat. Res.*, **127**, 81–89

177. Denny, W. A., Roberts, P. B., Anderson, R. F., Brown, J. M. and Denny, W. A. (1991). NLA-1: a 2-nitroimidazole radiosensitiser targeted to DNA by intercalation. *Int. J. Radiat. Oncol. Biol. Phys.*, **22**, 553–556

178. Wilson, W. R., Denny, W. A., Twigden, S. J., Baguley, B. C. and Probert, J. C. (1984). Selective toxicity of nitracrine to hypoxic mammalian cells. *Br. J. Cancer*, **49**, 215–223

179. Denny, W. A., Wilson, W. R., Atwell, G. J., Boyd, M., Pullen, S. M. and Anderson, R. F. (1990). Nitroacridines and nitroquinolines as DNA-affinic hypoxia-selective cyotoxins. In Adams, G.E. (ed.) *Activation of Drugs by Redox Processes*. NATO Advanced Study Series, **198**, 149–158

180. Wilson, W. R., Thompson, L. H., Anderson, R. F. and Denny, W. A. (1989). Hypoxia-selective antitumor agents. 2. Electronic effects of 4-substituents on the mechanisms of cytotoxicity and metabolic stability of nitracrine analogues. *J. Med. Chem.*, **32**, 31–38

181. Denny, W. A., Atwell, G. J., Roberts, P. B., Anderson, R. F., Boyd, M., Lock, C. J. L. and Wilson, W. R. (1992). 4-Alkylaminonitroquinolines, a new class of hypoxia-selective cytotoxic agents. *J. Med. Chem.*, submitted

182. Sebolt, J. S., Scavone, S. V., Pinter, C. D., Hamelehle, K. I., von Hoff, D. D. and Jackson, R. C. (1987). Pyrazoloacridines, a new class of anticancer agents with selectivity against solid tumors *in vivo. Cancer Res.*, **47**, 4299–4304

183. Alston, T. A., Porter, D. J. T. and Bright, H. J. (1983). Enzyme inhibition by nitro and nitroso compounds. *Acc. Chem. Res.*, **16**, 418–424

184. Connors, T. A. (1983) In Reinhoudt, D. N., Connors, T. A., Pinedo, H. M. and van der Poll, K. W. (eds.) *Structure–activity Relationships of Antitumor Agents*, pp 47–59, (The Hague: Nijihoff)

185. Lewis, D. F. V. (1989). Molecular orbital calculations on tumour-inhibitory aniline mustards: QSARs. *Xenobiotica*, **19**, 243–251

186. Palmer, B. D., Wilson, W. R., Pullen, S. M. and Denny, W. A. (1990). Hypoxia-selective antitumor agents. 3. Relationships between structure and cytotoxicity against cultured tumor cells for substituted N,N-bis(2-chloroethyl)anilines *J. Med. Chem.*, **33**, 112–121

187. Stratford, I. J., Williamson, C., Hoe, S. and Adams, G. E. (1981). Radiosensitising and cytotoxicity studies with CB 1954 (2,4-dinitro-5-aziridinyl)benzamide. *Radiat. Res.*, **88**, 502–509

188. Sartorelli, A. C. (1988). Therapeutic attack of hypoxic cells of solid tumours: Presidential address. *Cancer Res.*, **48**, 775–778

189. Weissberg, J. B., Son, Y. H., Papac, R. J., Sasaki, C., Fischer, D. B., Lawrence, R., Rockwell, S. A., Sartorelli, A. C. and Fischer, J. J. (1989). Randomised clinical trial of mitomycin C as an adjunct to radiotherapy in head and neck cancer. *Int. J. Radiat. Oncol. Biol. Phys.*, **17**, 3–9

190. Rauth, A. M., Mohindra, J. I. K. and Tannock, I. F. (1983). Activity of mitomycin C for aerobic and hypoxic cells *in vitro* and *in vivo. Cancer Res.*, **43**, 4154–4358

191. Borowy-Borowski, H., Lipman, R., Chowdary, D. and Tomasz, M. (1990). Duplex oligodeoxyribonucleotides cross-linked by mitomycin C at a single site: synthesis, properties and cross-link reversibility. *Biochemistry*, **29**, 2992–2999

192. Fisher, J. F. and Aristoff, P. A. (1988). The chemistry of DNA modification by antitumor antibiotics. *Prog. Drug Res.*, **32**, 411–498

193. Zeman, E. M., Brown, J. M., Lemmon, M. J., Hirst, V. K. and Lee, W. W. (1986). SR 4233: a new bioreductive agent with high selective toxicity for mammalian cells. *Int. J. Radiat. Oncol. Biol. Phys.*, **12**, 1239–1242

194. Baker, M. A., Zeman, E. M., Hirst, V. K. and Brown, J. M. (1988). Metabolism of SR 4233 by Chinese hamster ovary cells: basis of selective hypoxic cytotoxicity. *Cancer Res.*, **48**, 5947–5952

195. Atwood, J. D. (1989). *Inorganic and Organometallic Reaction Mechanisms*, p. 87. (Monterey, USA: Brooks/Cole)

196. Simic, M. and Lilie, J. (1974). Kinetics of ammonia detachment from reduced Co(III) complexes based on conductimetric pulse radiolysis. *J. Am. Chem. Soc.*, **96**, 291–292

197. Ware, D. C., Siim, B. G., Robinson, K. J., Brothers, P. J., Clark, G. R. and Denny, W. A. (1991). Synthesis and characterisation of aziridine complexes of cobalt (III) and chromium (III) and the X-ray crystal structure of *trans*-[Co(Az)$_4$(NO$_2$)$_2$]Br.H$_2$O.LiBr. *Inorg. Chem.*, **30**, 3750–3757

198. Ware, D. C., Wilson, W. R., Denny, W. A. and Rickards, C. E. F. (1991). Design and symthesis of cobalt (III) nitrogen mustard complexes as hypoxia-selective cytotoxins. The X-ray crystal structure of bis(3-chloro-2,4-pentanedionate)RS-*N,N*'-bis(2-chloroethyl) ethylenediamine) cobalt(III)perchlorate, Co[(Clacacc)$_2$(BCE)]ClO$_4$. *J. Chem. Soc. Chem. Commun.*, 1171–1173

199. Gatenby, R. A., Kessler, H. B., Rosenblum, J. S., Coia, L. R., Moldofsky, P. J., Hartz, W. H. and Brodler, G. J. (1988). Oxygen distribution in squamous cell carcinoma metastases and its relationship to outcome of radiation therapy. *Int. J. Radiat. Oncol. Biol. Phys.*, **14**, 831–838

200. Adams, G. E., Clarke, E. D., Flockhart, I. R., Jacobs, R. S., Sehmi, D. S., Stratford, I. J., Wardman, P., Watts, M. E., Parrick, J.,Wallace, R. G. and Smithen, C. E. (1979). Structure–activity relationships in the development of hypoxic cell radiosensitizers. I. Sensitization efficiency. *Int. J. Radiat. Biol.*, **35**, 133–150

201. Adams, G. E., Clarke, E. D., Gray, P., Jacobs, R. S., Stratford, I. J., Wardman, P., Watts, M. E., Parrick, J., Wallace, R. G. and Smithen, C. E. (1979). Structure–activity relationships in the development of hypoxic cell radiosensitizers. II. Cytotoxicity and therapeutic ratio. *Int. J. Rad. Biol.*, **35**, 151–166

202. Overgaard, J., Hansen, H. S., Anderson, A. P., Hjelm-Hansen, H., Jorgensen, K., Sandberg, E., Berthelsen, A., Hammer, R. and Pedersen, M. (1989). Misonidazole combined with split-course radiotherapy in the treatment of invasive carcinoma of larynx and pharynx: report from the DAHANCA 2 study. *Int. J. Radiat. Oncol. Biol. Phys.*, **16,** 1065–1068

203. Dische, S. (1989). Hypoxic cell sensitisers: clinical developments. *Int. J. Radiat. Oncol. Biol. Phys.*, **16**, 1057–1060

204. Brown, D. M., Parker, E. and Brown, J. M. (1982). Structure–activity relationships of 1-substituted-2-nitroimidazoles: effect of partition coefficient and sidechain hydroxyl groups on radiosensitisation *in vitro*. *Radiat. Res.*, **90**, 98–108

205. Brown, J. M. (1989). Hypoxic cell sensitizers: where next? *Int. J. Radiat. Oncol. Biol. Phys.*, **16**, 987–993

206. Adams, G. E., Ahmed, I., Sheldon, P. W. and Stratford, I. J. (1984). Radiation sensitisation and chemopotentiation: RSU-1069, a compound more efficient than misonidazole *in vitro* and *in vivo*. *Br. J. Cancer*, **40**, 571–577

207. Ahmed, I., Jenkins, T. C., Walling, J. M., Stratford, I. J., Sheldon, P. W., Adams, G. E. and Fielden, E. M. (1986). Analogies of RSU-1069: radiosensitisation and toxicity *in vitro* and *in vivo*. *Int. J. Radiat. Oncol. Biol. Phys.*, **12**, 1079–1081

208. Roberts, P. B., Denny, W. A., Wakelin, L. P. G., Anderson, R. F. and Wilson, W. R. (1990). Radiosensitisation of mammalian cells *in vitro* by nitroacridines. *Radiat. Res.*, **123**, 153–164

209. Skov, K. A. (1987). Modification of radiation response by metal complexes: a review with emphasis on non-platinum studies. *Radiat. Res.*, **112**, 217–242

3
In vitro systems for anticancer drug testing

G. J. FINLAY

INTRODUCTION

Once a cancer has metastasized widely, chemotherapy would be expected to offer the best hope for control. However, there are few agents with a high degree of efficacy against the common cancers, and continued drug discovery remains a priority in cancer research. The development of new methods for testing anticancer drugs constitutes a rapidly evolving and, at times, controversial field. The frustrations experienced in identifying useful new compounds arise in part from the subtlety of the biochemical differences between normal and neoplastic cells, and the difficulties encountered in developing model systems for screening and testing experimental compounds[1–4]. *In vivo* screens, using rapidly growing transplantable murine tumours such as the P388 and L1210 leukaemias, in general have proved disappointing in identifying agents effective in the treatment of carcinomas. Whereas these classical murine tumours have identified agents active against rapidly proliferating tumours, there has been little impact on long-term survival rates for patients with the common malignancies which are characterized by low growth fractions.

It is to be hoped that drug discovery will benefit from the availability of an increasing diversity of well-characterized testing systems. A large number of such systems have been developed, and these run the gamut of cell-free biochemical tests to long-term assays in mice (Figure 3.1). Molecular biological studies are identifying many regulatory proteins which are aberrantly expressed in neoplastic cells, including growth factors, growth factor receptors, protein kinases and other oncogene products involved in signal transduction. Such key regulatory proteins could well be targets for chemotherapeutic agents[5], and extensive use of cell-free systems to identify such compounds seems inevitable. The next level of complexity, the use of intact cells in culture, has received widespread attention[6–9], and is the subject of this review. Cell culture methods have found extensive use in the random screening of large collections of synthetic compounds, of fermentation beers[10,11] and of other natural products isolated from plants and animals. In rational synthesis programmes, they provide a first-line testing system ideally suited to rapid feedback of information

55

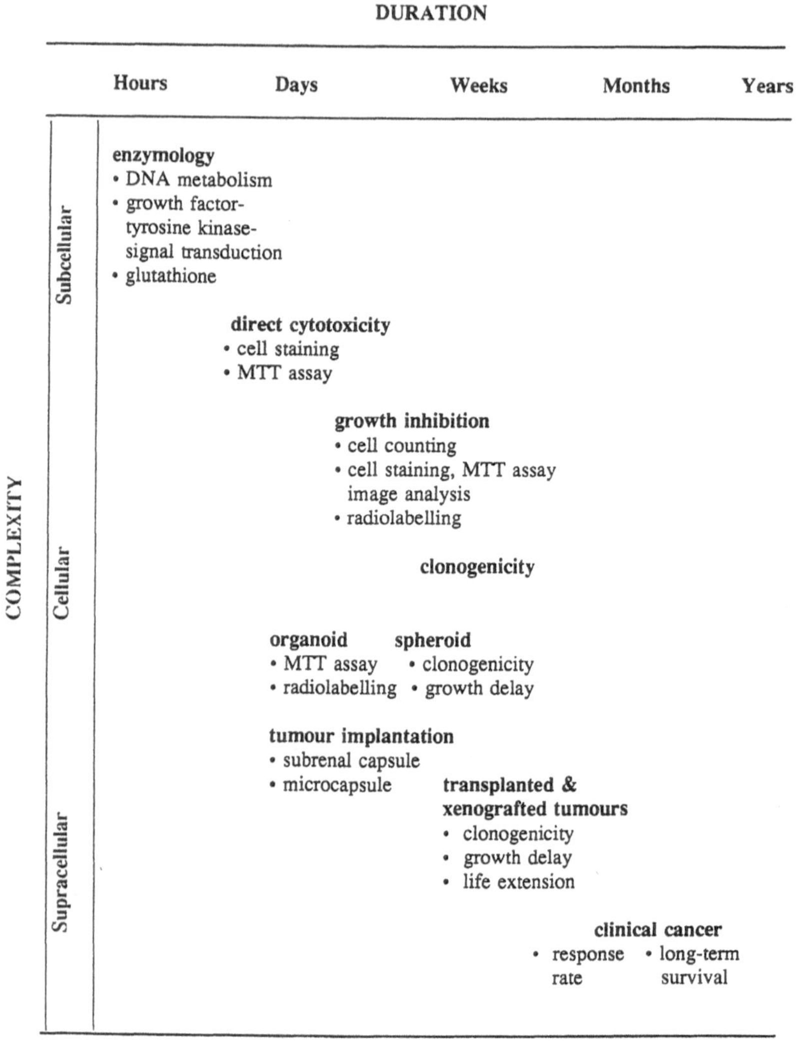

Figure 3.1 Tests for anticancer drugs

regarding structure–activity relationships. Compounds of known activity have been tested against panels of tumour cells of different histological types to investigate selectivity of effect (the so-called '*in vitro* phase II trial'). The availability of mutant cell lines or of cells selected for drug resistance has resulted in the widespread use of *in vitro* assays for mechanistic studies and for the identification of new compounds[12,13] which can bypass inherent or acquired resistance to antineoplastic compounds. Considerable effort has also been expended to develop *in vitro* assays using tumour cells recovered freshly from cancer patients, in order to identify those agents which will maximally benefit the patient[9,14–16]. Although such predictive tests are not in the immediate purview of this survey, they involve the same methodology as many of the assays being developed for drug discovery programmes. The success of the latter will ultimately depend on their ability to correlate with clinical experience and thus both preclinical and clinical applications of *in vitro* testing will be discussed. At the risk of merely reflecting fashion, new trends over the last five years will be emphasized.

Short-term assays bridging cell culture and transplantable tumour systems have been developed. The effects of anticancer drugs have been investigated on human tumour samples implanted into mice intraperitoneally in microcapsules[17] or under the renal capsule[18], although the latter method remains controversial[19]. Finally, transplantable syngeneic[2] and xenogeneic (human) tumours will continue to play an important role in drug discovery programmes. Xenografted human tumours serve as a convenient abundant source of human tumour cells for *in vitro* work[1,20–26], as well as allowing the testing of anticancer compounds against human tumours growing *in vivo*[1,20–22,25].

CLONOGENIC ASSAYS

Clonogenic assays have long been regarded as the method of choice for assessing the effect of cytotoxic drugs in culture[27]. Typically, cells are exposed to the investigational agent for one hour. The short drug treatment attempts to reproduce conditions of transient drug exposure. The cells are washed free of drug and placed into culture for surviving cells to develop into colonies. The proportion of cells retaining the ability to proliferate into a macroscopic colony is determined after sufficient time has elapsed for discrimination to be made between abortive colonies (up to 5 divisions) and those with unlimited proliferative potential. This growth time must make allowance for the fact that many drug-treated cells with proliferative integrity will have sustained damage requiring a substantial lag period during which repair occurs prior to the resumption of active cell division. Under such conditions, clonogenic assays are ideally suited to distinguishing between cytotoxic and cytostatic effects. Clonogenic assays have been performed on cell lines from non-human and human sources, on cells recovered from human tumours passaged as xenografts, and on cells recovered from freshly excised clinical cancers. These will be discussed in order.

Cell lines

Much has been written regarding the use of primary cultures in drug development. However, continuous cell lines, or cells from established transplantable tumours, will always possess important advantages. Established lines can be characterized in detail for cytogenetic, isozyme, and drug sensitivity profiles. An unlimited supply of cells and facile adaptation to different culture conditions allows the use of such cells in a range of assays and mode of action studies. Data can be compared by independent laboratories over extended periods of time in screening or structure–activity studies on large series of compounds.

Full survival curves are highly informative, yielding data that cannot be obtained by most non-clonogenic assays. This includes the extent to which cells can tolerate sublethal damage (as indicated by the presence of a shoulder), the total extent of cytotoxicity, and the presence of resistant subpopulations, as manifested by the presence of a plateau region where increasing drug concentrations fail to effect a constant decrement in survival[28]. This approach has been used to investigate the effects of drugs on cycling and non-cycling cells[29], and also the effects of pH, temperature, hypoxia, radiation and drug interactions on the cytotoxicity of chemotherapeutic agents.

Large-scale screening has been performed on well-established tumour cells using clonogenic assays in agar[30]. Cells of two tumour types are plated together and a paper disc impregnated with the test compound is placed on the agar. The selectivity of the compound (leukaemia vs carcinoma; murine vs human) is determined by comparing the zones of inhibition of colony growth of the two cell types plated. A very small proportion of compounds was found to be selectively toxic for either carcinoma (relative to leukaemia) or human (relative to murine) cells. Of 11 (out of 1472) compounds shown to be carcinoma-selective, 6 (including 4 of one structural class) were shown to be active against solid tumours *in vivo* [31].

Human tumours maintained as xenografts

Xenografted human tumours have been used extensively as a source of cells for clonogenic assays of anticancer drugs. They retain the phenotype of the tumours of origin, provide an essentially unlimited supply of well-characterized tissue for repeated assays, and cells recovered from them retain the relevant cytokinetic features characteristic of malignant tissue growing *in vivo*. Cryopreservation of early passage xenografted cells minimizes the hazards of genetic drift. The effects of drugs can be studied *in vivo*[20,22,25] and compared with clonogenic assays on freshly isolated tumour cells[20–25] and on derived cell lines[23,24], which can be established from xenografts with greater ease than from fresh surgical explants. In the large-scale screening programme of Fiebig and co-workers[25], investigational agents are first studied by clonogenic assays using cells recovered from a large panel (twenty) of well-characterized xenografts. The two most responsive tumours in this system are then studied by growth-delay experiments *in vivo* using a drug concentration equal to the LD_{10}. Agents with even minimal activity are then tested in a disease-oriented panel of 60 xenografts.

The use of xenografted cells for *in vitro* assays has been validated by several criteria. In their elegant series of experiments on xenografted human melanomas, Tveit and co-workers[20,21] established that there was an excellent correspondence between the response to chemotherapy *in vivo* (in athymic mice) and results obtained using the clonogenic assay for several drugs. Such *in vitro–in vivo* correlations were generally but not always observed by others[22,25]. Moreover, when cells from patients' melanomas were tested for chemosensitivity using the clonogenic assay, it was shown that a drug demonstrating *in vitro* activity equivalent to an expected growth delay of at least 2 tumour doubling times (as defined by its activity in the xenograft panel) would demonstrate some efficacy in the patient[21] (Figure 3.2). Results from clonogenicity assays on cells recovered from xenografts correlated well with the effects of chemotherapy on the patients from whom the tumour cells were derived[26].

The frequency with which established anticancer agents satisfy the criterion of being active against cells from different melanoma xenografts *in vitro* is consonant with the response rate of those drugs in the clinic[21]. Clonogenic assays of cells from human xenografts (but not standard murine long-term transplantable tumours) were able to predict the clinical inactivity of the experimental compounds 1,2,4-triglycidylurazol and tiazofurin. The predictive superiority of human xenografted tumours was taken as evidence of the critical role of growth kinetics for accurate drug sensitivity testing[25], a conclusion supported by Taetle and Abramson[1].

Repeated testing of cells from xenografts and cell lines derived from them showed that cell lines generally but not always retain the drug sensitivity of the original xenograft[24]. Thus, the greater convenience and reproducibility offered by cell lines must be weighed against the probability (10% in this study) of a cell line deviating greatly from its parent tumour with respect to its sensitivity to an agent.

Fresh human tumour cells in agar

Clonogenic assays using cells recovered directly from freshly extirpated human tumours have been the subject of intensive investigation, despite the technical difficulties involved and the limited availability of material from any one patient which generally precludes repeated assays. Many workers have been prepared to brave the methodological difficulties because of the knowledge that such cells are the closest available to those actually responsible for clinical disease.

Assays for testing anticancer drugs on freshly isolated human tumour cells were developed independently in the late 1970s by Hamburger and Salmon[32] and by Courtenay and co-workers[33]. Selective tumour growth was obtained by culturing the cells in agar. The method of Courtenay was shown to be superior in cultures of melanoma[34] and breast carcinoma[35] cells. This superiority was manifested by a higher proportion of tumours which formed colonies *in vitro*, by a higher plating efficiency of those that did generate colonies, and, in some cases, by an increased colony size. The critical features of the Courtenay procedure that promoted growth were the presence of rat erythrocytes and the use of reduced oxygen concentration to minimize the toxicity due to reactive oxygen species[34,36]. Subsequent work showed that excellent survival curves were obtained when human tumour cells were X-irradiated[37] and when melanoma[38] and breast cancer cells[35] were treated with chemotherapeutic agents. For the melanoma cells, there was close correspondence between *in vitro* sensitivity and the effect of chemotherapy in the respective patients, based on the 'expected growth delay' calibration previously established for melanoma

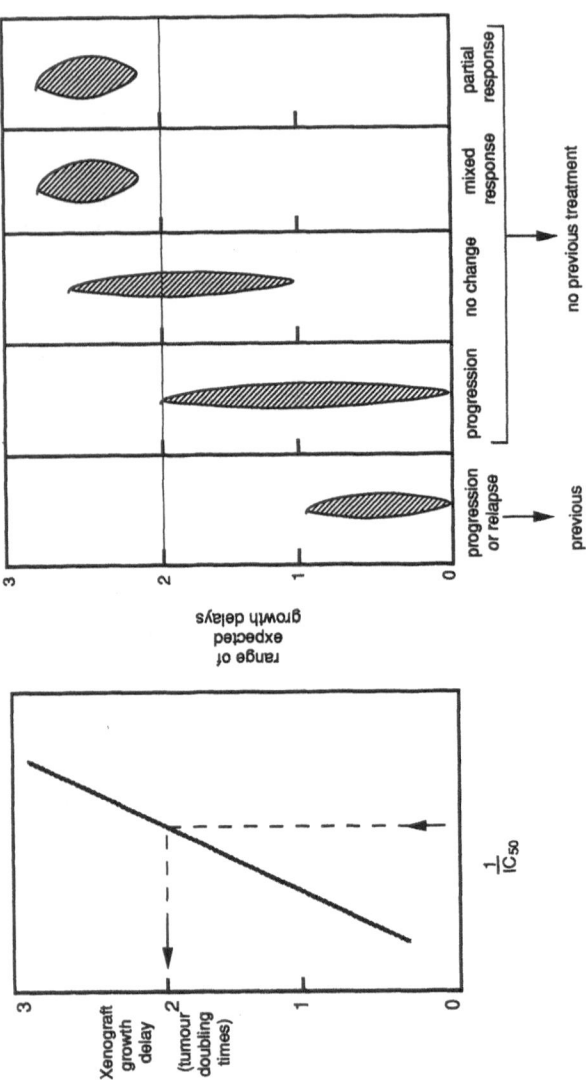

Figure 3.2 Use of growth delays of tumour xenografts in athymic mice to relate *in vitro* clonogenic assays to patient responses. The *left-hand panel* indicates how a correlation was established between the *in vitro* and *in vivo* activities of an agent against a series of tumours. Activity *in vitro* is expressed as the reciprocal of the IC50 (the drug concentration which reduces clonogenicity to 50% of control values), and the activity against xenografted tumours in athymic mice is given as drug-induced delay of tumour growth, expressed as tumour doubling times. The *right-hand panel* depicts the relationship (shaded ellipses) between calculated xenograft growth delays (expressed as tumour doubling times) and responses in patients with melanoma who were treated with chemotherapy. The growth delays were calculated from *in vitro* results (clonogenic assays for a large number of melanoma samples from five categories of patients) using the regression line obtained in the left-hand panel. The *in vitro* sensitivities of tumours from patients who had already failed on treatment corresponded to a growth delay of less than one doubling time. In contrast, *in vitro* sensitivities equivalent to a growth delay of at least two tumour doubling times were manifested by samples from patients who responded to treatment (adapted from References 20, 21, 34)

xenografts[20,21] which translates *in vitro* data into an expected clinical outcome[38] (Figure 3.2).

Most work using fresh tumour cells has been performed by the procedure of Hamburger and Salmon[32]. A recent innovation introduced capillary tubes for colony growth[39–41], which increased colony-forming efficiency several-fold, thus reducing the number of cells required for each assay. The basis of this beneficial effect has not been elucidated but may be related to a reduction in oxygen concentration within the cultures.

Over the last decade, many studies have been performed to compare the sensitivity of cells in this assay and the response to chemotherapy in the clinic. Sensitivity *in vitro* has been defined as a drug-induced decrease in colony number of at least 50–70% using no more than one-tenth of the pharmacologically achievable drug concentration. This criterion of sensitivity has been justified by statistical treatments of preliminary clinical correlations[42] (Figure 3.3). For 2300 patients for whom both culture data and clinical responses were available, the *in vitro* assay was able to identify correctly 79% of the tumours which were sensitive to the respective drug *in vivo*, and 89% of the tumours which were resistant[9,14]. Prospective correlations have also supported the validity of the *in vitro* human tumour cloning assay. When patients with advanced metastatic cancers were treated with the drugs identified as active *in vitro* against their tumours, improved response rates were observed, although this was not translated into survival[41]. Similar results were obtained with melanoma patients in the study of Tveit *et al.* [38].

A multicentre collaborative trial was performed (before the advent of capillary tube cultures) to investigate the potential of the colony assay for drug screening[43]. Four quality-control criteria had to be satisfied before an assay was considered acceptable. There had to be no more than 47 colony-sized clumps in

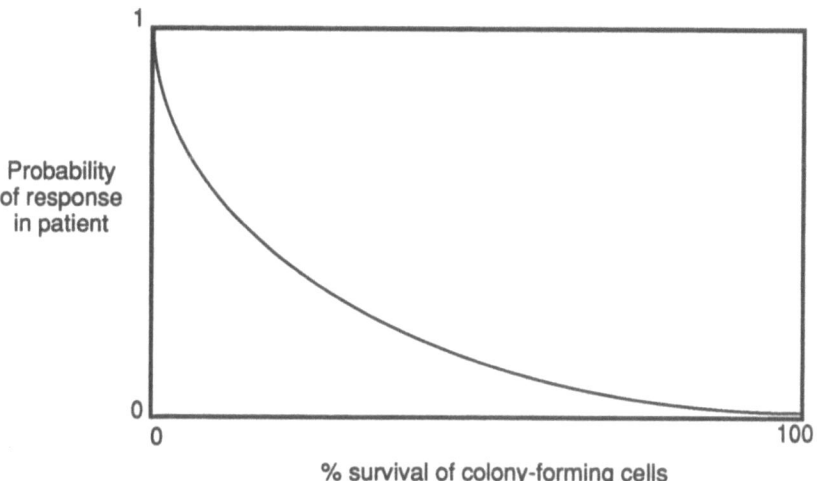

Figure 3.3 Correlation of sensitivity of clonogenic cells from patients' tumours with clinical responses (adapted from Reference 42)

each culture at the commencement of the experiment and a mean increase of at least 70 colonies in control cultures at the termination of the assay. The coefficient of variation of colony number in control cultures had to be less than 50%. Finally, the presence of a toxic positive control substance had to reduce colony numbers to below 30% of control. Under these conditions, 30% of all tumour samples received were evaluable for drug sensitivity. A compound was considered active if it reduced the number of colonies to less than 30% of control values in at least 20% of the tumours at a drug concentration of $10 \, \mu g \, ml^{-1}$. One hundred compounds which were inactive in the *in vivo* P388 screen were tested. At the time of publication, six were shown to possess activity in the system. Their clinical efficacy is not yet known.

Other studies have tested investigational new drugs against panels of tumours representing several histological types. These results have proved to predict subsequent clinical experience with modest success[3,9]. Despite the demonstrable clinical correlations, the routine use of fresh human tumour cells in clonogenic assays for the testing of new drugs is premature[44].

An assay specifically designed for breast cancer

Breast cancers represent a special problem for cell culture because they are often fibrotic and yield few tumour cells. Smith and co-workers[45] have developed an elegant method whereby tumour tissue is disaggregated enzymatically and clumps of epithelial cells cultured in medium specifically designed for the growth of breast epithelial cells. After a few days, cells are recovered by partial trypsinization and seeded on fibroblast monolayers for clonogenic assays.

This method gives excellent plating efficiencies (up to 50%), survival curves, and clinical correlations for anthracyclines and vinblastine[46]. Breast cancer cells have been shown to range widely in sensitivity to doxorubicin with the drug concentration producing an equitoxic effect varying from ten-fold[45] to one thousand-fold[47] in different studies, as was also found in the agar assay[35]. Resistance has been correlated with expression of the P170 glycoprotein efflux pump, and, in some cases, with high amounts of the anionic isozyme of glutathione-S-transferase[47]. This method thus represents a well-characterized and reproducible approach to the *in vitro* testing of anticancer drugs.

NON-CLONOGENIC ASSAYS

Despite the fact that clonogenic assays have long been regarded as the drug-testing method of choice[27], it has been argued more recently that non-clonogenic methods are at least as relevant for anticancer drug testing[6]. The labour-intensive nature of clonogenic assays, and their requirement for punctilious attention to quality control (at least for cells in primary culture), as well as theoretical considerations, have been cited to promote the use of methods measuring drug-induced growth inhibition or loss of metabolic integrity in the treated cell population[6].

Early evidence of cell damage manifested in short-term non-clonogenic assays may reliably predict the extent of tumour cell kill as defined by full-length clonogenic assays. Weisenthal and Lippman[6] have argued that many studies demonstrating lack of agreement between clonogenic and non-clonogenic assays allowed insufficient time for cell damage to become apparent in the latter case. Moreover, the preparation of single cell suspensions required for clonogenic assays disrupts intercellular communication characteristic of epithelial tissues from which most neoplastic disease arises.

With freshly resected tumour samples, the cells capable of forming colonies *in vitro* may not be equivalent to those which act as stem cells *in vivo*. As an extreme example, a well-established transplantable tumour (P388) has a stem cell composition approaching 100% when assayed in an *in vivo* tumorigenicity assay, but a colony-forming efficiency of 0.2% when assayed in culture[48]. Clonogenic cells may also fail to represent the chemosensitivity of cells which are in a G_0 state *in vivo* and contribute poorly to colony formation *in vitro*. Assays investigating clonogenic cells cannot take account of cells with limited proliferative potential which can, nevertheless, contribute to morbidity.

The critical criterion for the validity of any cell culture method is its correspondence to clinical experience. A variety of assays, whether based on cell metabolism, membrane integrity, DNA precursor incorporation, or clonogenic growth, have been shown to improve the probability of selecting an agent active *in vivo* 2–3-fold (given that clinical responses have been obtained in 25–30% of those cancer patients whose tumours have been tested for chemosensitivity[6,14,49]) while having little effect on the already high probability of administering an inactive agent[6]. Thus, there seems to be ample justification for the current emphasis on drug testing using cell growth inhibition (as measured by radiometric, colorimetric and fluorimetric end-points) and direct killing of cells as assessed by differential staining of viable and non-viable cells.

Growth inhibition assays: DNA precursor incorporation

Radiolabelled substrates, including thymidine[23], uridine[50], leucine[51] and glucose[52,53], have been used as markers of ongoing macromolecular synthesis and metabolism following treatment of cell lines with cytotoxic agents. For drug screening and evaluation with cell lines, highly efficient non-radioactive alternative methods are now available, and it is expected that these will displace radioactive approaches for routine work.

Radiolabelled thymidine incorporation into DNA allows very sensitive quantification of proliferation. For this reason, [³H]thymidine uptake has been widely used in testing methods using tumour cells in primary culture in which net increases in cell number are not detected readily. At the time when the clonogenic assay was attracting intense interest, various workers recognized that culturing tumour cells in[54] or on[55] soft agar offered a method supporting selective tumour cell proliferation, but that [³H]thymidine incorporation had several advantages over the clonogenic end-point. It would eliminate the exacting requirement for single cell suspensions; it would reduce greatly the assay duration from at least 2 weeks down to 4 days; and it would yield an end-point less ambiguous than colony counting which requires discrimination between colonies of various sizes, clumps and debris. Experience with the method which has been miniaturized[56] showed that an increased proportion of specimens satisfied the criteria for an evaluable assay[54–57], and that the early end-point was an excellent predictor of chemosensitivity results obtained subsequently from a full-length colony assay[54,55,57]. Moreover, the approach was validated by clinical correlations equivalent to those obtained by the clonogenic method[58].

In a further innovation, cells were cultured in agarose which was placed over a Millipore filter. To harvest the cells after labelling with [^{3}H]thymidine, the agarose was melted and drawn through the filter under negative pressure, which allows the cells to be collected directly[59]. This simplified procedure yields chemosensitivity data consistent with those described above, in which the acid-precipitable isotope was harvested from each culture[54,58].

An alternative method of promoting selective growth of tumour cells is to seed the cell suspensions on to confluent contact-inhibited fibroblast monolayers, of which Balb/3T3 A31 cells have been used widely. Non-neoplastic cells fail to grow in the absence of available sites for adherence (e.g. a plastic surface). The preformed monolayers support the growth both of cell lines which normally grow poorly in vitro, and of neoplastic cells prepared from patients' tumours[60–62]. Effects of oestrogen[62] and of cytotoxic drugs[60] have been investigated in assays of short duration (3–4 days).

The ultimate short-term assay measures the effect of cytotoxic drugs on radiolabelled thymidine incorporated by cells undergoing DNA synthesis at the time of tumour resection, thus obviating the requirement for selective growth conditions. Freshly disaggregated ovarian carcinoma cells were incubated with cis-platinum for three hours and thymidine uptake determined over the third hour. The inhibition of radiolabel incorporation correlated with three-year patient survival[63], a remarkable result in view of the generally transient benefit obtained when patients were treated with agents identified as active by more conventional culture techniques[38,41,64]. Whether this assay identifies tumours which are generally sensitive to chemotherapy[65], or identifies the superior activity of individual drugs against particular tumours, is not clear. The validity of such assays for sensitivity testing remains to be established.

Growth inhibition assays: semi-automated colorimetric approaches

Development of the methodology

Screening of large numbers of compounds for antitumour activity is best performed by the use of continuous cell lines, for which growth inhibition can be measured simply, economically and reproducibly, and without the need for highly sensitive approaches, such as radiolabelled thymidine uptake. Assays using rapidly growing murine leukaemia cells for which growth is quantitated efficiently by electronic particle counting[66] are convenient but inappropriate for identifying agents effective against solid tumours, most of which are cyto-kinetically very different from leukaemias. The cell counting assay was adapted for adherent lines such as Chinese hamster fibroblasts[67], murine Lewis lung cells[68] and human carcinoma lines[69,70] in which cells were harvested by trypsinization. Some human carcinoma cells possessing strong intercellular bonds required further disaggregation by the time-consuming and hazardous practice of irrigating them through a hypodermic needle[69], and alternative strategies were sought to turn such adherent (cell–cell, cell–substrate) properties to advantage.

The cytotoxicity of cytokines on confluent monolayers of L929 cells has been measured by staining surviving cells with crystal violet and quantitating the results spectrophotometrically[71,72] using 96-well ELISA plate readers. This method was adapted to the culture of exponentially-growing human adherent tumour cells exposed to cytotoxic compounds present continuously in culture. Surviving (adherent) cells present at the end of the culture period were stained and fixed with methylene blue in 50% aqueous ethanol, and absorbances determined using a 96-well plate reader. Excellent correlations were obtained between cell number and absorbance, and between IC_{50} values (drug concentrations inhibiting cell growth to 50% of that in control cultures) obtained by cell counting and spectrophotometric means[73].

This highly efficient method has been used for many purposes, including the study of oxygen toxicity in culture[74], the interactions between cytostatic cytokines and growth factors[75], the structure–activity relationships in extensive congeneric series of synthetic experimental anticancer acridines[76,77], and the screening fermentation broths for antitumour antibiotics[10,11]. With respect to the latter application, the concentration of antibiotic producing a given growth-inhibitory effect correlated well with potency as defined by clonogenicity assays[11]. The growth inhibition assays using mammalian tumour cell lines identified as active a spectrum of fermentation broths different from that identified by traditional antimicrobial screens. Every cell line possessed superior predictive value (relative to antimicrobial screens) for antitumour activity against the P388 leukaemia *in vivo*[10]. The miniaturization and automation afforded by microculture plate technology has also made feasible very large-scale screening for new anticancer drugs which will provide the basis of the drug discovery programme of the National Cancer Institute[78,79].

In addition to methylene blue staining, biomass or protein contents of cultures have been quantitated by Giemsa[11] and crystal violet[10,75]. In their systematic search for optimal staining methods, the NCI workers have chosen sulphorhodamine B which is very sensitive and yields absorbance values which vary linearly with cell number and protein content[78,79]. It also fluoresces with laser excitation at 488 nm and thus is amenable to fluorimetric measurement. Several other fluorochromes have been described as stains for sensitive and efficient drug assays including hydroethidine[80,81] and Hoechst DNA minor groove binders[82,83].

Ironically, the application of this extremely efficient 'solid-phase' assay for drug-induced growth inhibition of adherent cells meant that non-adherent cells, such as the classical murine leukaemia lines, were now much less efficiently assayed. Thus, alternative microplate approaches were sought by which leukaemic cells could be used for drug testing with comparable efficiency. Again the impetus was provided by techniques developed in immunological research.

In 1983, Mosmann described an automated method by which living cells metabolized the tetrazolium salt, MTT, to a dark-coloured insoluble formazan product which could be dissolved by organic solvents and quantitated spectrophotometrically to give an extremely rapid assay of cell proliferation[84]. In 1986, it was shown that MTT could be used to quantitate the effects of cytotoxic drugs on the growth of adherent and non-adherent (leukaemia, small-cell lung cancer) cells in microcultures[85,86]. Subsequent studies confirmed the widespread applicability of the method[50,87–92] and investigated technical improvements, such as the use of better solvents to dissolve the formazan crystals[50,87,89,92,93], the use of tetrazolium substrates that yield soluble products upon reduction[94,95] and interfacing of microplate readers with computers for efficient data capture, analysis and display[96,97].

The MTT assay gives drug sensitivity data compatible with those obtained by electronic particle counting[86,89], protein or biomass staining[79,86], clonogenic survival[87,88], visual counting of dye-excluding viable cells[87,88,90], and metabolic labelling[50]. Its general applicability cannot be assumed, however, as not all cells metabolize MTT[98], whereas others lose the ability to do so at high density[86]. Artefactual results can also be obtained in high-density cultures containing conditioned (acidified) growth medium. This latter anomaly was shown to result in an underestimation of the growth inhibitory effects of cytotoxic drugs[93] and particularly of interferons[99].

Application of automated drug screening

The advent of microculture assays represents a watershed in screening for anticancer drugs. The NCI has embarked on a disease-oriented programme of drug discovery based on a large panel of well-characterized human tumour cell lines representative of histotypes important in clinical disease: lung, colon, renal, and ovarian carcinoma, CNS tumours, melanoma and leukaemia[92,100]. As a primary screen, it will process at least 10 000 compounds per year, requiring the use of several million individual cultures. This is feasible only with microculture automation, and, after investigating the MTT assay, the NCI workers chose the sulphorhodamine B protein stain as the method of preference[78,79,92, 94].

Fundamental to this strategy is the rationale that cell lines will manifest the diverse phenotypes (particularly the determinants of drug sensitivity) characteristic of the tumour histotypes from which they were derived. Compounds will be advanced for further testing (in xenografts) on the basis of selective toxicity in the cell line panel[100].

Growth inhibition assays have given results for different cell lines consistent with clinical experience. In small series of cell lines, colon carcinomas were found to be more resistant than breast carcinoma and much more resistant than leukaemias to topoisomerase II-directed drugs (intercalators, etoposide), but not 5FU, bleomycin and mitomycin C[69,70,86]. Similarly, using the MTT assay, Park and co-workers[101] showed that colon carcinomas were more resistant than gastric carcinomas to doxorubicin but not to 5FU or 5FUdR. The colon cancer lines showed a wide range of sensitivities to 5FU, and the observation that the lower IC_{50} values occurred within a clinically achievable concentration was consistent with the clinical activity of this agent. No other agent tested was active by these criteria[102].

With respect to lung cancer lines, SCLC (smal-cell lung cancer) was shown to be more sensitive than NSCLC (non-small-cell lung cancer) to 7 out of 8 drugs tested[103] as well as to radiation[104]. Horiuchi and co-workers found a similar trend in a series of compounds with the difference being significant in four of eight drugs[105]. SCLC lines derived from treated patients were more resistant than those from non-treated patients[103,106].

A 'disease-oriented panel' of 11 head and neck tumour cell lines has been used to test 10 anticancer drugs to ascertain whether they were sensitive (as defined by low IC_{50}:peak plasma concentration ratios) to those drugs known to be clinically active against this tumour type[107]. In general, clinically active (methotrexate, *cis*-platinum) and inactive (BCNU, CCNU, deoxyazacytidine) agents performed *in vitro* as expected. Other compounds (vindesine, amsacrine, etoposide) performed better *in vitro* than clinical experience would have predicted. Although these results are encouraging, this study did not address the question of whether *non*-head and -neck tumours would have performed differently under the same assay conditions.

Data from the NCI also support the contention that cell lines in growth inhibition assays demonstrate drug sensitivity profiles concordant with clinical experience: generally, leukaemia and SCLC lines are most sensitive, NSCLC lines are heterogeneous, and renal carcinoma lines are resistant. BCNU manifested high activity against leukaemia and SCLC lines but was relatively inactive against those from colon and renal carcinoma; bleomycin was active against renal lines and relatively inactive against leukaemia; and doxorubicin demonstrated selective toxicity towards leukaemia cells and heterogeneous activity against those from solid tumours[96,100].

It remains to be seen whether continuous cell lines, which are composed of relatively homogeneous populations of undifferentiated cells possessing the capacity of unlimited proliferation, retain the potential chemotherapeutic targets of their tissues of origin. Such tissue-specific targets would have to be expressed in a high proportion of cell lines to ensure that small (6-member) panels of lines would reliably identify growth-inhibitory agents interacting with them. Many workers have shown that cell lines display a wide range of sensitivities to drugs, but these may simply reflect variations in a small number of critical biochemical features shared to a greater or lesser degree by all cells. The most obvious variable that might affect cell sensitivity is growth rate. At least in this case it can be said with confidence that differential sensitivities of cell lines are not simply a reflection of cell doubling times[69,70,86,103,106] although cloning efficiency in agar (stem cell character) has been associated with sensitivity[1,102]. Determinants of activity shared by all cell lines could include the P170 efflux pump responsible for classical multidrug resistance, glutathione-S-transferase, and other ubiquitous detoxifying systems. For example, a dozen cell lines of diverse origin demonstrated variation in sensitivity to a series of topoisomerase II-reactive drugs which was largely accounted for by the extent to which the cells manifested naturally occurring classical MDR-like character[77]. Moreover, several leukaemia lines selected for resistance to doxorubicin or amsacrine exhibit a few discrete patterns of cross-resistance when tested against a panel of key indicator drugs[12]. This again indicates that there are a discrete number of recurring loci responsible for drug resistance. It is possible that a small panel of six cell lines carefully chosen to represent such key features known to confer resistance to cytotoxic agents may be as effective as a large panel of sixty. The NCI's initiative, described as a "massive experiment"[108], will at the least greatly increase our knowledge of the factors determining drug sensitivity in cell lines. Whether it will also identify new anticancer drugs will become known in time.

A new application of the MTT assay: primary cultures

The MTT assay has also been applied to predictive drug sensitivity testing on cells freshly isolated from patients. The basis of the MTT procedure, as applied to the drug testing of primary tumours, is fundamentally different from that underlying the use of continuous lines. The latter are proliferating whereas the vast majority of neoplastic cells in primary culture are non-proliferating and, indeed, are viable for a limited time, necessitating an early (2–4 day) end-point. A short-term assay which measures drug-induced acceleration of cell death in a quiescent population may not be appealing, but there is evidence supporting its validity[6]. It is especially valuable for many leukaemias for which growth in clonal assays is often unattainable, and thus may be the most effective means of testing new drugs on fresh leukaemia cells. It has been used with specimens of CLL[109], ALL[110–112], AML and CML[112–114], and is finding an increasing role in the testing of solid tumours, including gastric, colon, liver[115–117], ovarian[118] and renal[119] carcinomas.

Shimoyama and co-workers[120] have used cells recovered from xenografts to show essential agreement between the 2-day MTT assay and a full clonogenicity assay in their ability to predict the activity of mitomycin C, 5FU and cis-platinum on xenografted tumours. Clinical correlations have shown that the assay is able to identify agents which are active in patients[112–114] and the extent of cell kill in vitro reflects the cytoreductive effect of a drug in vivo[114]. Progressive loss of sensitivity in vitro as patients relapse has been demonstrated[110–112]. In a series of renal cancers, several calcium antagonists were tested for their ability to counteract the MDR (multidrug resistance) phenotype. The specimens most resistant to vinblastine demonstrated the greatest increase in sensitivity when the calcium antagonists were present, and also stained for the MDR-associated P170 efflux pump[119].

The adhesive tumour cell culture system

Although primary cultures of tumour cells generally do not proliferate vigorously, a system has been described in which cells from a wide variety of solid tumours are cultured as monolayers on a cell adhesive matrix, a complex of biopolymers including fibronectin and fibrinopeptides[121,122], the precise nature of which has not been disclosed. The medium, serum[123], and growth factor requirements[124] have been optimized to give successful growth in at least

80% of the tumours received, and a cloning efficiency of 1–3%. The basis of the tumour cell growth has not been elucidated but presumably resides in the constituents of the adhesive matrix. Although clonal growth can be determined, an efficient crystal violet staining method in conjunction with image analysis has been used to quantitate cell proliferation.

Clinical correlations equivalent to those obtained by other methods have been presented[125]. An experimental compound is said to be active if its IC_{50} against tumour samples in at least 30% of cases is lower than the IC_{90} of a reference normal haematopoietic population. On this basis, taxol was postulated to be clinically active[126]. The activities of bleomycin and two analogues have been compared[127]. Tallisomycin S10b appeared to have an improved selectivity compared with bleomycin for tumour cells relative to bone marrow cells, but IC_{90} values of the two drugs were highly correlated against the series of tumours tested. On the other hand, liblomycin (which is known to possess some bone marrow toxicity in preclinical studies) demonstrated preferential cytotoxicity towards tumour cells relative to haematopoietic cells with 70% of the tumours tested, and a lack of correlation with bleomycin in terms of their IC_{90} values. This suggests that it is an effective compound with a dissimilar spectrum of activity. A similar analysis has been performed on *cis*-platinum and several derivatives[128]. Before this system is more widely applied, however, it will first be necessary to elucidate the basis of the discrepant published findings[129,130]. Other workers have been unable to replicate the high cloning efficiencies and selective growth claimed for the adherent tumour cell culture system by the group at Houston.

Microscopic estimation of cell death

Weisenthal and Lippman have argued strongly that the overall degree of cytotoxicity in all the cells of a tumour population is as valid a measure of drug efficacy as any that quantitates loss of clonogenic or proliferative capacity[6]. They have developed a microscopic method in which differential staining is used to assess whether cells retain metabolic activity sufficient for the maintenance of membrane integrity[131]. At the end of the culture period, viable and non-viable cells are stained differentially, cytospins are prepared, and the number of surviving cells from control and drug-treated cultures counted. Cell counts from different cytospin slides are normalized by adding a constant number of duck erythrocytes to all samples. This method depends on there being sufficient time for mortally injured cells to die following drug exposure (at least 4 days). Results are compatible in general with those measuring clonogenic survival[131] and the method is applicable to cells recovered freshly from patients for which proliferation is unattainable. Correlations with clinical results have been demonstrated[132,133].

The dye exclusion assay has also been applied to cell lines in proliferating cultures[64,87,88] for which correlation with the MTT assay has been demonstrated. Both assays are based upon cellular metabolism and, as the dye exclusion assay is highly labour intensive, its future use will probably be restricted largely to the study of those clinical specimens for which cytological assessment is necessary to enable discrimination between neoplastic cells and large numbers of contaminating normal cells.

In a method analogous to the differential cell staining assay, cells are exposed to drugs and then growth rates measured 1–3 days later. Cells are stained with fluorescein diacetate (viable cells) and ethidium (dead cells), and the number of viable cells determined relative to a known number of fluorescent beads by flow cytometry. The early end-point yields excellent concordance with clonogenic assays but the method suffers from the requirement for regular sampling[134].

LIMITATIONS OF THE CELL CULTURE APPROACH

Despite the versatility of cell culture methods, there are limitations, both in practice and in principle, in the way they can be applied to the search for anticancer agents. Practical dangers include the effect of culture conditions on apparent drug effectiveness. The presence of nucleosides in serum can make antimetabolites, such as methotrexate, ineffective[43]. The presence or absence of ascorbate in various media formulations affects rates of oxidative degradation of certain drugs, leading to great variations in apparent potency in assays where the drugs are present in culture for the duration of several halflives[76]. Cells cultured under conditions suboptimal for growth may be less able to tolerate sublethal damage and will then manifest greater sensitivity to drugs than when assayed under more optimal conditions *in vitro* [34] or *in vivo* [48].

There are more serious problems inherent to the reductionist approach of cell culture. Firstly, the ability of a drug to distribute through bulky tumour tissues which are heterogeneous microenvironmentally and cytokinetically, cannot be reflected by conditions in conventional monolayer cell cultures where cells are bathed in a large volume of medium, presenting no barriers to the delivery of oxygen, nutrients or drug. Secondly, *in vitro* assays will not reflect the activity of those compounds which are metabolically activated or detoxified by host tissues, such as the liver. Thirdly, anticancer agents may exert their effects indirectly, via host cells such as those of the immune system. Finally, the toxicity of experimental drugs for cultured cancer cells needs to be related to their toxicity towards those host tissues which will ultimately limit the dose of drug that can be administered *in vivo*. Special applications are available in strictly *in vitro* settings by which these considerations can be at least partially addressed. These are discussed in the order given above.

Distribution of drugs through 3-dimensional arrays of cells can be studied by the use of spheroid models[135–137]. Durand[138] has recently used spheroids of V79 fibroblasts to resolve a long-standing paradox: why is doxorubicin such an effective anticancer drug when it distributes within tissues very poorly? Doxorubicin-treated spheroids were washed to remove free drug and then maintained for varying periods of time before disaggregation and colony assay for cell survival. Doxorubicin was initially bound only to the cells at the periphery of the spheroid and would have failed to reach more central cells if the spheroid had been disaggregated immediately after the 1 h exposure to the drug. However, if disaggregation of the spheroid was delayed, the drug slowly penetrated the spheroid, killing cells which would otherwise have been inaccessible to it. Spheroids also model tumour nodules by representing the dynamic interplay that exists between fractionated therapy, cytotoxicity, cytokinetics and regrowth[139]. Cell cycle status varies with distance from the surface of the spheroid, and the size and clonogenic cell content of populations of spheroids can be determined over extended periods of time during which repeated cytotoxic treatments can be administered.

The metabolism of anticancer drugs *in vivo* is often mediated by liver enzymes. *In vitro* assays are available in which either viable hepatocytes[140] or the postmitochondrial supernatant from hepatocytes (which contains the appropriate oxidative enzymes)[141] is added together with drugs in cultures of target tumour cells. Cyclophosphamide is the classical example of drugs of this class. It must be enzymatically hydroxylated before it is biologically active, and either of these procedures increases its cytotoxicity at least 200-fold.

Where it is anticipated that a compound may exert its anticancer effect via a host cell type, co-cultures of effector and target (tumour) cells have been used to test drug action. Flavone acetic acid is very active against many murine tumours and was postulated to act indirectly when it proved to be unexpectedly non-toxic in culture[142]. It was subsequently shown that this compound could induce the cytotoxic activity of macrophages in culture[143], and co-cultures of peritoneal macrophages and tumour cells have been used to investigate the activity of analogues. Co-cultures of hepatocytes and tumour cells have also been used to show that the antitumour effects of α/β interferon on Friend erythroleukaemia cells is mediated by a protein secreted by the hepatocytes[144].

Studies on the selectivity of those anticancer drugs for which the most sensitive host tissue is known can be performed in culture. When the efficacy of a class of agents is known to be limited by haematopoietic toxicity, assays comparing the relative sensitivities of normal GM-CFUs and tumour cells may point to those compounds possessing the most favourable therapeutic index[22,25,145]. This rationale is analogous to that used in studies investigating the ability of cytotoxic drugs to purge bone marrows of leukaemic cells so they can be used for autologous transplantation[146-148]. Drug treatments may need to kill 10^8 leukaemic cells (which may be present in a bone marrow harvested from a patient in complete remission) whilst killing no more than 99% of the GM-CFUs[147].

In an extensive study, Hug and co-workers[149] compared the effects of a series of anthraquinone derivatives with normal bone marrow GM-CFUs and breast cancer colony-forming cells. Comparisons were made in terms of both the surviving fraction of breast cancer cells at the IC_{50} for GM-CFUs and the areas enclosed by the respective survival curves at 40% survival (Figure 3.4A–C). When doxorubicin was considered to be selectively toxic for an individual tumour *in vitro*, it was, in general, found to be active in the patient from whom the tumour was taken (Figure 3.4, lower panels). This approach was further validated by the demonstration that drugs which are bone marrow sparing *in vivo* (bleomycin, *cis*-platinum) were less toxic to GM-CFUs than to most tumours of a range of histological types *in vitro*, whereas drugs to which haematopoietic cells are highly sensitive (doxorubicin, etoposide) were not toxic for many of the tumour specimens at the IC_{90} for GM-CFUs[125,126] (Figure 3.5). On this basis, the experimental compounds, spirogermanium and caracemide,

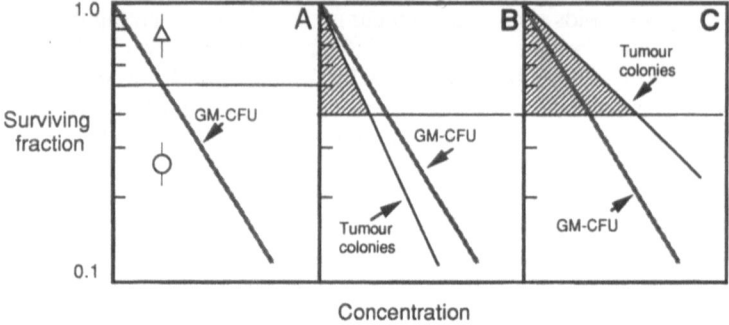

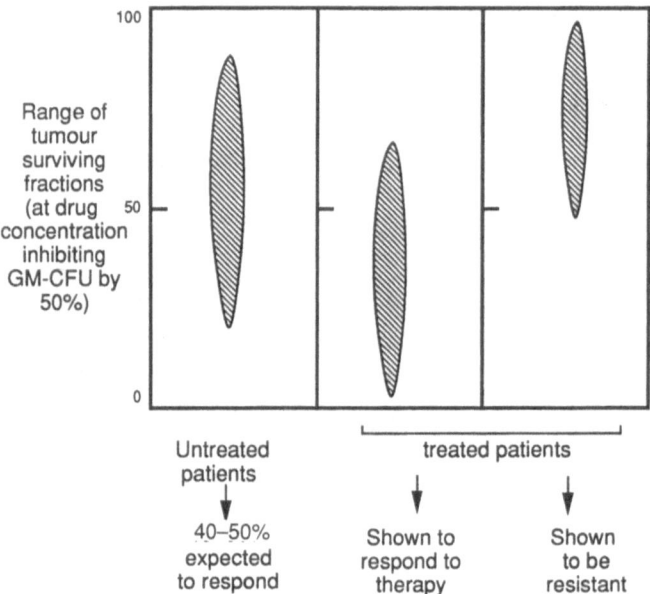

Figure 3.4 Use of the relative *in vitro* sensitivity of cultures of GM-CFUs and cultures of patients' tumour cells to predict clinical responses. *Upper panel*: **A**: Survival curve of GM-CFUs compared with the surviving fraction of cells from a resistant tumour (Δ) and a sensitive tumour ($\bigcirc$) at the GM-CFU IC$_{50}$. **B,C**: Comparison of survival curves of GM-CFUs and sensitive (**B**) and resistant (**C**) tumours (adapted from Reference 149). The relative areas bounded by the ordinate, the horizontal line corresponding to a surviving fraction of 40%, and the survival curves for tumour cells (shaded) and GM-CFUs have been taken to indicate sensitivity or resistance. *Lower panel*: Correlations between *in vitro* sensitivity and clinical responses of breast cancer patients (adapted from Reference 149). The shaded ellipses represent the distribution of *in vitro* sensitivities of a series of tumour specimens, expressed as surviving fractions at a doxorubicin concentration which reduces GM-CFU colony formation by 50% (as depicted in **A**, upper panel). The patients were divided into three groups: those who had not been treated at the time of *in vitro* assay (of whom 40–50% would be expected to respond to doxorubicin), and treated patients who were judged by clinical criteria to have either sensitive or resistant tumours

72

were predicted to be ineffective therapeutically, whereas taxol was expected to be active[126], a prediction that has been realized in phase II clinical trials[150]. More recently, an IL-3-dependent permanent murine haematopoietic progenitor cell line has been used as a convenient source of proliferating bone marrow-derived cells for use as a basis of drug-sensitivity comparisons[127].

Non-haematological toxicity is more difficult to assess *in vitro*. The most that can be said for those drugs which are selectively toxic for tissues other than the haematopoietic system is that an unfavourable relative activity towards bone marrow (a non-dose-limiting tissue) *in vitro* will strongly indicate a lack of therapeutic benefit[126]. Other workers have related *in vitro* cytotoxicities to the peak plasma concentration in humans as this value reflects the maximum drug dose tolerated by the individual[41,52,53,107]. For many experimental compounds, this concentration will not be known. In such cases, a value related to the LD_{50} in mice has been adopted as the reference concentration[53,105].

However, it has been shown that knowledge of the pharmacologically attainable serum concentration cannot adequately account for drug distribution in the body nor its penetration or halflife within individual tissues[3]. The response of a tumour to chemotherapy can vary widely depending on its site of implantation[3,68], demonstrating the unpredictable role of pharmacokinetics. Often there is a lack of correlation between *in vitro* chemosensitivity and *in vivo* response for a cell line[3,48]. Whether such anomalies reflect pharmacokinetic factors, differences in tumour cell cytokinetics or physiology between culture and whole animal environments is not clear. The drug sensitivities of cells recovered from a rapidly growing subcutaneous mouse tumour are equivalent to those of quiescent cells at saturation density *in vitro*[151], suggesting that cytokinetics may be an important factor.

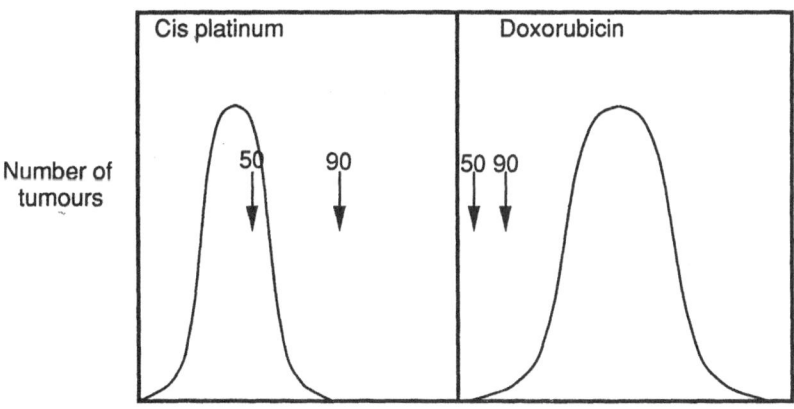

Drug concentration inhibiting growth by 50%

Figure 3.5 Relationship of *in vitro* sensitivity of patients' tumour cells to that of GM-CFUs for two clinical drugs with different dose-limiting toxicity. The distribution of IC_{50} values for a large series of tumour cell preparations treated with *cis*-platinum (left panel) and doxorubicin is depicted. Arrows indicate the IC_{50} and IC_{90} values of normal GM-CFUs when treated with the respective drugs (adapted from Reference 126).

In view of such considerations, it has been stressed that *in vitro–in vivo* correlations need to be established empirically for each drug[20,46,149]. Where this is not possible, as with any programme investigating large numbers of experimental compounds, *in vitro* assays reflecting inherent sensitivity should be considered a first approximation of cytotoxicity and used in conjunction with other approaches to determine antitumour activity. With clinical predictive assays, the *in vitro* criteria of activity can be modified depending on whether the aim is to identify any drugs which may be active[112] or rigorously exclude all drugs which will be inactive[49]. The same choice faces those using cell cultures for the identification and evaluation of compounds with anticancer activity.

NOVEL APPLICATIONS AND FUTURE DIRECTIONS

As far as the development of new cytotoxic drugs is concerned, the cell culture strategy in general, and individual methods in particular, will be judged by the clinical performance of the compounds that have been selected by large screening programmes. Of particular interest are those based on clonogenic assays of cells derived from xenografts[25] or clinical tumours[43] and the disease-oriented cell-line panel[100].

Greater understanding of the requirements of cells for survival and proliferation, including the role of the ever-increasing range of growth factors, will facilitate the application of assays using cells in primary culture. The use of basement membrane-like substrates, such as those derived from corneal endothelial cells[152] and the extracellular matrix elaborated by the murine Engelbreth-Holm-Swarm tumour[153], may well promote growth and the differentiated character of cells by producing a more authentic environment.

Many tumours proliferate well as 3-dimensional aggregates when seeded as clumps on[154,156] or in[157,158] an appropriate collagen gel. This represents a more natural form of growth than is afforded by monolayer cultures as it maintains intercellular connections, facilitates retention of differentiated character, and provides cytokinetic and drug-penetration barriers more akin to those of complex tissues. Application of such 'organoid' cultures represents a radically different strategy from that which has long prevailed using single cell suspensions to quantitate clonogenic survival precisely. Although it is not readily apparent how such organoid cultures can be used for large-scale drug screening, the introduction of fluorimetric and colorimetric means of estimating drug effects on growth has made this approach very attractive. Thus, Rotman and co-workers have seeded organoids on collagen gels supported by cellulose mesh[159]. They monitored drug effects by sequentially investigating the viability of cells in the tissue fragments by a non-destructive method involving uptake of the vital stain, fluorescein acetate[159]. Growing organoids have also been cultured in alginate microbeads. This attractive approach which has been used with cell lines allows quantitation of drug effects by the MTT assay[160].

The full potential of cell lines has not yet been realized. There have been calls for greater reliance on the development of anticancer drugs directed towards specific biochemical targets[108], the use of cell lines manifesting particular characteristics (such as dependence on an oncogene product), either naturally or fol-

74

lowing selection or engineering, should find an ever-increasing place in drug discovery. Hitherto, *in vitro* systems have been discussed solely in relation to the identification of cytotoxic agents. The versatility of cell culture has made possible the development of assays for substances which counteract neoplastic growth by interfering with various processes involved in carcinogenic development. Compounds identified may lead in time to the pharmaceutical treatment of neoplastic disease by an increasing variety of strategies. These are listed below.

Cultures of tumour cells have been used to test for agents which induce stasis in the absence of direct cytotoxicity. These include peptides[161,162] and tyrosine kinase inhibitors[163] which interact with components of the signal transduction pathway. Other agents, such as herbimycin[164] and oxanosine[165] have been shown to effect reversion to the normal phenotype of oncogene-transformed cells.

Culture methods have also been used to test for anticarcinogens (chemo-preventive compounds). Early passage hamster embryo fibroblasts have been used to detect natural products which inhibit the activation of benz[a]pyrene[166]. Screening for compounds which induce the protective detoxifying enzyme, NAD(P)H:quinone reductase, has been performed in a miniaturized 96-well plate assay using mouse hepatoma cells[167]. Several classes of anticarcinogens (including compounds that increase glutathione levels, display nucleophilic activity, or promote conjugation, cytochrome P450 expression, or cell differentiation) and antipromoters (retinoic acid, fluocinolone acetate and bryostatin-1) were identified in long-term transformation assays using benz[a]pyrene-treated rat tracheal epithelial cells[168] and phorbol ester-treated co-cultured normal and initiated mouse keratinocytes[169], respectively.

There is scope for studying inhibitors of angiogenesis in culture. Neoplastic cells require an adequate blood supply before they can grow into macroscopic tumours. Although angiogenic factors and inhibitors of neovascularization are assayed conveniently using *in vivo* systems, the selective inhibition of endothelial cell proliferation by compounds such as α-difluoromethyl-ornithine[170] and fumagillin[171] *in vitro* shows that endothelial cell cultures have a place in the study of agents inhibiting capillary development.

The ability of cells to penetrate a reconstituted basement membrane (Matrigel) supported on a polycarbonate filter has been used to test for inhibitors of invasion and metastasis[172]. The effect of pharmacologically active agents or randomly selected compounds on this process was tested by exposing cells to non-toxic concentrations of test compound, either prior to or during cultivation on the Matrigel. Retinoic acid[173] and staurosporine[174] have been found to inhibit tumour cell migration through Matrigel by suppressing protease secretion[173] and motility[173,174].

Differentiation inducers which promote the re-expression of the normal dif-ferentiated phenotype in neoplastic cells possess antitumour activity. An elegant 96-well plate assay for the screening of such inducers uses the inducible human promyelocytic leukaemia cell line HL-60[175]. When appropriately induced, HL-60 cells acquire the ability to produce superoxide in response to phorbol ester. Superoxide is measured spectrophotometrically by the reduction of cytochrome C. More detailed evaluations of differentiating agents, such as butyrate, DMSO, *N*-methylformamide and hexamethylene bisacetamide, have been performed using cell lines and cells from tumours[155].

Chemopotentiators and radiation sensitizers have been studied extensively in culture. Cancer cells often manifest inherent or acquired drug-resistance phenotypes. The efflux pump operated by the membrane glycoprotein P170 is a classical mechanism of resistance, and methods have featured in the search for compounds which can negate this resistance mechanism and potentiate cytotoxic agents through other routes[176]. New cell culture methods permit highly efficient screening for potential radiosensitizers and protectors[88].

CONCLUSION

For large-scale testing of potential cytotoxic compounds, highly efficient, economical and reproducible methods are now available. The procedure of choice employs microcultures in 96-well plates with colorimetric quantitation of cell growth. However, this approach can investigate only the toxicity of a compound, and the assessment of antitumour activity still requires an indication of selectivity.

For detailed investigation of a limited number of compounds of demonstrated interest, a range of assays should be utilized to measure drug effects on the clonogenic, proliferative or metabolic integrity of cultured cells, as well as the use of *in vivo* (murine) screens. Cell lines are the most convenient for such studies, but, since their relevance to clinical cancer is still controversial, fresh cells from clinical tumours are being increasingly used, both as xenografts and in culture in conjunction with assays using normal haematopoietic progenitor cells, as a measure of tumour selectivity. Rules for translating *in vitro* effects into *in vivo* responses in mice may be derived in many cases, but need to be established empirically for each compound. Ultimately, the decision to advance a compound to clinical trial should be based on as wide a range of different assays as practicable.

Acknowledgements

I would like to express my gratitude to Professors B. C. Baguley and W. A. Denny of the Auckland Cancer Research Laboratory for their help in the preparation of this manuscript and Ms Wendy Hodgson for secretarial assistance.

References

1. Taetle, R and Abramson, I (1988). Drug screening and biological systems. *J. Natl. Cancer Inst.*, **80**, 720–721
2. Double, J. A. and Bibby, M. C. (1989). Therapeutic index: a vital component in selection of anticancer agents for clinical trial. *J. Natl. Cancer Inst.*, **81**, 988–994
3. Phillips, R. M., Bibby, M. C. and Double, J. A. (1990). A critical appraisal of the predictive value of *in vitro* chemosensitivity assays. *J. Natl. Cancer Inst.*, **82**, 1457–1468
4. Grindey, G. B. (1990). Current status of cancer drug development: failure or limited success? *Cancer Cells*, **2**, 163–171

5. Tritton, T. R. and Hickman, J. A. (1990). How to kill cancer cells: membranes and cell signalling as targets in cancer chemotherapy. *Cancer Cells*, **2**, 95–105
6. Weisenthal, L. M. and Lippman, M. E. (1985). Clonogenic and nonclonogenic *in vitro* chemosensitivity assays. *Cancer Treat. Rep.*, **69**, 615–632
7. Carney, D. N. and Winkler, C. F. (1985). *In vitro* assays of chemotherapeutic sensitivity. In De Vita, V. T., Hellman, S. and Rosenberg, S.A. (eds). *Important Advances in Oncology*, pp. 78–103. (Philadelphia: J. B. Lippincott Company)
8. Hill, B. T. (1987). *In vitro* screening of new drugs and analogues – specificity and selectivity. *Cancer Treat. Rev.*, **14**, 197–202
9. Von Hoff, D. D. (1988). Human tumour cloning assays: applications in clinical oncology and new antineoplastic agent development. *Cancer Metastasis Rev.*, **7**, 357–371
10. Catino, J. J., Francher, D. M., Edinger, K. J. and Stringfellow, D. A. (1985). A microtitre cytotoxicity assay useful for the discovery of fermentation-derived antitumour agents. *Cancer Chemother. Pharmacol.*, **15**, 240–243
11. Mirabelli, C. K., Bartus, H., Bartus, J. O. L., Johnson, R., Mong, S. M., Sung, C. P. and Crooke, S. T. (1985). Application of a tissue culture microtitre test for the detection of cytotoxic agents from natural products. *J. Antibiotics*, **38**, 758–766
12. Finlay, G. J., Baguley, B. C., Snow, K. and Judd, W. (1990). Multiple patterns of resistance of human leukaemia cell sublines to amsacrine analogues. *J. Natl. Cancer Inst.*, **82**, 662–667
13. Coley, H. M., Twentyman, P. R. and Workman, P. (1990). 9-Alkyl, morpholinyl anthracyclines in the circumvention of multidrug resistance. *Eur. J. Cancer*, **26**, 665–667
14. Von Hoff, D. D. (1990). He's not going to talk about *in vitro* predictive assays again, is he? *J. Natl. Cancer Inst.*, **82**, 96–101
15. Mitchell, J. B. (1988). Potential applicability of nonclonogenic measurements to clinical oncology. *Radiat. Res.*, **114**, 401–414
16. Veerman, A. J. P. and Pieters, R. (1990). Drug sensitivity assays in leukaemia and lymphoma. *Br. J. Haematol.*, **74**, 381–384
17. Gorelik, E., Ovejera, A., Shoemaker, R., Jarvis, A., Alley, M., Duff, R., Mayo, J., Herberman, R. and Boyd, M. (1987). Microencapsulated tumour assay: new short term assay for *in vivo* evaluation of the effects of anticancer drugs on human tumour cell lines. *Cancer Res.*, **47**, 5739–5747
18. Bogden, A. E., Griffin, W., Reich, S. D., Costanza, M. E. and Cobb, W. R. (1984). Predictive testing with the subrenal capsule assay. *Cancer Treatment Rev.*, **11** (Suppl.), 113–124
19. Tueni, E. A., Dumont, P., Jacobovitz, D., Atassi, G., Rocmans, P., Lejeune, F., de Franquen, P., Semal, P. and Klastersky, J. (1987). Subrenal capsule assay for fresh human tumours in immunocompetent mice; an inappropriate technique for non-small-cell lung cancer. *Eur. J. Cancer Clin. Oncol.*, **23**, 1163–1167
20. Tveit, K. M., Fodstad, O., Olsnes, S. and Pihl, A. (1980). *In vitro* sensitivity of human melanoma xenografts to cytotoxic drugs. Correlation with *in vivo* chemosensitivity. *Int. J. Cancer*, **26**, 717–722
21. Tveit, K. M., Fodstad, O., Lotsberg, J., Vaage, S. and Pihl, A. (1982). Colony growth and chemosensitivity *in vitro* of human melanoma biopsies. Relationship to clinical parameters. *Int. J. Cancer*, **29**, 533–538
22. Taetle, R., Howell, S. B., Giuliani, F. C., Koziol, J. and Koessler, A. (1982). Comparison of the activity of doxorubicin analogues using colony-forming assays and human xenografts. *Cancer*, **50**, 1455–1461
23. Taetle, R., Honeysett, J. M., Rosen, F. and Shoemaker, R. (1986). Use of nude mouse xenografts as preclinical drug screens. Further studies on *in vitro* growth of xenograft tumour colony-forming cells. *Cancer*, **58**, 1969–1978
24. Taetle, R., Jones, O. W., Honeysett, J. M., Abramson, I., Bradshaw, C. and Reid, S. (1987). Use of nude mouse xenografts as preclinical screens. Characterization of xenograft-derived melanoma cell lines. *Cancer*, **60**, 1836–1841
25. Fiebig, H. H., Schmid, J. R., Bieser, W., Henss, H. and Lohr, G. W. (1987). Colony assay with human tumour xenografts, murine tumours and human bone marrow. Potential for anticancer drug development. *Eur. J. Cancer Clin. Oncol.*, **23**, 937–948
26. Scholz, C. C., Berger, D. P., Winterhalter, B. R., Henss, H. and Fiebig, H.-H. (1990). Correlation of drug response in patients and in the clonogenic assay with solid human tumour xenografts. *Eur. J. Cancer*, **26**, 901–905

27. Roper, P. R. and Drewinko, B. (1976). Comparison of *in vitro* methods to determine drug-induced cell lethality. *Cancer Res.*, **36**, 2182–2188
28. Drewinko, B., Roper, P. R. and Barlogie, B. (1979). Patterns of cell survival following treatment with antitumour agents *in vitro*. *Eur. J. Cancer*, **15**, 93–99
29. Drewinko, B., Patchen, M., Yang, L.-Y. and Barlogie, B. (1981). Differential killing efficacy of twenty antitumour drugs on proliferating and nonproliferating human tumour cells. *Cancer Res.*, **41**, 2328–2333
30. Corbett, T. H. (1984). A selective two-tumour soft assay for drug discovery. *Proc. Am. Assoc. Cancer Res.*, **25**, 325
31. Bissery, M. C., Wozniak, A. J., Heilbrun, L. and Corbett, T. H. (1988). Evaluation of synthetic agents by a selective multiple tumour soft agar assay. *Proc. Am. Assoc. Cancer Res.*, **29**, 492
32. Hamburger, A. W. and Salmon, S. E. (1977). Primary biossay of human tumour stem cells. *Science*, **197**, 461–463
33. Courtenay, V. D., Selby, P. J., Smith, I. E., Mills, J. and Peckham, M. J. (1978). Growth of human tumour cell colonies from biopsies using two soft-agar techniques. *Br. J. Cancer*, **38**, 77–81
34. Tveit, K. M., Endresen, L., Rugstad, H. E., Fodstad, O. and Pihl, A. (1981). Comparison of two soft-agar methods for assaying chemosensitivity of human tumours *in vitro*: malignant melanomas. *Br. J. Cancer*, **44**, 539–544
35. Ottestad, L., Tveit, K. M., Hoifodt, H. K., Nesland, J. M., Vaage, S., Hoie, J., Lund, E. and Pihl, A. (1988). Cultivation of human breast carcinoma in soft agar. Experience with 237 fresh tumour specimens. *Br. J. Cancer*, **58**, 8–12
36. Tveit, K. M., Fodstad, O. and Pihl, A. (1981). Cultivation of human melanomas in soft agar. Factors influencing plating efficiency and chemosensitivity. *Int. J. Cancer*, **28**, 329–334
37. Rofstad, E. K., Wahl, A. and Brustad, T. (1987). Radiation sensitivity *in vitro* of cells isolated from human tumour surgical specimens. *Cancer Res.*, **47**, 106–110
38. Tveit, K. M., Gundersen, S., Hoie, J. and Pihl, A. (1988). Predictive chemosensitivity testing in malignant melanoma: reliable methodology – ineffective drugs. *Br. J. Cancer*, **58**, 734–737
39. Von Hoff, D. D., Forseth, B. J., Huong, M., Buchok, J. B. and Lathan, B. (1986). Improved plating efficiencies for human tumours cloned in capillary tubes versus petri dishes. *Cancer Res.*, **46**, 4012–4017
40. Ali-Osman, F. and Beltz, P. A. (1988). Optimization and characterization of the capillary human tumour clonogenic cell assay. *Cancer Res.*, **48**, 715–724
41. Von Hoff, D. D., Sandbach, J. F., Clark, G. M., Turner, J. N., Forseth, B. F., Piccart, M. J., Colombo, N. and Muggia, F. M. (1990). Selection of cancer chemotherapy for a patient by an *in vitro* assay versus a clinician. *J. Natl. Cancer Inst.*, **82**, 110–116
42. Moon, T. E., Salmon, S. E., White, C. S., Chen, H.-S. G., Meyskens, F. L., Durie, B. G. M. and Alberts, D. S. (1981). Quantitative association between the *in vitro* human tumour stem cell assay and clinical response to cancer chemotherapy. *Cancer Chemother. Pharmacol.*, **6**, 211–218
43. Shoemaker, R. H., Wolpert-DeFilippes, M. K., Kern, D. H., Lieber, M. M., Makuch, R. W., Melnick, N. R., Miller, W. T., Salmon, S. E., Simon, R. M., Venditti, J. M. and Von Hoff, D. D. (1985). Application of a human tumour colony-forming assay to new drug screening. *Cancer Res.*, **45**, 2145–2153
44. Bertoncello, I. and Bradley, T. R. (1987). Human cell cultures for screening anti-cancer drugs. *Trends Pharm. Sci.* **8**, 249–251
45. Smith, H. S., Lan, S., Ceriani, R., Hackett, A. J. and Stampfer, M. R. (1981). Clonal proliferation of cultured non-malignant and malignant human breast epithelia. *Cancer Res.*, **41**, 4637–4643
46. Smith, H. S., Zoli, W., Volpi, A., Hiller, A., Lippman, M., Swain, S., Mayall, B., Dollbaum, C., Hackett, A. J. and Amadori, D. (1990). Preliminary correlations of clinical outcome with *in vitro* chemosensitivity of second passage human breast cancer cells. *Cancer Res.*, **50**, 2943–2948
47. Keith, W. N., Stallard, S. and Brown, R. (1990). Expression of mdr-1 and gst-π in human breast tumours: comparison to *in vitro* chemosensitivity. *Br. J. Cancer*, **61**, 712–716
48. Mirabelli, C. K., Sung, C.-M., McCabe, F. L., Faucetti, L. F., Crooke, S. T. and Johnston, R. K. (1988). A murine model to evaluate the ability of *in vitro* clonogenic assays to predict the response to tumours *in vivo*. *Cancer Res.*, **48**, 5447–5454

49. Kern, D. H. and Weisenthal, L. M. (1990). Highly specific prediction of antineoplastic drug resistance with an *in vitro* assay using suprapharmacologic drug exposures. *J. Natl. Cancer Inst.*, **82**, 582–588

50. Ford, C. H. J., Richardson, V. J. and Tsaltas, G. (1989). Comparison of tetrazolium colorimetric and [³H]-uridine assays for *in vitro* chemosensitivity testing. *Cancer Chemother. Pharmacol.*, **24**, 295–3015

51. Merry, S., Courtney, E. R., Fetherston, C. A., Kaye, S. B. and Freshney, R. I. (1987). Circumvention of drug resistance in human non-small cell lung cancer *in vitro* by verapamil. *Br. J. Cancer*, **56**, 401–405

52. Arteaga, C. L., Forseth, B. J., Clark, G. M. and Von Hoff, D. D. (1987). A radiometric method for evaluation of chemotherapy sensitivity: results of screening a panel of human breast cancer cell lines. *Cancer Res.*, **47**, 6248–6253

53. Scheithauer, W., Moyer, M. P., Clark, G. M. and Von Hoff, D. D. (1988). Application of a new preclinical drug screening system for cancer of the large bowel. *Cancer Chemother. Pharmacol.*, **21**, 31–34

54. Tanigawa, N., Kern, D. H., Hikasa, Y. and Morton, D. L. (1982). Rapid assay for evaluating the chemosensitivity of human tumours in soft-agar culture. *Cancer Res.*, **42**, 2159–2164

55. Friedman, H. M. and Glaubiger, D. L. (1982). Assessment of *in vitro* drug sensitivity of human tumour cells using [³H]thymidine incorporation in a modified human tumour stem cell assay. *Cancer Res.*, **42**, 4683–4689

56. Kern, D. H., Drogemuller, C. R., Kennedy, M. C., Hildebrand-Zanki, S. U., Tanigawa, N. and Sondak, V. K. (1985). Development of a miniaturized improved nucleic acid precursor incorporation assay for chemosensitivity testing of human solid tumours. *Cancer Res.*, **45**, 5436–5441

57. Tsushima, K., Podratz, K. C., Stanhope, C. R. and Lieber, M. M. (1987). *In vitro* chemotherapy sensitivity testing of human ovarian carcinoma: comparison of optical colony counting and [³H]thymidine incorporation assays. *Gynecol. Oncol.*, **28**, 170–180

58. Kern, D. H., Sondak, V. K., Morgan, C. R. and Hildebrand-Zanki, S. U. (1987). Clinical application of the thymidine incorporation assay. *Ann. Clin. Lab. Sci.*, **17**, 383–838

59. Wada, T., Akiyoshi, T. and Nakamura, Y. (1988). A simplified tritiated thymidine incorporation assay for chemosensitivity testing of human tumours. *Eur. J. Cancer Clin. Oncol*, **24**, 1421–1424

60. Nakayama, M., Nakano, S., Koga, T. and Niho, Y. (1989). Development of a rapid chemo-sensitivity test for anticancer drugs with contact-sensitive monolayers of Balb/3T3 cells. *J. Natl. Cancer Inst.*, **81**, 153–157

61. Matsuoka, H., Ueo, H. and Sugimachi, K. (1990). Growth of cells superinoculated onto irradiated and nonirradiated confluent monolayers. *Semin. Surg. Oncol.*, **6**, 48–52

62. Matsuoka, H., Ueo, H., Yano, K., Kido, Y., Shirabe, K., Mitsudomi, T. and Sugimachi, K. (1990). Estradiol sensitivity test using contact-sensitive plates of confluent BALB/c 3T3 cell monolayers. *Cancer Res.*, **50**, 2113–2118

63. Khoo, S. K., Hurst, T., Webb, M. J., Dickie, G., Kearsley, J., Parsons, P. G. and MacKay, E. V. (1988). Cisplatin chemotherapy of ovarian cancer: is short-term *in vitro* chemosensitivity predictive of long-term patient survival? *Aust. NZ J. Obstet. Gynaecol.*, **28**, 313–317

64. Gazdar, A. F., Steinberg, S. M., Russell, E. K., Linnoila, R. I., Oie, H. K., Ghosh, B. C., Cotelingam, J. D., Johnson, B. E., Minna, J. D. and Ihde, D. C. (1990). Correlation of *in vitro* drug-sensitivity testing results with response to chemotherapy and survival in extensive-stage small cell lung cancer: a prospective clinical trial. *J. Natl. Cancer Inst.*, **82**, 117–124

65. Volm, M., Drings, P., Hahn, E. W. and Mattern, J. (1988). Prediction of the clinical chemotherapeutic response of Stage III lung adenocarcinoma patients by an *in vitro* short term test. *Br. J. Cancer*, **57**, 198–200

66. Baguley, B. C. and Nash, R. (1981). Antitumour activity of substituted 9-anilinoacridines – comparison of *in vivo* and *in vitro* testing systems. *Eur. J. Cancer*, **17**, 671–679

67. Wilson, W. R., Tapp, S. M. and Baguley, B. C. (1984). Differential growth inhibition of cultured mammalian cells: comparison of clinical antitumour agents and amsacrine derivatives. *Eur. J. Cancer Clin. Oncol.*, **20**, 383–389

68. Baguley, B. C. and Wilson, W. R. (1987). Comparison of *in vivo* and *in vitro* drug sensitivities of Lewis lung carcinoma and P388 leukaemia to analogues of amsacrine. *Eur. J. Cancer Clin. Oncol.*, **23**, 607–613

69. Finlay, G. J. and Baguley, B. C. (1984). The use of human cancer cell lines as a primary screening system for antineoplastic compounds. *Eur. J. Cancer Clin. Oncol.*, **20**, 947–954
70. Ozawa, S., Yasuda, T. and Inaba, M. (1988). Comparison of cellular basis of drug sensitivity of human colon, pancreatic and renal carcinoma cell lines with that of leukaemia cell lines. *Cancer Chemother. Pharmacol.*, **22**, 41–46
71. Ruff, M. R. and Gifford, G. E. (1980). Purification and physico-chemical characterization of rabbit tumour necrosis factor. *J. Immunol.*, **125**, 1671–1677
72. Alexander, R. B., Nelson, W. G. and Coffey, D. S. (1987). Synergistic enhancement by tumour necrosis factor of *in vitro* cytotoxicity from chemotherapeutic drugs targeted at DNA topoisomerase II. *Cancer Res.*, **47**, 2403–2406
73. Finlay, G. J., Baguley, B. C. and Wilson, W. R. (1984). A semiautomated microculture method for investigating growth inhibitory effects of cytotoxic compounds on experimentally growing carcinoma cells. *Anal. Biochem.*, **139**, 272–277
74. Alexander, P. and Senior, P. V. (1986). Toxicity of oxygen at atmospheric concentration for newly explanted cancer cells. *Biochem. Pharmacol.*, **35**, 91–92
75. Sugarman, B. J., Lewis, G. D., Eessalu, T. E., Aggarwal, B. B. and Shepard, H. M. (1987). Effects of growth factors on the antiproliferative activity of tumour necrosis factors. *Cancer Res.*, **47**, 780–786
76. Baguley, B. C. and Finlay, G. J. (1988). Derivatives of amsacrine: determinants required for high activity against Lewis lung carcinoma. *J. Natl. Cancer Inst.*, **80**, 195–199
77. Baguley, B. C. and Finlay, G. J. (1988). Relationship between the structure of analogues of amsacrine and their degree of cross-resistance to adriamycin-resistant P388 leukaemia cells. *Eur. J. Cancer Clin. Oncol.*, **24**, 205–210
78. Skehan, P., Storeng, R., Scudiero, D., Monks, A., McMahon, J., Vistica, D., Warren, J. T., Bokesch, H., Kenney, S. and Boyd, M. R. (1990). New colorimetric cytotoxicity assay for anticancer-drug screening. *J. Natl. Cancer Inst.*, **82**, 1107–1112
79. Rubinstein, L. V., Shoemaker, R. H., Paull, K. D., Simon, R. M., Tosini, S., Skehan, P., Scudiero, D. A., Monks, A. and Boyd, M. R. (1990). Comparison of *in vitro* anticancer-drug-screening data generated with a tetrazolium assay versus a protein assay against a diverse panel of human tumour cell lines. *J. Natl. Cancer Inst.*, **82**, 1113–1118
80. Saiki, I., Bucana, C. D., Tsao, J. Y. and Fidler, I. J. (1986). Quantitative fluorescent microassay for identification of antiproliferative compounds. *J.Natl. Cancer Inst.*, **77**, 1235–1240
81. Bowles, A. P., Pantazis. C. G., Wansley, W. and Allen, M. B. (1990). Chemosensitivity testing of human gliomas using a fluorescent microcarrier technique. *J. Neuro-Oncol.*, **8**, 103–112
82. McCaffrey, T. A., Agarwal, L. A. and Weksler, B. B. (1988). A rapid fluorometric DNA assay for the measurement of cell density and proliferation *in vitro*. *In Vitro Cell. Devel. Biol.*, **24**, 247–252
83. Begg, A. C. and Mooren, E. (1989). Rapid fluorescence-based assay for radiosensitivity and chemosensitivity testing in mammalian cells *in vitro*. *Cancer Res.*, **49**, 565–569
84. Mosmann, T. (1983). Rapid colorimetric assay for cellular growth and survival: application to proliferation and cytotoxicity assays. *J. Immunol. Meth.*, **65**, 55–63
85. Cole, S. P. C. (1986). Rapid chemosensitivity testing of human lung tumour cells using the MTT assay. *Cancer Chemother. Pharmacol.*, **17**, 259–263
86. Finlay, G. J., Wilson, W. R. and Baguley, B. C. (1986). Comparison of *in vitro* activity of cytotoxic drugs towards human carcinoma and leukaemia cell lines. *Eur. J. Cancer Clin. Oncol.*, **22**, 655–662
87. Carmichael, J., DeGraff, W. G., Gazdar, A. F., Minna, J. D. and Mitchell, J. B. (1987). Evaluation of a tetrazolium-based semiautomated colorimetric assay: assessment of chemo-sensitivity testing. *Cancer Res.*, **47**, 936–942
88. Carmichael, J., DeGraff, W. G., Gazdar, A. F., Minna, J. D. and Mitchell, J. B. (1987). Evaluation of a tetrazolium-based semiautomated colorimetric assay: assessment of radio-sensitivity. *Cancer Res.*, **47**, 943–946
89. Twentyman, P. R. and Luscombe, M. (1987). A study of some variables in a tetrazolium dye (MTT) based assay for cell growth and chemosensitivity. *Br. J. Cancer*, **56**, 279–285
90. Ruben, R. L. and Neubauer, R. H. (1987). Semiautomated colorimetric assay for *in vitro* screening of anticancer compounds. *Cancer Treat. Rep.*, **71**, 1141–1149
91. Romijn, J. C., Verkoelen, C. F. and Schroeder, F. H. (1988). Application of the MTT assay to human prostate cancer cell lines *in vitro*: establishment of test conditions and assessment of hormone-stimulated growth and drug-induced cytostatic and cytotoxic effects. *Prostate*, **12**, 99–110

92. Alley, M. C., Scudiero, D. A., Monks, A., Hursey, M. L., Czerwinski, M. J., Fine, D. L., Abbott, B. J., Mayo, J. G., Shoemaker, R. H. and Boyd, M. R. (1988). Feasibility of drug screening with panels of human tumour cell lines using a microculture tetrazolium assay. *Cancer Res.*, **48**, 589–601

93. Plumb, J. A., Milroy, R. and Kaye, S. B. (1989). Effects of the pH dependence of 3-(4,5-dimethylthiazol-2-yl)-2,5-diphenyltetrazolium bromide-formazan absorption on chemosensitivity determined by a novel tetrazolium-based assay. *Cancer Res.*, **49**, 4435–4440

94. Scudiero, D. A., Shoemaker, R. H., Paull, K. D., Monks, A., Tierney, S., Nofziger, T. H., Currens, M. J., Seniff, D. and Boyd, M. R. (1988). Evaluation of a soluble tetrazolium/ formazan assay for cell growth and drug sensitivity in culture using human and other tumour cell lines. *Cancer Res.*, **48**, 4827–4833

95. Bernabei, P. A., Santini, V., Silvestro, L., Dal Pozzo, O., Bezzini, R., Viano, I., Gattei, V., Saccardi, R. and Rossi Ferrini, P. (1989). *In vitro* chemosensitivity testing of leukaemic cells: development of a semiautomated colorimetric assay. *Hematol. Oncol.*, **7**, 243–253

96. Paull, K. D., Shoemaker, R. H., Hodes, L., Monks, A., Scudiero, D. A., Rubinstein, L., Plowman, J. and Boyd, M. R. (1989). Display and analysis of patterns of differential activity of drugs against human tumour cell lines: development of mean graph and COMPARE algorithm. *J. Natl. Cancer Inst.*, **81**, 1088–1092

97. Reile, H., Birnbock, H., Bernhardt, G., Spruss, T. and Schonenberger, H. (1990). Computerized determination of growth kinetic curves and doubling times from cells in microculture. *Anal. Biochem.*, **187**, 262–267

98. Einspahr, J., Alberts, D. S., Gleason, M., Dalton, W. S. and Leibovitz, A. (1988). Pharmacologic pitfalls in the use of the MTT (versus human tumour clonogenic-HTCA) assay to quantitate chemosensitivity of human tumour cell lines. *Proc. Am. Assoc. Cancer Res.*, **29**, 492

99. Jabbar, S. A. B., Twentyman, P. R. and Watson, J. V. (1989). The MTT assay underestimates the growth inhibitory effects of interferons. *Br. J. Cancer*, **60**, 523–528

100. Shoemaker, R. H., Monks, A., Alley, M. C., Scudiero, D. A., Fine, D. L., McLemore, T. L., Abbott, B. J., Paull, K. D., Mayo, J. G. and Boyd, M. R. (1988). Development of human tumour cell line panels for use in disease-oriented drug screening. *Prog. Clin. Biol. Res.*, **276**, 265–286

101. Park, J.-G., Kramer, B. S., Lai, S.-L., Goldstein, L. J. and Gazdar, A. F. (1990). Chemosensitivity patterns and expression of human multidrug resistance-associated MDR1 gene by human gastric and colorectal carcinoma cell lines. *J. Natl. Cancer Inst.*, **82**, 193–198

102. Park, J.-G., Kramer, B. S., Steinberg, S. M., Carmichael, J., Collins, J. M., Minna, J. D. and Gazdar, A. F. (1987). Chemosensitivity testing of human colorectal carcinoma cell lines using a tetrazolium-based colorimetric assay. *Cancer Res.*, **47**, 5875–5879

103. Carmichael, J., Mitchell, J. B., DeGraff, W. G., Gamson, J., Gazdar, A. F., Johnson, B. E., Glatstein, E. and Minna, J. D. (1988). Chemosensitivity testing of human lung cancer cell lines using the MTT assay. *Br. J. Cancer*, **57**, 540–547

104. Carmichael, J., DeGraff, W. G., Gamson, J., Russo, D., Gazdar, A. F., Levitt, M. L., Minna, J. D. and Mitchell, J. B. (1989). Radiation sensitivity of human lung cancer cell lines. *Eur. J. Cancer Clin. Oncol.*, **25**, 527–534

105. Horiuchi, N., Nakagawa, K., Sasaki, Y., Minato, K., Fujiwara, Y., Nezu, K., Ohe, Y and Saijo, N. (1988). *In vitro* antitumour activity of mitomycin C derivative (RM-49) and new anticancer antibiotics (FK973) against lung cancer cell lines determined by tetrazolium dye (MTT) assay. *Cancer Chemother. Pharmacol.*, **22**, 246–250

106. Hida, T., Ueda, R., Takahashi, T., Watanabe, H., Kato, T., Suyama, M., Sugiura, T., Ariyoshi, Y. and Takahashi, T. (1989). Chemosensitivity and radiosensitivity of small cell lung cancer cell lines studied by a newly developed 3-(4,5-dimethylthiazol-2-yl)-2,5-diphenyltetrazolium bromide (MTT) hybrid assay. *Cancer Res.*, **49**, 4785–4790

107. Schroyens, W., Tueni, E., Dodion, P., Bodecker, R., Stoessel, F. and Klatersky, J. (1990). Validation of clinical predictive value of *in vitro* colorimetric chemosensitivity assay in head and neck cancer. *Eur. J. Cancer*, **26**, 834–838

108. Johnson, R. K. (1990). Screening methods in antineoplastic drug discovery. *J. Natl. Cancer Inst.*, **82**, 1082–1083

109. Twentyman, P. R., Fox, N. E. and Rees, J. K. H. (1989). Chemosensitivity testing of fresh leukaemia cells using the MTT colorimetric assay. *Br. J. Haematol.*, **71**, 19–24

110. Pieters, R., Huismans, D. R., Leyva, A. and Veerman, A. J. P. (1989). Comparison of the rapid automated MTT-assay with a dye exclusion assay for chemosensitivity testing in childhood leukaemia. *Br. J. Cancer*, **59**, 217–220

111. Pieters, R., Loonen, A. H., Huismans, D. R., Broekema, G. J., Dirven, M. W. J., Heyenbrok, M. W., Hahlen, K. and Veerman, A. J. P. (1990). *In vitro* drug sensitivity of cells from children with leukaemia using the MTT assay with improved culture conditions. *Blood*, **76**, 2327–2336

112. Hongo, T., Fujii, Y. and Igarashi, Y. (1990). An *in vitro* chemosensitivity test for the screening of anti-cancer drugs in childhood leukaemia. *Cancer*, **65**, 1263–1272

113. Santini, V., Bernabei, P. A., Silvestro, L., Dal Pozzo, O., Bezzini, R., Viano, I., Gattei, V., Saccardi, R. and Rossi Ferrini, P. (1989). *In vitro* chemosensitivity testing of leukaemia cells: prediction of response to chemotherapy in patients with acute non-lymphocytic leukaemia. *Hematol. Oncol.*, **7**, 287–293

114. Sargent, J. M. and Taylor, C. G. (1989). Appraisal of the MTT assay as a rapid test of chemosensitivity in acute myeloid leukaemia. *Br. J. Cancer*, **60**, 206–210

115. Suto, A., Kubota, T., Shimoyama, Y., Ishibiki, K. and Abe, O. (1989). MTT assay with reference to the clinical effect of chemotherapy. *J. Surg. Oncol.*, **42**, 28–32

116. Kanematsu, T., Maehara, Y., Kusumoto, T. and Sugimachi, K. (1988). Sensitivity to six antitumour drugs differs between primary and metastatic liver cancers. *Eur. J. Cancer Clin. Oncol.*, **24**, 1511–1513

117. Maehara, Y., Kohnoe, S. and Sugimachi, K. (1990). Chemosensitivity test for carcinoma of digestive organs. *Semin. Surg. Oncol.*, **6**, 42–47

118. Wilson, J. K., Sargent, J. M., Elgie, A. W., Hill, J. G. and Taylor, C. G. (1990). A feasibility study of the MTT assay for chemosensitivity testing in ovarian malignancy. *Br. J. Cancer*, **62**, 189–194

119. Mickisch, G. H., Kossig, J., Keilhauer, G., Schlick, E., Tschada, R. K. and Alken, P. M. (1990). Effects of calcium antagonists in multidrug resistant primary human renal cell carcinomas. *Cancer Res.*, **50**, 3670–3674

120. Shimoyama, Y., Kubota, T., Watanabe, M., Ishibiti, K. and Abe, O. (1989). Predictability of *in vivo* chemosensitivity by *in vitro* MTT assay with reference to the clonogenic assay. *J. Surg. Oncol.*, **41**, 12–18

121. Baker, F. L., Spitzer, G., Ajani, J. A., Brock, W. A., Lukeman, J., Pathak, S., Tomasovic, B., Thielvoldt, D., Williams, M., Vines, C. and Tofilon, P. (1986). Drug and radiation sensitivity measurements of successful primary monolayer culturing of human tumour cells using cell-adhesive matrix and supplemented medium. *Cancer Res.*, **46**, 1263–1274

122. Baker, F. L., Spitzer, G., Ajani, J. A. and Brock, W. A. (1988). Drug and radiation sensitivity testing of primary human tumour cells using the adhesive-tumour-cell culture system (ATCCS). *Prog. Clin. Biol. Res.*, **276**, 105–117

123. Baker, F. L., Ajani, J., Spitzer, G., Tomasovic, B. J., Williams, M., Finders, M. and Brock, W. A. (1988). High colony-forming efficiency of primary human tumour cells cultured in the adhesive-tumour-cell culture system: improvements with medium and serum alterations. *Int. J. Cell Cloning*, **6**, 95–105

124. Singletary, S. E., Baker, F. L., Spitzer, G., Tucker, S. L., Tomasovic, B., Brock, W. A., Ajani, J. A. and Kelly, A. M. (1987). Biological effect of epidermal growth factor on the *in vitro* growth of human tumours. *Cancer Res.*, **47**, 403–406

125. Ajani, J. A., Baker, F. L., Spitzer, G., Kelly, A., Brock, W., Tomasovic, B., Singletary, S. E., McMurtrey, M. and Plager, C. (1987). Comparison between clinical response and *in vitro* drug sensitivity of primary human tumours in the adhesive tumour culture system. *J. Clin. Oncol.*, **5**, 1912–1921

126. Fan, D., Ajani, J. A., Baker, F. L., Tomasovic, B., Brock, W. A. and Spitzer, G. (1987). Comparison of antitumour activity of standard and investigational drugs at equivalent granulocyte-macrophage colony-forming cell inhibitory concentrations in the adhesive tumour cell culture system: an *in vitro* method of screening new drugs. *Eur. J. Cancer Clin. Oncol.*, **23**, 1469–1476

127. Tueni, E. A., Newman, R. A., Baker, F. L., Ajani, J. A., Fan, D. and Spitzer, G. (1989). *In vitro* activity of bleomycin, tallysomycin S10b, and liblomycin against fresh human tumour cells. *Cancer Res.*, **49**, 1099–1102

128. Fan, D., Baker, F. L., Khokhar, A. R., Ajani, J. A., Tomasovic, B., Newman, R. A., Brock, W. A., Tueni, E. and Spitzer, G. (1988). Antitumour activity against human tumour samples of *cis*-diamminedichloroplatinum (II) and analogues at equivalent *in vitro* myelotoxic concentrations. *Cancer Res.*, **48**, 3135–3139

129. Head, J. F., Paolini, J. H. and Foster, L. B. (1989). Growth of normal cells in the adhesive tumour cell culture system. *Proc. Am. Assoc. Cancer. Res.*, **30**, 29

130. Parkins, C. S. and Steel, G. G. (1990). Growth and radiosensitivity testing of human tumour cells using the adhesive tumour cell culture system. *Br. J. Cancer*, **62**, 935–941

131. Weisenthal, L. M., Dill, P. L., Kurnick, N. B. and Lippman, M. E. (1983). Comparison of dye exclusion assays with a clonogenic assay in the determination of drug-induced cytotoxicity. *Cancer Res.*, **43**, 258–264

132. Bird, M. C., Bosanquet, A. G. and Gilby, E. D. (1985). *In vitro* determination of tumour chemosensitivity in haematological malignancies. *Haematol. Oncol.*, **3**, 1–10

133. Bird, M. C., Bosanquet, A. G., Forskitt, S. and Gilby, E. D. (1988). Long-term comparison of results of a drug sensitivity assay *in vitro* with patient response in lymphatic neoplasms. *Cancer*, **61**, 1104–1109

134. Ellwart, J. W., Kremer, J.-P. and Dormer, P. (1988). Drug testing in established cell lines by flow cytometric vitality measurements versus clonogenic assay. *Cancer Res.*, **48**, 5722–5725

135. Sutherland, R. M. (1988). Cell and environment interactions in tumour microregions: The multicell spheroid model. *Science*, **240**, 177–184

136. Carlsson, J. and Nederman, T. (1989). Tumour spheroid technology in cancer therapy research. *Eur. J. Cancer Clin. Oncol.*, **25**, 1127–1133

137. Kerr, D. J., Wheldon, T. E., Kerr, A. M. and Kaye, S. B. (1987). *In vitro* chemosensitivity testing using the multicellular tumour spheroid model. *Cancer Drug Deliv.*, **4**, 63–73

138. Durand, R. E. (1990). Slow penetration of anthracyclines into spheroids and tumours: a therapeutic advantage? *Cancer Chemother. Pharmacol.*, **26**, 198–204

139. Durand, R. E. and Vanderbyl, S. L. (1990). Schedule dependence for cisplatin and etoposide multifraction treatments of spheroids. *J. Natl. Cancer Inst.*, **82**, 1841–1845

140. Alley, M. C., Powis, G., Appel, P. L., Kooistra, K. L. and Lieber, M. M. (1984). Activation and inactivation of cancer chemotherapeutic agents by rat hepatocytes co-cultured with human tumour cell lines. *Cancer Res.*, **44**, 549–556

141. Lebsanft, J., McMahon, J. B., Steinmann, G. G. and Shoemaker, R. H. (1989). A rapid *in vitro* method for the evaluation of potential antitumour drugs requiring metabolic activation by hepatic S9 enzymes. *Biochem. Pharmacol.*, **38**, 4477–4483

142. Finlay, G. J., Smith, G. P., Fray, L. M. and Baguley, B. C. (1988). Effect of flavone acetic acid (NSC 347512) on Lewis lung carcinoma: Evidence for an indirect effect. *J. Natl. Cancer Inst.*, **80**, 241–245

143. Ching, L.-M., and Baguley, B. C. (1988). Enhancement of *in vitro* cytotoxicity of mouse peritoneal exudate cells by flavone acetic acid (NSC 347512). *Eur. J. Cancer Clin. Oncol.*, **24**, 1521–1525

144. Yasui, H., Proietti, E., Vignaux, F., Eid, P. and Gresser, I. (1990). Inhibition by mouse α/β-interferon of the multiplication of α/β-interferon-resistant Friend erythroleukemia cells co-cultured with mouse hepatocytes. *Cancer Res.*, **50**, 3533–3539

145. Ching, L.-M., Finlay, G. J., Joseph, W. R. and Baguley, B. C. (1990). Comparison of the cytotoxicity of amsacrine and its analogue CI-921 against cultured human and mouse bone marrow and tumour cells. *Eur. J. Cancer. Clin. Oncol.*, **26**, 49–54

146. Chang, T.-T., Gulati, S., Chou, T.-C., Colvin, M. and Clarkson, B. (1987). Comparative cytotoxicity of various drug combinations for human leukaemic cells and normal hematopoietic precursors. *Cancer Res.*, **47**, 119–122

147. Jones, R. J., Colvin, O. M. and Sensenbrenner, L. L. (1988). Prediction of the ability to purge tumour from murine bone marrow using clonogenic assays. *Cancer Res.*, **48**, 3394–3397

148. Singer, C. R. J. and Linch, D. C. (1987). Comparison of the sensitivity of normal and leukaemic myeloid progenitors to *in vitro* incubation with cytotoxic drugs: a study of pharmacological purging. *Leukemia Res.*, **11**, 953–959

149. Hug, V., Thames, H., Blumenschein, G. R., Spitzer, G. and Drewinko, B. (1984). Normalization of *in vitro* sensitivity testing of human tumour clonogenic cells. *Cancer Res.*, **44**, 923–928

150. Einzig, A. I., Wiernik, P. H., Sasloff, J., Garl, S., Runowicz, C., O'Hanlan, K. A. and Goldberg, G. (1990). Phase II study of taxol (T) in patients (pts) with advanced ovarian cancer. *Proc. Am. Assoc. Cancer. Res.*, **31**, 187

151. Finlay, G. J., Wilson, W. R. and Baguley, B. C. (1987). Cytokinetic factors in drug resistance of Lewis lung carcinoma: comparison of cells freshly isolated from tumours with cells from exponential and plateau-phase cultures. *Br. J. Cancer*, **56**, 755–762

152. Bulbul, M. A., Pavelic, K., Slocum, H. K., Frankfurt, O. S., Rustum, Y. M., Huben, R. P. and Bernacki, R. J. (1986). Growth of human urologic tumours on extracellular matrix. *J. Urol.*, **136**, 512–516

153. Fridman, R., Giaccone, G., Kanemoto, T., Martin, G. R., Gazdar, A. F. and Mulshine, J. L. (1990). Reconstituted basement membrane (Matrigel) and laminin can enhance the tumorigenicity and the drug resistance of small cell lung cancer cell lines. *Proc. Natl. Acad. Sci. USA*, **87**, 6698–6702

154. Schroy, P. C., Cohen, A., Winawer, S. J. and Friedman, E. A. (1988). New chemotherapeutic drug sensitivity assay for colon carcinomas in monolayer culture. *Cancer Res.*, **48**, 3236–3244

155. Schroy, P. C., Carnright, K., Winawer, S. J. and Friedman, E. A. (1988). Heterogeneous responses of human colon carcinomas to hexamethylene bisacetamide. *Cancer Res.*, **48**, 5487–5494

156. Willson, J. K. V., Bittner, G. N., Oberley, T. D., Meisner, L. F. and Weese, J. L. (1987). Cell culture of human colon adenomas and carcinomas. *Cancer Res.*, **47**, 2704–2713

157. Freeman, A. E. and Hoffman, R. M. (1986). *In vivo*-like growth of human tumours *in vitro*. *Proc. Natl. Acad. Sci. USA*, **83**, 2694–2698

158. Vescio, R. A., Connors, K. M., Youngkin, T., Bordin, G. M., Robb, J. A., Umbreit, J. N. and Hoffman, R. M. (1990). Cancer biology for individualized therapy: correlation of growth fraction index in native-state histoculture with tumour grade and stage. *Proc. Natl. Acad. Sci. USA*, **87**, 691–695

159. Rotman, B., Teplitz, C., Dickinson, K. and Cozzolino, J. P. (1988). Individual human tumours in short-term micro-organ cultures: chemosensitivity testing by fluorescent cytoprinting. *In Vitro Cell Dev. Biol.*, **24**, 1137–1146

160. Kupchik, H. Z., Collins, E. A., O'Brien, M. J. and McCaffrey, R. P. (1990). Chemotherapy screening assay using 3-dimensional cell culture. *Cancer Lett.*, **51**, 11–16

161. Woll, P. J. and Rozengurt, E. (1988). Bombesin and bombesin antagonists: studies in Swiss 3T3 cells and human small cell lung cancer. *Br. J. Cancer*, **57**, 579–586

162. Layton, J. E., Scanlon, D. B., Soveny, C. and Morstyn, G. (1988). Effects of bombesin antagonists on the growth of small cell lung cancer cells *in vitro*. *Cancer Res.*, **48**, 4783–4789

163. Yaish, P., Gazit, A., Gilon, C. and Levitzki, A. (1988). Blocking of EGF-dependent cell proliferation by EGF receptor kinase inhibitors. *Science*, **242**, 933–935

164. Uehara, Y., Murakami, Y., Sugimoto, Y. and Mizuno, S. (1989). Mechanism of reversion of Rous Sarcoma Virus transformation by herbimycin A: reduction of total phosphotyrosine levels due to reduced kinase activity and increased turnover of p60^{v-src}. *Cancer Res.*, **49**, 780–785

165. Itoh, O., Kuroiwa, S., Atsumi, S., Umezawa, K., Takeuchi, T. and Hori, M. (1989). Induction by the guanosine analogue oxanosine of reversion toward the normal phenotype of K-*ras*-transformed rat kidney cells. *Cancer Res.*, **49**, 996–1000

166. Cassady, J. M., Zennie, T. M., Chae, Y.-H., Ferin, M. A., Portuondo, N. E. and Baird, W. M. (1988). Use of a mammalian cell culture benzo(a)pyrene metabolism assay for the detection of potential anticarcinogens from natural products: inhibition of metabolism by biochanin A, an isoflavone from *Trifolium pratense L. Cancer Res.*, **48**, 6257–6261

167. Prochaska, H. J. and Santamaria, A. B. (1988). Direct measurement of NAD(P)H: quinone reductase from cells cultured in microtitre wells: a screening assay for anticarcinogenic enzyme inducers. *Anal. Biochem.*, **169**, 328–336

168. Steele, V. E., Kelloff, G. J., Wilkinson, B. P. and Arnold, J. T. (1990). Inhibition of transformation in cultured rat tracheal epithelial cells by potential chemopreventive agents. *Cancer Res.*, **50**, 2068–2074

169. Hennings, H., Robinson, V. A., Michael, D. M., Pettit, G. R., Jung, R. and Yuspa, S. H. (1990). Development of an *in vitro* analogue of initiated mouse epidermis to study tumour promoters and antipromoters. *Cancer Res.*, **50**, 4794–4800

170. Takigawa, M., Enomoto, M., Nishida, Y., Pan, H.-O., Kinoshita, A. and Suzuki, F. (1990). Tumour angiogenesis and polyamines: α-difluoromethylornithine, an irreversible inhibitor of ornithine decarboxylase, inhibits B16 melanoma-induced angiogenesis *in ovo* and the proliferation of vascular endothelial cells *in vitro*. *Cancer Res.*, **50**, 4131–4138

171. Ingber, D., Fujita, T., Kishimoto, S., Sudo, K., Kanamaru, T., Brem, H. and Folkman, J. (1990). Synthetic analogues of fumagillin that inhibit angiogenesis and suppress tumour growth. *Nature (London)*, **348**, 555–557

172. Welch, D. R., Lobl, T. J., Seftor, E. A., Wack, P. J., Aeed, P. A., Yohem, K. H., Seftor, R. E. B. and Hendrix, M. J. C. (1989). Use of the Membrane Invasion Culture System (MICS) as a screen for anti-invasive agents. *Int. J. Cancer*, **43**, 449–457

173. Hendrix, M. J. C., Wood, W. R., Seftor, E. A., Lotan, D., Nakajima, M., Misiorowski, R. L., Seftor, R. E. B., Stetler-Stevenson, W. G., Bevacqua, S. J., Liotta, L. A., Sobel, M. E., Raz, A. and Lotan, R. (1990). Retinoic acid inhibition of human melanoma cell invasion through a reconstituted basement membrane and its relation to decreases in the expression of proteolytic enzymes and motility factor receptor. *Cancer Res.*, **50**, 4121–4130

174. Schwartz, G. K., Redwood, S. M., Ohnuma, T., Holland, J. F., Droller, M. J. and Liu, B. C.-S. (1990). Inhibition of invasion of invasive human bladder carcinoma cells by protein kinase C inhibitor staurosporine. *J. Natl. Cancer Inst.*, **82**, 1753–1756

175. Catino, J. J. and Miceli, L. A. (1988). Microtiter assay useful for screening of cell-differentiation agents. *J. Natl. Cancer Inst.*, **80**, 962–966

176. Stewart, D. J. and Evans, W. K. (1989). Non-chemotherapeutic agents that potentiate chemotherapy efficacy. *Cancer Treat. Rev.*, **16**, 1–40

4
Tumour hypoxia: challenges for cancer chemotherapy

W. R. WILSON

INTRODUCTION

The development of new anticancer drugs has, throughout the history of cancer chemotherapy, struggled with a fundamentally difficult problem, namely that the biochemical differences between neoplasms and normal tissues are subtle ones. The essence of this problem was expressed in a despairing analogy by a participant at an early conference on cancer chemotherapy[1]: "It is almost, not quite but almost, as hard as finding some agent that will dissolve away the left ear, say, yet leave the right ear unharmed, so slight is the difference between the cancer cell and its normal ancestor". Since that time, much has been achieved in cancer chemotherapy without a complete understanding of the unique biochemical features of neoplasia, but the selectivity of existing anticancer agents still leaves much to be desired. Almost all agents in clinical use owe their limited utility to a selective toxicity towards proliferating cells, and, as a consequence, are toxic to normal tissues with high rates of cell turnover.

The dramatic advances of molecular biology in identifying gene products involved in neoplastic transformation have raised hopes that this pessimistic picture will soon change. But enthusiasm for the 'rational' design of drugs directed against oncogene products must be tempered by the realization that many are components of ubiquitous signal transduction and regulatory pathways. Oncology has not yet arrived at that golden age where receptor targeting can form the cornerstone of drug discovery. In a recent review, Moolten[2] pointed out that major therapeutic improvements will need to exploit properties of neoplastic cells which are *tumour specific* rather than *proliferation specific*, and has argued that no exploitable tumour-specific features (including oncogenes and tumour suppressor genes) are currently known. This is not to deny that genetic changes in specific tumours may prove to be exploitable. The activity of all-*trans* retinoic acid in acute promyelocytic leukaemia, which expresses aberrant forms of the retinoic acid receptor-α gene, appears to be a first instance of the exploitation of a tumour-specific genetic abnormality, although this development was entirely serendipitous[3].

It is salutary to remember, at a time when selectivity is increasingly being sought at the level of specific single gene products, that fundamental (and potentially exploitable) differences between normal and tumour tissue have been known for many decades. If we view the tumour at a higher level than the biochemical, i.e. at the tissue and organ levels of organization, then quite general differences between tumours and their normal counterparts emerge. Most conspicuous among these is the inefficient vascular system within solid tumours, a feature which determines many aspects of tumour biology. The hypoxic microenvironments which result from a spatially and temporally disorganized blood supply are characteristic of solid tumours of diverse origin and histology, and have important implications for cancer treatment[4].

Tumour hypoxia can be viewed as a two-edged sword in the context of cancer therapy. On the one hand, there is evidence that cells in such environments are resistant to many existing therapeutic agents. On the other, severely hypoxic microenvironments are largely restricted to tumours and hence offer potential for the development of selective anticancer agents. Other peculiarities of tumours arising from their disorganized vasculature, including low extracellular pH, might similarly be exploitable in anticancer drug development[5]. In this sense, hypoxia represents only the first, and currently best understood, of a new class of targets for anticancer drug design which are based on peculiarities of tumour physiology rather than biochemistry.

This essay outlines current understanding of tumour hypoxia, its importance in the resistance of solid tumours to therapeutic agents, and, particularly, the development of hypoxia-selective cytotoxins (HSC) as chemotherapeutic agents. Several earlier reviews on aspects of the latter topic are available[6–11].

TUMOUR HYPOXIA

Oxygen has long been known to sensitize almost all biological structures to ionizing radiation[12]. It is thus hardly surprising that most of our knowledge of tumour hypoxia stems from the radiobiological literature. Powers and Tolmach[13] were the first to demonstrate a subpopulation of viable (clonogenic) cells in an environment sufficiently hypoxic to cause radioresistance within a solid tumour. Radioresistant hypoxic cells have since been demonstrated in almost all murine solid tumours[14,15] and human tumour xenografts[16] which have been investigated.

Irreversible ('chronic') hypoxia

Prior to the experimental demonstration of tumour hypoxia, a seminal study by Thomlinson and Gray[17] had already suggested the existence of hypoxic regions in solid tumours as a consequence of oxygen diffusion limitations. Their model was built on indirect evidence, resting on the demonstration that the distance from the vascularized stroma to the onset of necrosis in human bronchial carcinomas (approximately 150 μm) was consistent with the estimated diffusion range of oxygen.

The inference that a population of viable radiobiologically hypoxic cells lies at the edge of the necrotic zone in murine tumours has since received strong support from many sources. One of the more direct is provided by flow cytometry studies with the fluorescent bisbenzimidazole, Hoechst 33342. The high DNA affinity of this minor groove binder ensures slow diffusion from vessels, and provides labelling of perivascular cells which is sufficiently stable to survive enzymatic dissociation of the tumour. Chaplin et al.[18,19] showed, after labelling with H33342 and irradiating in vivo, that brightly fluorescent (perivascular) cells in the SCCVII tumour were radiosensitive and that dimly fluorescent cells distant from functional vessels were radioresistant. These cells are sensitized by oxygen-mimetic drugs in vivo, confirming that radioresistance is due to hypoxia. Hypoxic cells have also been visualized in histological sections of tumours following treatment in vivo with 2-nitroimidazoles. These drugs are metabolized to form covalently bound products in the absence of oxygen, and can be detected using autoradiographic or immunohistochemical methods, displaying a pattern in accord with the Thomlinson–Gray model in some (but not all) tumours[20–23].

Reversible ('acute') hypoxia

Thomlinson–Gray hypoxia is a consequence of oxygen *diffusion* limitations, and leads to zones of chronically hypoxic cells. Recent studies have demonstrated that tumour hypoxia can also arise through transient *perfusion* defects. Cinemicrographic examination of blood flow in tumours growing between transparent windows in the rabbit ear or rat skin show that flow is temporally as well as spatially disorganized, with temporary cessation (and even reversal) of flow in some vessels[24]. The potential for such fluctuating blood flow to contribute to tumour hypoxia has been a source of speculation for many years[25], but recent investigations have clearly established its contribution to hypoxia in murine tumours.

One of the clearest indications that diffusional hypoxia is not the sole contributor comes, once again, from flow cytometry of SCCVII tumours stained in vivo with H33342[18,19]. The pattern noted above (radioresistance of cells with low fluorescence intensity) was observed only when H33342 was administered *during* irradiation. No such relationship was evident if tumours were irradiated 20 minutes after injection of the rapidly cleared[26] vascular marker. This observation, since confirmed with other experimental tumours[27], indicates that cells near functional vessels can become hypoxic within minutes, a finding which suggests frequent vessel closure and hence fluctuating blood flow.

The existence of such fluctuations was soon demonstrated more directly by double-label fluorescence microscopy, with two vascular markers administered a few minutes apart[19,28]. In large SCCVII tumours, about 8% of blood vessels appear to open or close over a 20-minute period[29]. It is not yet clear whether this fluctuation in blood flow represents an infrequent change in the flow status of most vessels, or whether a subset open and close frequently.

Multiple mechanisms

There are almost certainly other mechanisms which contribute to tumour hypoxia. Imaging of hypoxia with [³H]misonidazole often demonstrates confluent labelling on a scale too large to be readily accounted for by either of the above mechanisms alone[20]. This macroregional hypoxia is usually more pronounced in the centre of tumours and may reflect, in part, decreased blood flow and irreversible collapse of vessels as a result of high central interstitial pressure[30]. In addition, a population of acutely hypoxic cells may result from transient decreases in flow (as distinct from transient vessel closure). This would differ from total cessation of flow in that a gradient of oxygen concentration from the vessel would be present. Such hypoxia would, in this respect, resemble that described by Thomlinson and Gray, but would differ by being reversible through blood flow fluctuations.

The above mechanistic distinctions are important in that they have implications for the development of hypoxia-selective cytotoxins and radiosensitizers, particularly regarding the accessibility of hypoxic cells to drugs and the duration of drug contact under hypoxia. In addition, fluctuating blood flow, if it affects the majority of vessels in a tumour at some time, provides a possible basis for exploiting hypoxia to achieve a much greater kill than just the instantaneous hypoxia fraction[31]. In terms of therapeutic significance, the distinction between acute and chronic hypoxia might be less useful than that between reversible and irreversible hypoxia. The latter may be considered to apply to cells which cannot reoxygenate *in the unperturbed (untreated) tumour*. If effective treatment results in debulking and improved blood flow, then hypoxia arising through all the above mechanisms will be diminished.

Hypoxia in human tumours

Human tumours, like those in rodents, are heterogeneous structures limited by their blood supply[32]. There is abundant evidence from a wide variety of sources, reviewed recently[33], that hypoxic cells exist in human tumours. What is less clear is the extent to which these cells limit response to radiotherapy. One problem is that the available techniques do not determine whether the hypoxic cells detected are clonogenic. The second is that fractionated radiotherapy, with its small cell kill each day, will not be limited by hypoxia if there is efficient reoxygenation between treatments. However, several therapeutic studies in which attempts have been made to overcome the putative hypoxia problem have shown clinical benefit. These include such diverse techniques as breathing of hyperbaric oxygen during radiotherapy[34], use of oxygen-mimetic radiosensitizers[35] and transfusion of anaemic patients[35,36]. Further, a prospective study in which oxygen tensions in lymph node metastases of head and neck tumours were measured with oxygen electrodes prior to radiotherapy showed a strong correlation between the estimated volume of hypoxic tissue and treatment failure[37]. These investigations provide strong support for the view that hypoxia does limit the outcome of conventional fractionated radiotherapy, although the evidence is clearer for squamous cell carcinomas of the head and neck than for most other tumour types.

HYPOXIC CELL RADIOSENSITIZERS VERSUS HYPOXIA-SELECTIVE CYTOTOXINS

The search for ways of overcoming the hypoxia problem in radiotherapy has been one of the most active themes in radiobiology over the last three decades. The initial drug development approach was to seek agents which would radiosensitize hypoxic cells by acting as oxygen mimetics, replicating either the radical-addition properties of the oxygen biradical or its capacity for oxidizing radiation-induced radicals by electron transfer. The former mechanism was exploited by nitroxyls, such as the piperidin-1-oxyl (TAN;**1**); although these agents proved to have insufficient metabolic stability for use *in vivo*[9]. The nitro(hetero)arenes, in contrast, appear to act primarily as one-electron radical oxidants[38]. The distinction may, however, be less clear than first thought since addition of nitroarenes to DNA radicals may also contribute, either as an intermediate step in one-electron transfer[39] or as an intermediate in oxygen transfer to DNA sugar radicals[40]. Whatever the mechanism, some nitro-heterocycles with one-electron reduction potentials in an appropriate range (−350 to −500 mV) are active as radiosensitizers of hypoxic cells in tumours. Most work has focused on the 5- and 2-nitroimidazoles and the 3-nitro-1,2,4-triazoles, illustrated by metronidazole (**2**), misonidazole (**3**), and AK 2146 (**4**) respectively, since these ring systems have reduction potentials in the desired range and have relatively low toxicities *in vivo*. Misonidazole has shown limited activity in clinical radiotherapy[35], but an unanticipated cumulative peripheral neuropathy[41] has limited the dose to such an extent that only marginal sensitization could be expected[42]. The more hydrophilic 2-nitroimidazoles, pimonidazole (**5**) and etanidazole (**6**), currently under clinical evaluation were developed to optimize pharmacokinetics, providing more rapid excretion after irradiation and reduced uptake by nervous tissue[43,44].

1 : TAN   **2** : metronidazole   **3** : misonidazole

4 : AK 2146   **5** : pimonidazole   **6** : etanidazole

Initial attempts to develop drugs against radioresistant hypoxic cells focused on strictly oxygen-mimetic mechanisms, and any cytotoxicity was seen as disadvantageous. Later, it was found that preincubation of cells with misonidazole under hypoxia caused additional radiosensitization[45]. The mechanism was clearly different from the classical oxygen-mimetic radiosensitization in that the effect was not 'dose-modifying' as it reduced only the shoulder of the radiation survival curve. This new mechanism required drug metabolism and appeared to be related to the recently discovered selective toxicity of the nitroimidazole radiosensitizers themselves under hypoxic conditions.

The discovery of this hypoxia-selective cytotoxicity was presaged by Sutherland's observation in 1974 that metronidazole was selectively toxic to cells in the central regions of multicellular spheroids[46]. Several groups soon demonstrated that metronidazole and misonidazole are selectively toxic to tumour cells in culture under hypoxic conditions[47-49] and this was inferred to be the reason for the sensitivity of cells in spheroids[50].

The discovery (or rediscovery) of the hypoxia-selective cytotoxicity of nitroimidazole seems, in retrospect, hardly surprising since such compounds were already well known in antimicrobial chemotherapy for the treatment of anaerobic infections. But the selectivity of the latter compounds was generally considered to reflect a change in reduction potential in anaerobic microbes rather than absence of oxygen *per se*, so its relevance for tumour biology was not obvious. Although the mechanism of the new-found hypoxic cytotoxicity of misonidazole was not immediately apparent, its potential significance for cancer treatment was quickly appreciated by the radiobiological community and intensive investigation of this new phenomenon soon followed.

Initially an unplanned by-product of radiosensitizer development, hypoxia-selective cytotoxicity is now recognized as offering an alternative strategy for eliminating radioresistant hypoxic cells, and drugs with such properties can act as 'radiosensitizers' *in vivo*[51]. There is currently a perception that killing hypoxic cells with a cytotoxin might be preferable to sensitizing them to radiation, and that optimization of hypoxia-selective cytotoxicity should now be the key objective in the design of drugs to overcome the oxygen problem in radiotherapy. There are several arguments in support of this view:

(1) Hypoxia-selective cytotoxins (HSCs) offer potential for *exploiting* hypoxia. A hypoxic cell radiosensitizer, acting as a purely oxygen-mimetic agent, can do no more than eliminate the hypoxia problem. Hypoxic cell cytotoxins can turn it to advantage if either of two conditions are met.

   (a) A high proportion of cells in tumours spend *some* of their time in a hypoxic state (e.g. as a consequence of cycling hypoxia associated with fluctuating blood flow) and can thus be eliminated by frequent and protracted treatment with an HSC. Classical radiosensitizers are less active when radiation is delivered in small daily fractions if reoxygenation occurs[52]. Brown and Koong[31] have shown theoretically that the converse would be true for an HSC if 'rehypoxiation' brings additional cells into the hypoxic pool throughout treatment. They have suggested that fluctuating blood flow could provide a mechanism for the required redistribution of hypoxic and oxic cells, with both reoxygenation and rehypoxiation being manifestations of this same phenomenon. The significance of this interesting analysis is not yet clear as it has not been shown that fluctuating blood flow occurs in human tumours or that a high proportion of cells in rodent tumours transit through the hypoxic compartment. But support for the argument has been obtained in studies demonstrating the superiority of the hypoxic cytotoxin, SR 4233, over the hypoxic cell radiosensitizer, etanidazole, in fractionated radiotherapy when the drugs are administered with each of 8 radiation fractions of 2.5 Gy, although the data indicate this superiority for only two of the four tumours examined[51].

(b) Bioactivation of the HSC in hypoxic microenvironments produces an active species which can diffuse to surrounding oxic cells. Maximization of this would appear to be a key goal for further development of HSCs and is discussed further below.

(2) HSCs can avoid problems resulting from inhibition of tumour blood flow after drug administration, which is observed with many sensitizers when used at high doses in mice[53]. The induction of hypoxia in this manner is suspected to be the reason for a worse outcome in the pimonidazole-treated arm than in the control arm in a recent clinical trial of this sensitizer[54]. Adams[55] has pointed out that, in the context of an HSC, the induction of hypoxia in this manner can be an advantage, with the drug enhancing its own antitumour action.

(3). HSCs have potential application in chemotherapy as well as radiotherapy if hypoxic cells are commonly resistant to available chemotherapeutic agents (see below), or if they can be exploited as noted above to provide tumour-selective killing. It should be noted in this context that micrometastases can have a significant hypoxic fraction[56-58] so the utility of HSCs in chemotherapy may extend to disseminated disease.

The above potential advantages of HSCs do not imply that further development of 'classical' hypoxic cell radiosensitizers is unwarranted. The latter still offer two key advantages over HSCs in the context of radiotherapy. Firstly, they need to be present in the target cells at the time of irradiation only, unlike HSCs which require some minimum contact time under hypoxia. If cells transit rapidly through a hypoxic state, then an appreciable fraction may be hypoxic at the time of irradiation, but spared from killing by an HSC because of a subthreshold duration of hypoxia. Secondly, classical hypoxic cell radiosensitization does not require drug metabolism. It may thus be the preferred strategy in tumours with low activity of the reductase(s) responsible for HSC activation. The lack of requirement for metabolism also offers possibilities for development of non-toxic radiosensitizers if toxigenic biotransformation can be prevented by appropriate drug design. The development of HSCs with low toxicity is a more subtle challenge since sensitivity to reductive metabolism must be retained, and such activation must be made strictly selective for cells at oxygen tensions below about 1–5%. Thus, despite calls to the contrary[59], the new enthusiasm for HSCs in radiotherapy should not preclude continuing innovation in sensitizer development; it is important that the challenging problem of tumour hypoxia should continue to be addressed on as broad a front as possible.

DRUG RESISTANCE OF HYPOXIC CELLS IN SOLID TUMOURS

Hypoxic cells are widely considered to be resistant to many available anticancer agents, as well as to radiation, and this problem is frequently cited as part of the rationale for development of HSCs. While a therapeutic role for HSCs in chemotherapy does not necessarily depend on such resistance (hypoxia, for example, could still be exploited to achieve additional cell killing), it is appropriate to review the evidence for this contention and to outline contributing mechanisms.

Direct enhancement of cytotoxicity by oxygen

Although the cell sterilizing potency of ionizing radiation is increased 2–3-fold in the presence of oxygen, early surveys of cytotoxic drugs in acutely hypoxic cultures indicated that few were subject to analogous resistance under hypoxia[60,61]. An exception is the oxygen-dependent antitumour antibiotic neocarzinostatin (NCS), a targeted diradical which is a true radiomimetic agent. NCS selectively generates C-5' deoxyribose radicals in DNA, oxidation of which by oxygen or oxygen-mimetic radiosensitizers results in DNA breakage[62]. The cytotoxicity of other cytotoxins is depressed under hypoxic conditions because cell killing depends on generation of reduced oxygen species. Bleomycin, the best-understood example, forms a complex with DNA, ferrous ion and oxygen. Reduction of the latter by Fe^{2+} generates reactive oxygen species[63]. Cytotoxicity by bleomycin is enhanced by oxygen *in vitro*[61] as is its antitumour effect *in vivo*[64].

Cytokinetic resistance in hypoxic regions

Indirect consequences of the hypoxic microenvironment, such as changes in cytokinetics, are probably more important than the absence of oxygen *per se* as determinants of drug resistance. Tannock[65] first demonstrated that the growth fraction of corded solid tumours decreases with distance from blood vessels, suggesting that chronically hypoxic cells may exist predominantly in a non-cycling state. Evidence to support this view was obtained by Pallavicini *et al.*[66] who showed that 85% of the hypoxic radiation survivors in the KHT fibrosarcoma have a G_1-phase DNA content. A decreasing gradient in [³H]thymidine incorporation with distance from functional blood vessels has also been demonstrated by flow cytometric sorting after Hoechst 33342 labelling *in vivo*[67]. Studies with severely hypoxic tumour cells in culture have also demonstrated cell cycle arrest[68–71] and the pre-DNA-synthetic arrest has been interpreted[72] as an adaptive response of mammalian cells to prevent the rapid cell death seen when early- and mid-S-phase cells are trapped in a hypoxic state[71,72]. Microenvironmental factors other than lack of oxygen *per se*, such as acidosis or nutrient deprivation, may also contribute to cytokinetic changes in hypoxic regions of tumours[73]. Low-growth-fraction regions, therefore, may not correspond exactly to chronically hypoxic regions, but if a high proportion of hypoxic cells are non-cycling they would certainly be expected to be resistant to many conventional cytotoxic agents, the majority of which are selective for cycling cells[74].

The hypoxic microenvironment as a pharmacological sanctuary

It is now widely appreciated that the inefficient blood supply in solid tumours limits the delivery of many cytotoxic drugs and can spare cells distant from functional vessels[75,76]. The problem is particularly severe for physical DNA binders, such as intercalators, since only the free drug in equilibrium provides a driving force for diffusion, and the high DNA concentration in cells can reduce the effective diffusion coefficient by orders of magnitude[77]. The penetration of DNA intercalators such as Adriamycin[78] and amsacrine[79] into spheroids is severely restricted, and may contribute to the patchy distribution of fluorescence[80] and resistance of hypoxic cells[81] to Adriamycin in murine tumours. Durand[82] has demonstrated in studies with spheroids that the problem is partially offset by correspondingly slow efflux from regions distant from vessels, so the contribution of diffusion limitation to resistance of hypoxic cells is not yet clear. However, even for relatively stable agents with little tissue binding, such as melphalan, for which good microregional distribution may be expected, there is a macroregional heterogeneity in drug delivery which contributes to drug resistance[83].

Acidosis in the hypoxic compartment

Extracellular pH values (pH_e), as recorded with microelectrodes, are highly heterogeneous in tumours, with a mean lower by approximately 0.5 units than in normal tissues[5]. It is assumed, although not yet proven, that the lowest pH values derive from chronically hypoxic regions from which metabolic acids are cleared inefficiently. Several lines of evidence indicate that intracellular pH (pH_i) is actively regulated and will not fall as low as pH_e in hypoxic zones[5]. Denny and Wilson[84] have pointed out that the presumed reversal of the pH gradient across the plasma membrane will lead to the exclusion of weak bases from cells in acidic microenvironments. Many clinical antitumour agents are weak bases, and are expected to be less toxic to cells in hypoxic micro-environments through this mechanism. The uptake of Adriamycin is inhibited at low pH_e as predicted by this model[85], and mitoxantrone is dramatically less cytotoxic at pH_e values below 7.4 in the BICR-MIR$_{k-d}$ rat mammary carcinoma cell line[86]. Reliance on basic functionality in drug development to improve water solubility and potency (which it often does in culture where $pH_i < pH_e$) may exacerbate problems of hypoxic cell resistance. An attractive feature of mitomycin C is that it undergoes an acid-catalysed, as well as a reductive, activation to an alkylating agent and is more toxic to tumour cells at low pH[87,88], although this effect is small over the physiological pH range.

Hypoxia-mediated generation of drug resistance

Rice et al.[89] showed that hypoxic Chinese hamster ovary cells became resistant to methotrexate following reoxygenation, apparently because of reinitiation of DNA replication and amplification of the dihydrofolate reductase gene. Subsequently, Young et al.[90] demonstrated, using cultures of the B16F10 melanoma and KHT fibrosarcoma, that reoxygenation after protracted hypoxia increased metastatic frequency as assayed by lung colony formation following intravenous injection of cells. This group also reported enhancement of Adriamycin and methotrexate resistance after hypoxic incubation of KHT cells for 24 hours[90]. These interesting observations raised the possibility that hypoxia in tumours might generate resistance to anticancer agents. Further studies by Young and Hill[91] have shown a small increase in metastatic potential of cells isolated from hypoxic regions of the KHT tumour following reoxygenation in vitro, but no enhancement of Adriamycin or methotrexate resistance was observed. It thus remains unclear whether the conditions of hypoxia responsible for generating drug resistance in vitro can arise in solid tumours.

Hypoxia-induced changes in gene expression

The interference with progression through the cell cycle in nutrient-deprived tumour regions must necessarily lead to changes in gene expression. In addition, changes are observed in response to stresses, such as hypoxia and glucose deprivation, which appear to be separate from those due to proliferative changes. The glucose-[92] and oxygen-regulated[93] proteins (GRPs and ORPs, respectively) are not yet well characterized, but at least some members of these two sets of stress proteins are identical[94]. The induction of oxygen-regulated proteins in Chinese hamster cell cultures is coincident with the emergence of Adriamycin[93] and etoposide[95] resistance under hypoxia. These stress conditions also cause rapid depletion of topoisomerase II[96], the target for both Adriamycin and etoposide, which may account for the induction of resistance to this important class of antitumour agents.

In conclusion, a variety of mechanisms (which are not exhausted by the above) are suspected to contribute to the resistance of hypoxic cells to anticancer drugs. Several studies have confirmed such resistance in tumours, although it is seldom clear which of the above mechanisms is primarily responsible. Thus, the resistance of hypoxic cells in solid tumours to Adriamycin may include drug-diffusion limitations[78,76], resistance of non-cycling cells[78,97], decreased drug uptake at low pH[85] or induction of stress proteins[93].

A recent survey of the activity of cytotoxic agents in relation to distance from functional blood vessels, using the Hoechst 33342 flow cytometry method, indicated that the majority of available antitumour agents spare the presumptively hypoxic cells[98]. This suggests that resistance of hypoxic cells is likely to be a frequent problem in chemotherapy. However, the problem is not universal since similar activity against both aerobic and hypoxic cells has been found for 5-fluorouracil in KHT and 16/C tumours[99], diaziquone in 16/C tumours[100],

DTIC in KHT tumours[101] and cyclophosphamide in B16 melanomas[102] and 16/C tumours[81]. For some compounds (excluding HSCs), the micro-environmental features of hypoxic regions might actually increase drug sensitivity. Low pH improves uptake and toxicity of weak acids like chlorambucil[103,104]; low glutathione concentrations in cells distant from functional blood vessels[105] may increase drug sensitivity, and increased sensitivity of cells to radiation is seen if they are reoxygenated after prolonged periods of hypoxia[82].

It is clearly an oversimplification to consider that hypoxic tumour cells are necessarily resistant to chemotherapy, and it is not yet possible to assess to what extent they are spared by combination chemotherapy regimens in current use. Just how important this type of drug resistance is in the clinic will probably only become clear when effective HSCs, proven in the context of radiotherapy, are added to the existing chemotherapeutic armamentarium. However, the existence of a plethora of drug resistance mechanisms for cells in hypoxic micro-environments strongly suggests that these cells should be considered important targets for anticancer drug development.

MECHANISMS OF HYPOXIA-SELECTIVE CYTOTOXICITY

Agents which exploit hypoxic cell biochemistry

Two broad mechanisms for selective toxicity against hypoxic cells can be distinguished. The paradigm for the first class is provided by the glucose analogues 5-thio-D-glucose (7) and 2-deoxy-D-glucose (8) which inhibit glucose transport and, after phosphorylation, act as competitive inhibitors of hexose phosphate isomerase to block glucose utilization[106,107]. These drugs are selectively toxic to hypoxic cells[108,109], apparently because of the dependence of the latter on high rates of anaerobic glycolysis. While (8) is preferentially toxic to hypoxic cells in multicellular spheroids[110], no such activity could be achieved *in vivo* with either drug, even after depression of glucose levels by fasting[111] or insulin administration[110]. The doses which can be administered are limited by neurotoxicity as a consequence of the high glucose requirement of nervous tissue.

There are many other biochemical changes in hypoxic cells which have not yet been explored in detail in the context of HSC development. The redox status

7 : 5-thio-D-glucose   **8** : 2-deoxy-D-glucose

of hypoxic cells is altered as indicated by changes in ratios of oxidized to reduced nicotinamide nucleotides over the physiological range[112]. Despite the shift to a more reducing environment, hypoxic hepatocytes have a decreased glucose-6-phosphate concentration which lowers the steady-state NADPH supply and increases susceptibility to peroxides which are detoxified by the NADPH-dependent glutathione reductase/GSH peroxidase system[113,114]. Hypoxic hepatocytes are, for the same reason, also more sensitive to oxidative stress imposed by thiol oxidants, such as diamide[115].

A number of alkylating agents have been reported to be selectively cytotoxic to hypoxic tumour cells. The mechanism of this selectivity is unclear, but may reflect biochemical changes under a hypoxic environment. 1,3-Bis(2-chloroethyl)-1-nitrosourea (BCNU) shows such selectivity against hypoxic 9L rat brain tumour cells[116], 5-(3,3-dimethyl-1-triazeno)imidazole-4-carboxamide (DTIC) is selectively toxic to hypoxic Chinese hamster cells[99], and nitrogen mustards such as aniline mustard[117] and melphalan[118] have been reported to demonstrate hypoxic selectivity. Activated cyclophosphamide is selectively toxic to hypoxic V79 cells at pH 7.4 but not at lower pH[119]. This compound also showed modest selectivity for hypoxic cells in a C_3H mammary carcinoma although its selectivity was less than for high-dose misonidazole[120] and no hypoxic cell selectivity has been observed with other tumours[81,102]. Uncertainty as to the mechanisms responsible, and the low selectivity of these agents, makes them unattractive as leads for development of HSCs at present.

Bioreductive drugs: prodrugs activated by oxygen-inhibited pathways

Bioactivation of prodrugs by metabolic routes which are suppressed in oxygenated cells provides an alternative mechanism for hypoxia-selective cytotoxicity. This approach currently dominates HSC development and offers the important theoretical advantage (probably not yet realized) of diffusible products which can attack aerobic tumour cells surrounding hypoxic foci. HSCs of this class are widely referred to as bioreductive drugs since the biotransformation by which they are activated is, to date, invariably a reductive one. The original rationale[121] suggested that hypoxia in tumours might generate a reducing environment conducive to such reactions, and drew an analogy with the lower half-wave reduction potential of anaerobic compared with aerobic microbial cultures. Subsequently, it has become clear that, for most hypoxia-selective bioreductive agents, it is the presence of oxygen *per se* which is of critical importance through its inhibition of bioactivation.

Existing bioreductive agents make use of oxygen-sensitive biotransformation of four different types of functionality: nitro, quinone, N-oxide and transition metals, although the latter have only recently been reported in this context[122]. The biotransformation of these major functional groups and the therapeutic approaches based on drugs activated in this manner are discussed in the following sections.

NITRO(HETERO)ARENES

Many nitro(hetero)arenes are selectively toxic under hypoxic conditions because reduction of the nitro group to more toxic products is inhibited by oxygen (Scheme I). The latter inhibition is primarily due to reoxidation of the initial one-electron reduction product, the nitro radical anion, by molecular oxygen[123,124] which establishes a one-electron futile cycle in aerobic cells[125]. Under hypoxic conditions, net reduction to the hydroxylamine (4 electrons) or amine (6 electrons) oxidation level is observed. Hypoxia-selective cytotoxicity requires that the products of net nitroreduction be more toxic than the superoxide (and resulting toxic species, such as the hydroxyl radical) derived from the action of the one-electron futile cycle, and also more toxic than the diversion of reducing equivalents which the latter can cause[126]. These conditions are not always met. The common generalization that toxicity of nitro(hetero)arenes is hypoxia selective needs to be balanced against many exceptions where one-electron redox cycling exerts toxicological dominance over net nitroreduction (e.g. trinitrobenzene sulphonic acid[127]), or where the parent drug is toxic without requiring metabolism.

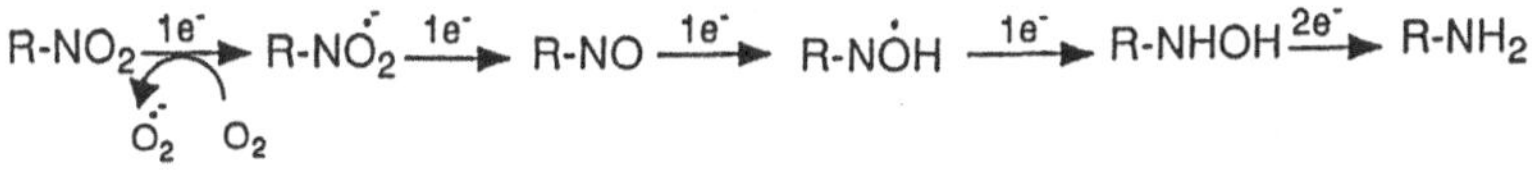

$$R\text{-}NO_2 \xrightarrow{1e^-} R\text{-}N\dot{O}_2^- \xrightarrow{1e^-} R\text{-}NO \xrightarrow{1e^-} R\text{-}N\dot{O}H \xrightarrow{1e^-} R\text{-}NHOH \xrightarrow{2e^-} R\text{-}NH_2$$
$$\dot{O}_2^- \quad O_2$$

Scheme I

Nitroreductases

A wide variety of enzymes can act as nitroreductases and many of these appear to have quite low substrate specificities. Thus, essentially all nitro(hetero)cycles with reduction potentials above about $-500\,mV$ are reduced metabolically at appreciable rates. Most catalyse one-electron reductions and, as a consequence, are effectively inhibited by oxygen through autoxidation of the one-electron adduct (Scheme I).

The major microsomal nitroreductases in liver are NADPH:cytochrome P450 reductase and the cytochrome P450s[128]. These appear to be the most important membrane-associated enzyme systems responsible for the reduction of the 2-nitroimidazole benznidazole to the corresponding amine[129]. Xanthine oxidase is considered a major cytosolic nitroreductase in liver[128], but aldehyde oxidase also has appreciable nitroreductase activity[130] and appears to be more important than xanthine oxidase in the reduction of benznidazole[129]. Neither of these molybdoflavoproteins appears to be active with substrates of low reduction potential, such as p-nitrobenzoic acid[130,131], this being reduced readily by cytochrome P450 and cytochrome P450 reductase[132,133]. The 'native' form of xanthine oxidase, xanthine dehydrogenase, also has nitroreductase activity although only one substrate, nitrofurazone, appears to have been investigated with this important enzyme[134]. NAD(P)H-quinone oxidoreductase (DT diaphorase), which is represented by multiple genes in human and rat liver[135,136], is best known in the context of quinone reduction[137] but also has limited nitroreductase activity. Its turnover number is lower with nitroaromatics than with most quinones, but known substrates include the dinitrophenylaziridine CB 1954[138], 4-nitroquinoline N-oxide[139] and 1,6-dinitropyrene[140]. An early report suggested that succinic dehydrogenase readily reduces trinitrotoluene[141] although that claim has been challenged and lipoyl dehydrogenase (Straub's 'diaphorase') proposed as an alternative trinitrotoluene nitroreductase[142]. The possible role of these dehydrogenases as nitroreductases appears not to have been investigated further.

Formation of cytotoxic species by nitroreduction

The identity of the proximal toxic species resulting from net nitroreduction is a matter of continuing controversy, and almost certainly differs between classes of nitro(hetero)arenes. Investigation has been dogged by the complex reduction chemistry of such compounds which is accompanied by rearrangements, ring fragmentation, autoxidation, disproportionation reactions, dimerizations and facile reaction with nucleophiles. The nitro radical anion itself appears to be insufficiently reactive to be responsible for the toxicity of nitroimidazoles[143,144] or nitrofurans[145]. This conclusion is supported by the finding that both 2-nitrosoimidazoles[146,147] and 5-nitrosoimidazoles[148] are highly toxic and thiol reactive, indicating the active species to be at or after the 2-electron reduction level. Similarly, 1-nitrosopyrene is much more toxic and mutagenic than 1-nitropyrene[149,150] although both give rise to the same major DNA adduct[151].

The hydroxylamines of many nitroarenes and arylamines appear to be responsible for their cytotoxic and mutagenic properties, often through formation of electrophilic nitrenes or nitrenium ions (Ar-N, Ar-NH+)[152–154]. These are readily formed after esterification of hydroxylamines by aminoacyl-tRNA synthetases[155], sulphotransferase or N,O-acyltransferase[156]. The hydroxylamines from reduction of 4-nitroquinoline N-oxide[155] or a variety of carcinogenic nitro-substituted polycyclic aromatic hydrocarbons[151,157–159] are known to be activated to DNA-reactive species by such acylation reactions. The carcinogenic 6-nitrophenanthrene aristolochic acid has a carboxyl *peri* to the nitro group which allows intramolecular acylation of the hydroxylamine to form a cyclic N-acylnitrenium ion as the DNA-reactive species[160].

In the case of misonidazole, radiolytic reduction proceeds with a 4-electron stoichiometry[161], but the unstable[162] hydroxylamine (9) fragments to form reactive and cytotoxic products such as glyoxal[163] (10; Scheme II). Glyoxal is also generated with a 25% yield on reduction of misonidazole by NADPH:cytochrome P450 reductase[164]. This reactive fragment rapidly forms an alkali-labile guanine adduct[165] (11), although glyoxal is clearly not the sole genotoxic product since it is formed from the C4 and C5 carbons yet [2-14C]misonidazole also gives rise to labelled nucleic acid adducts[166]. Despite their reactivity, the 2-hydroxylaminoimidazoles appear to lack cytotoxic activity[146,167]. Similarly, the N-acetyl and N,O-diacetyl derivatives of the hydroxylamine moiety of 1,2-dimethyl-5-hydroxylaminoimidazole do not appear to be cytotoxic, even in the presence of deacetylating enzymes[168]. An alternative candidate toxic species is the transient 3-electron reduction product,

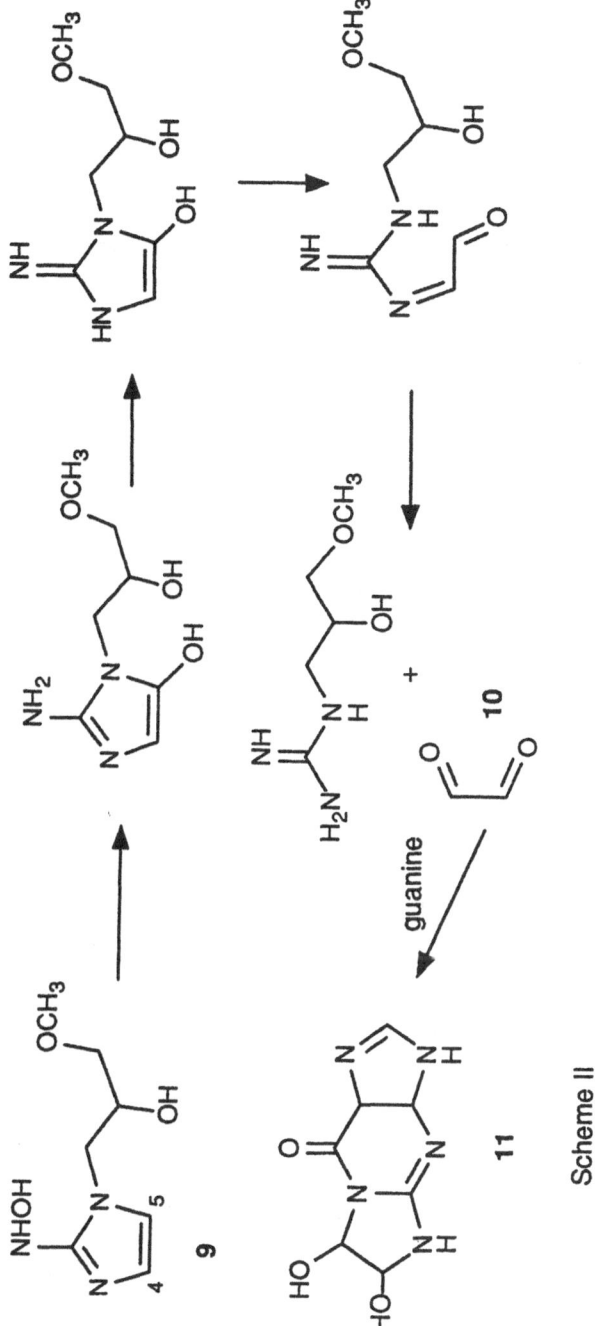

Scheme II

the nitroso radical anion. This intermediate in the reduction of the 5-nitro-imidazoles has been detected by ESR and suggested as a key cytotoxic species[169], which would be consistent with the high cytotoxicity of the nitrosoimidazoles noted above.

Therapeutic potential of the early nitroaromatic bioreductive agents

The most appropriate method for demonstrating hypoxia-selective cytotoxicity *in vivo* is to administer the drug immediately after a dose of radiation sufficient to kill essentially all oxic tumour cells. Under these conditions additional cell killing is seen with metronidazole and misonidazole in several tumour systems[170], but the required doses are close to the LD_{50} and effects are much smaller than the radiosensitization seen when the same drugs are administered before irradiation. In view of the minimal radiosensitization observed in clinical studies even when these compounds are given before irradiation, the nitroheterocycles first demonstrated as HSCs in tumour cell cultures appear to have little future as bioreductive drugs. This state of affairs is hardly surprising. The monofunctional nitroimidazoles were not designed as HSCs, and have very low potency in culture with significant toxicity only in the millimolar concentration range, even after several hours under hypoxic conditions.

Nonetheless, studies with 2-nitroimidazoles clearly indicate localization of reduction products, by covalent binding, in chronically hypoxic regions of spheroids and tumours[20–23]. Thus, these compounds can reach, and be selectively activated in, hypoxic cells. There is, then, a clear need for nitroheterocycles with much more toxic reduction products capable of turning this selective activation to therapeutic advantage. Enhancing toxicity of the products of net nitroreduction should also help to improve selectivity by minimizing the relative contribution of the one-electron redox cycle to toxicity[77].

Structure–activity relationships for nitro(hetero)arenes as hypoxia-selective cytotoxins

In a key study, Adams *et al.* demonstrated a good correlation between cytotoxic potency and one-electron reduction potential at pH 7 [E(1)] in Chinese hamster cell cultures under both aerobic and hypoxic conditions[171]. This suggests that nitroreduction is rate limiting for cell killing and that, taken together, mammalian cell nitroreductases are of sufficiently low specificity that E(1) is the main determinant of rates of reduction and toxicity. Quantitatively, the dependence on E(1) was consistent with a one-electron transfer process controlling this rate, and the similarity of this dependence for aerobic and hypoxic cytotoxicity implied that hypoxic selectivity is broadly similar for all nitroheterocycles. The observed relationship also implied that there are no marked differences between the cytotoxic potencies of the active reduction products. These conclusions are probably not valid outside the limited range of structural types investigated in this study (nitrobenzenes, nitroimidazoles and nitrofurans) and, since then, many compounds which do not fit the observed relationship have been described. In our own programme, aerobic and hypoxic cytotoxicity data and one-electron reduction potentials (determined by Dr R. F. Anderson, CRC Gray Laboratory) are available for 107 nitro(hetero)arenes, of which the largest groups are nitroquinolines, nitroacridines, nitrobenzenes and nitroimidazoles. While there are significant correlations with E(1) within some congeneric series, no clear overall relationship is apparent (unpublished data).

It would, indeed, be surprising if enzymatic nitroreduction kinetics were a simple matter of thermodynamics. Correlations between E(1) and rates of reduction of nitroimidazoles and nitrobenzenes by xanthine oxidase have been reported[172] and, at least for the nitroimidazoles, appear to be consistent with one-electron transfer controlling the rate. However, this enzyme is of notoriously low specificity, being a partially denatured derivative of the native dehydrogenase form of the enzyme[173,174]. Even with xanthine oxidase, significant differences in K_m values were observed within a congeneric series of nitroacridines, although the dependence of V_{max} on E(1) was in accord with Marcus theory[175]. The rate of reduction of nitroquinolines by hypoxic AA8 cells shows little relationship to E(1) (B.G. Siim, personal communication). It is not clear to what extent differences in ability to serve as substrates for reductases might underlie differences in nitro(hetero)arene cytotoxicity.

It is of interest that Wild[154] has recently reported a correlation between the bacterial mutagenic potencies of nitroarenes, the corresponding arylamines and their presumptive proximally active nitrenium ion derivatives, the latter being generated by photolysis of the corresponding arylazides. This study suggests that, at least in *Salmonella typhimurium*, the electrophilic reactivity of arylnitrenium ions, rather than their formation, is rate limiting for mutagenesis. Differences in proximal cytotoxins may be one of the factors contributing to the lack of correlation between reduction potential and cytotoxicity noted above.

Despite these qualifications, the generalization remains that nitroaromatics with E(1) values above about $-300\,\text{mV}$ lack activity *in vivo* as radiosensitizers, and this is probably a reflection of excessively rapid rates of metabolism. Thus, the development of more potent HSCs cannot proceed by elevating reduction potentials. A variety of other approaches to improving potency and hypoxic selectivity have been explored.

Alkylating 2-nitroimidazoles

Several approaches to enhancing potency of nitroreduction products currently offer promise. The 'mixed function' radiosensitizer, RSU 1069 (**12**), contains an alkylating aziridine moiety in the N1 side chain and is superior to non-alkylating 2-nitroimidazoles as a radiosensitizer of hypoxic cells in mouse tumours[176]. Although the alkylating group does enhance sensitizing potency[177], it appears that the excellent activity of this compound *in vivo* is primarily due to its superior hypoxic cytotoxicity[178]. RSU 1069 has much greater potency than misonidazole as an HSC in culture, apparently because nitroreduction generates a second alkylating centre to convert the monoalkylating aziridine into a much more toxic DNA cross-linking agent[179]. RSU 1069 also shows greater hypoxic selectivity than monofunctional 2-nitroimidazoles in culture, especially in cell lines defective in the repair of DNA interstrand cross-links[180], presumably because the products of net reduction are now much more toxic either than those due to the one-electron cycle in oxic cells, or than the unreduced mono-functional parent drug. An extensive analogue development programme has explored aziridine and other monofunctional alkylating moieties appended to a wide variety of other nitroheterocycles, but the high selectivity of RSU 1069 has not yet been matched[181].

12 : RSU 1069

13 : RB 6145

Modification of the aziridinyl side chain of RSU 1069 has also failed to produce a clearly superior agent, with the possible exception of a prodrug of RSU 1069, the bromoethylamino analogue, RB 6145 (**13**). The latter spontaneously ring closes to form RSU 1069 under physiological conditions, but the prodrug is less toxic than RSU 1069[182]. Despite an unfavourable early clinical study with RSU 1069[183], evaluation of RB 6145 as a bioreductive agent for use with radiotherapy is planned. A key factor in the viability of this proposal is the significant improvement in control of emesis, a severe problem with the use of RSU 1069[183], which has been made possible by the advent of 5-HT3 antagonists such as ondansetron[184]. RB 6145 offers the advantage of an oral clinical formulation. It is stable under acid conditions and has lower systemic toxicity but unchanged therapeutic activity when administered orally to mice[185].

Non-covalent DNA binders

If DNA reactivity can enhance the potency and selectivity of nitroheterocycles, can the same be achieved using reversible binding (e.g. intercalation) to target DNA? The paradigm for this approach is provided by the 1-nitroacridine nitracrine (**14**), developed in Poland as an antitumour agent[186]. Nitracrine binds to DNA by intercalation and is a hypoxia-selective cytotoxin with a potency in culture some 100 000-fold greater than misonidazole[187]. It lacks activity *in vivo*, and studies with spheroids suggest that this is a consequence of a rate of enzymatic reduction which is high in relation to its slow extravascular diffusion[188]. This problem is a critical one for development of HSCs endowed with affinity for DNA, but the association constant for nitracrine under physiological conditions is unusually low for an intercalator and in a range where diffusion times should be acceptable if the rate of nitroreduction can be lowered[77]. Electron-donating 4-substituents have been used to lower E(1)[189], resulting in lower rates of nitroreduction[175,190], but activity *in vivo* has not been achieved at non-toxic doses. 5-Nitroquinoline analogues of nitracrine (e.g. **15**) with lower DNA-binding affinity[191], improved spheroid penetration[192] and higher hypoxic selectivity[193] are currently under investigation.

14 : nitracrine   **15 : nitraquine**

Despite their high potency, the differential toxicity of DNA-binding nitroacridines towards hypoxic cells is no greater than that of the 2-nitroimidazoles[189,192]. This is also true of other DNA-binding nitroheterocycles, such as the pyrazoloacridine, PD 114,245 (**16**)[194], and intercalators with appended nitroimidazoles, such as NLP-1 (**17**)[195] and NLA-1 (**18**)[196]. Both of the limitations of the nitroacridines (modest hypoxic selectivity and poor extravascular transport) may, however, be surmountable through the design of prodrug forms with low DNA affinity as discussed below.

16 : PD 114,245   **17 : NLP-1**   **18 : NLA-1**

Activation of an alkylating agent by nitroreduction

In the above cases, the reduced nitro group can, itself, act as DNA-reactive species. A variety of attempts have been made to enhance the toxicity of reduction products by using nitroreduction to enhance the alkylating reactivity of a second centre in the molecule, or to generate such a centre *de novo*. One of the earliest such attempts[197] extended earlier studies on generation of reactive quinone methides by reduction of quinones[121], using nitroreduction as the trigger for methide generation (Scheme III). *o*-Nitrobenzyl halides, such as (**19**), showed moderate hypoxic selectivity to EMT6 cells *in vitro*, and were much more potent than nitroimidazoles of similar reduction potential.

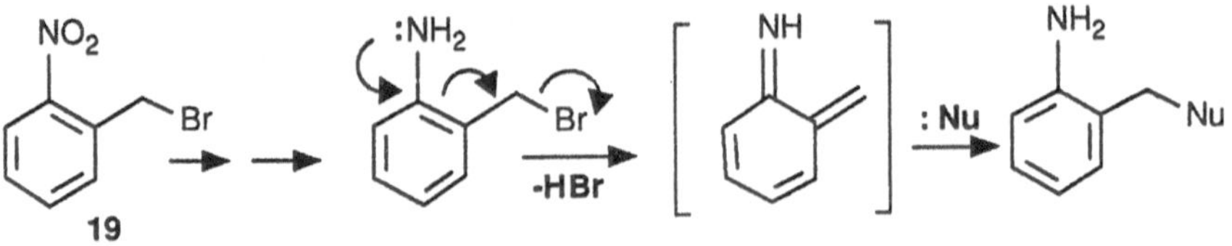

Scheme III

Denny and Wilson[84] suggested that nitroreduction could be used to activate aromatic nitrogen mustards. The reactivity of the latter is determined by the electron density on the mustard nitrogen, which is expected to be greatly enhanced on reduction of a strongly electron-withdrawing nitro group to an electron donating hydroxylamine or amine (Scheme IV).

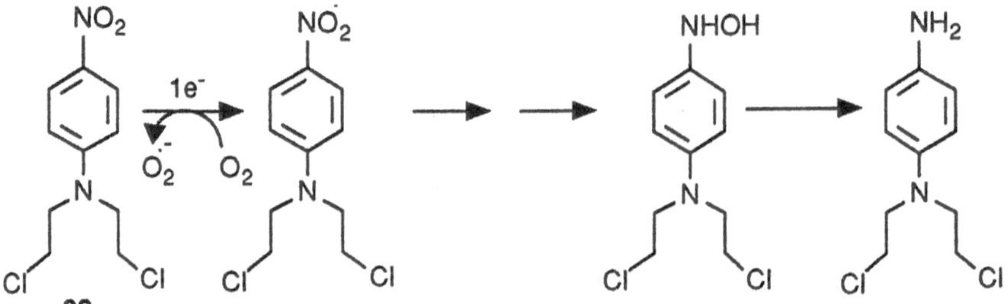

Scheme IV

Studies with aromatic nitrogen mustards confirmed the expected very large differences in reactivity and toxicity in culture (e.g. 20 000-fold between the p-nitro and p-amino mustards, **20** and **21**), but showed that mononitrophenyl mustards, such as **20**, have little hypoxic selectivity as the reduction potential is too low to allow appreciable reduction[198,199]. Recently, dinitrocarboxamide analogues with higher reduction potentials have been shown to offer excellent hypoxic selectivity in culture[199]. SN 23862 (**22**) is 70-fold more toxic to UV4 cells under hypoxic than under oxic conditions, and is an important new lead compound for further development. The superiority of SN 23862 over the corresponding aziridine compound, CB 1954 (**23**), is discussed below. The reductive bioactivation of the latter is primarily due to the generation of a second alkylating centre to form a DNA cross-linking agent[200,201]. The possibility that increased aziridine reactivity on reduction also contributes to bioactivation of CB 1954 appears not to have been considered, although alkylating reactivity of phenylaziridines is lowered considerably by electron-withdrawing ring substituents[202].

Wong et al.[203] suggested that 3-ethoxy-3(2-nitroimidazol-1-yl)-1-propene (**24**, NBK-50) might release acrolein from the N1 side chain on bioreduction, and provided evidence for acrolein formation on enzymatic reduction. Hypoxic selectivity was observed in B16 melanoma cell cultures, but with potency little

106

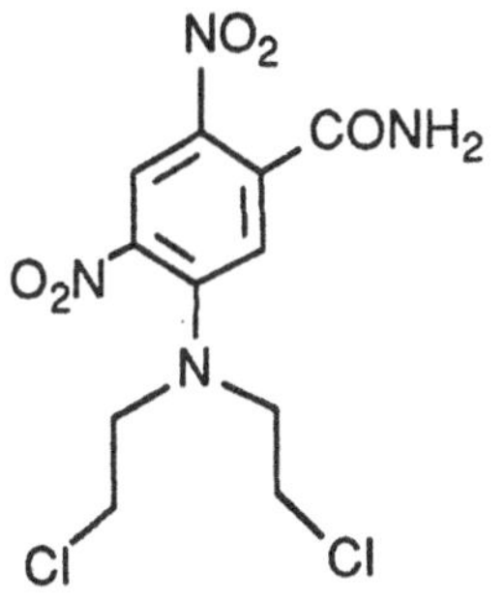

22 : SN 23862

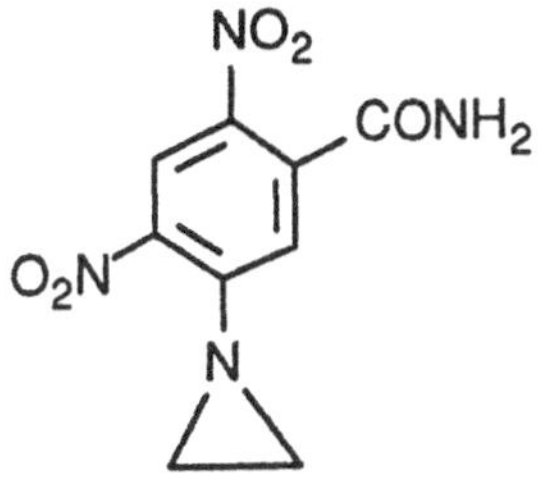

23 : CB 1954

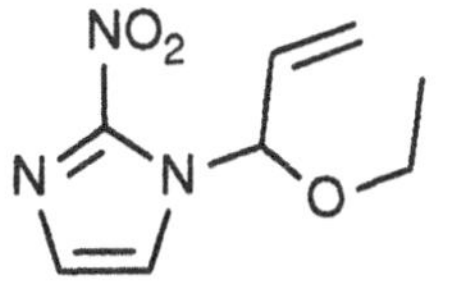

24 : NBK-50

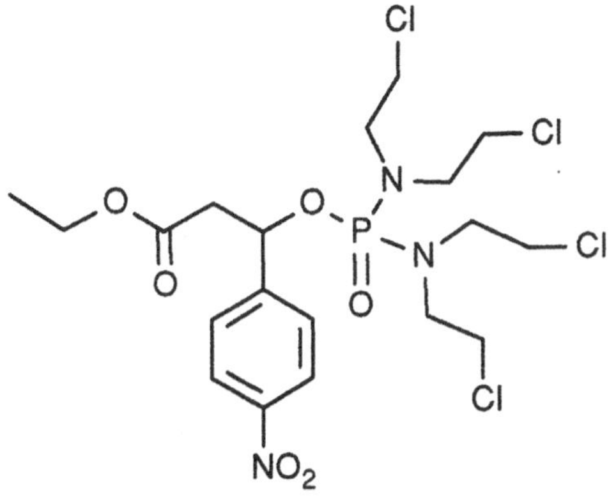

26 : JSD-231

different from a typical 2-nitroimidazole. A recent analogous example of alkylating agent release on nitroreduction is provided by the release of the much more toxic phosphoramide mustard following reduction of a 3-nitroquinoline. The increased basicity on reduction to the electron-donating hydroxylamine or amine is proposed as triggering intramolecular base-catalysed elimination of the phosphoramide mustard (Scheme V)[204]. Compound **25** was shown to be 11-fold more toxic to hypoxic than aerobic HT-29 cells, and DNA cross-linking under hypoxic conditions was demonstrated by alkaline elution. This is an interesting approach which is being pursued using other nitroaromatic systems, such as the nitrobenzyl phosphorodiamidate, JSD-231 (**26**), which also shows a hypoxic differential of approximately 10-fold[205].

Other novel approaches for using nitroreduction to generate highly cytotoxic products will no doubt be forthcoming. However, it is important to bear in mind that a large differential in toxicity between parent and reduced metabolites is not, in itself, sufficient to ensure a high hypoxic selectivity. A large differential in the rate of metabolic activation (high oxygen sensitivity of reduction) is also required, and this is probably the limiting factor for the activity of many nitro(hetero)arenes as HSCs.

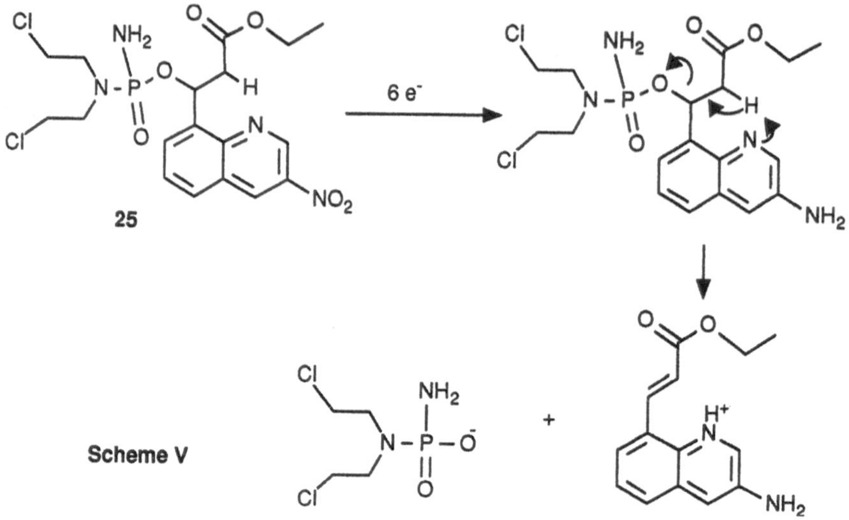

Scheme V

QUINONES AS HYPOXIA-SELECTIVE CYTOTOXINS

Reduction of variously-substituted 1,4-benzoquinones represents a second major biotransformation which can be inhibited by molecular oxygen. The basis for oxygen selectivity is analogous to that for nitroreduction in that the one-electron reduction intermediate, in this case the semiquinone, can be re-oxidized by oxygen to inhibit net reduction in aerobic cells (Scheme VI) although, in some cases, autoxidation of the dihydroquinone can also be appreciable[206]. As for the nitro(hetero)arenes, these futile 1-electron redox cycles generate potentially toxic reactive oxygen species[207]. Because the dihydroquinones are (usually) less prone to redox cycling, and are substrates for conjugation, the alternative 2-electron reduction route (Scheme VI) is generally considered a detoxification pathway.

In contrast to the situation with nitro compounds, the reduced quinones themselves generally have low toxicity (apart from their propensity for reducing oxygen). Those quinones with useful activity as HSCs therefore also bear potential alkylating functionality which is activated on reduction to the semi-quinone or dihydroquinone, thus providing the required increase in cytotoxicity on reduction. This approach to the development of HSCs was first articulated in 1972 with reference to synthetic benzoquinones capable of generating reactive methides on reduction[121] and the term 'bioreductive alkylation' was coined to describe this process. Subsequently, a wide variety of synthetic and naturally-occurring quinone methide precursors have been reported[208], although none appear to have useful activity as HSCs *in vivo*. Wilson *et al.*[209] have pointed out that the very high reactivity of many of these quinones with thiols may be one of the factors limiting activity *in vivo*.

The quinone-containing antitumour antibiotic, mitomycin C (MMC, **27**), was in clinical use as an anticancer agent well before the development of synthetic

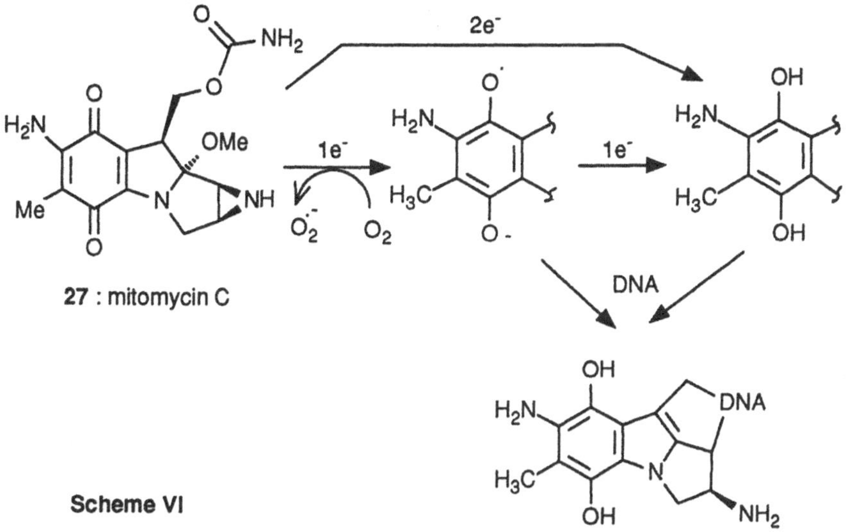

Scheme VI

quinones as bioreductive alkylating agents, and can be considered the prototype for this class since reduction to the semiquinone or dihydroquinone activates its alkylating activity[210] (Scheme VI). MMC is preferentially toxic to EMT6 cells under hypoxia[211], although with less selectively than the 2-nitroimidazoles. The hypoxic selectivity of MMC is dependent on culture conditions, being modified by ascorbate in the medium[212] and is markedly cell-line dependent[213], with selectivity reported to be lacking entirely in human tumour cell lines or biopsied human tumours[211]. It has similar activity against hypoxic and oxic cells in mouse tumours[210]. MMC has been shown to provide improved survival as an adjunct to radiotherapy of head and neck tumours[214], although it has not been established that its utility in this context is a consequence of hypoxic cytotoxicity.

The enzymology of MMC bioactivation is controversial. Cytochrome P450 reductase is considered the major one-electron reductase for MMC[215], but there is evidence[216–218] for competing two-electron reductive activation by DT diaphorase (Scheme VI). The latter process is not inhibited by oxygen, and may limit the hypoxic selectivity of MMC[217,218]. Rockwell et al.[219] have used dicoumarol, an inhibitor of DT diaphorase (DTD), to improve the efficacy of MMC against hypoxic cells in EMT6 tumours. The importance of DTD is challenged by the finding that a CHO-K1 mutant resistant to MMC has lowered cytochrome P450 reductase activity[220], and the apparent lack of reduction of MMC by purified DTD although reduction has now been observed at pH ≤ 7.0, which is lower than the pH optimum for other quinones[221].

The limited hypoxic differential of MMC has stimulated a search for more selective analogues. Porfiromycin (**28a**), the N-methyl aziridine analogue of MMC, has superior hypoxia-selective cytotoxicity as a result of a lowered aerobic cytotoxicity[215], and shows selective toxicity against hypoxic cells in

109

EMT6 tumours[216]. It received a preliminary trial as a chemotherapeutic agent in 1965[222], but has recently commenced clinical evaluation in combination with radiation at Yale University School of Medicine. A recently reported cyclic acetal derivative of porfiromycin, BMY-42355 (**28b**) showed very high hypoxic selectivity (approximately 100-fold) in EMT6 cell cultures but, disappointingly, did not demonstrate selective killing of hypoxic cells in EMT6 tumours[223].

Synthetic aziridinyl quinones have also been investigated as potential HSCs. Diaziquone (**29**, AZQ) is very similar to MMC, showing modest selectivity for hypoxic cells *in vitro* with the aziridine probably most active in the semiquinone form[224]. It is an efficient substrate for DT diaphorase[225] and has no greater activity against hypoxic than aerobic cells in the 16/C tumour[111]. A new aziridinylindoloquinone, EO9 (**30**), synthesized by Oostveen and Speckamp[226], has hypoxic selectivity much superior to MMC against KHT cells in culture (ratio 33 versus 2 respectively) and shows excellent hypoxia-selective toxicity *in vivo*[55] despite a very short halflife (about 2 min) in mice[227] and very efficient aerobic activation by rat and human DT diaphorases[228]. Clinical evaluation of EO9 under the auspices of EORTC is expected.

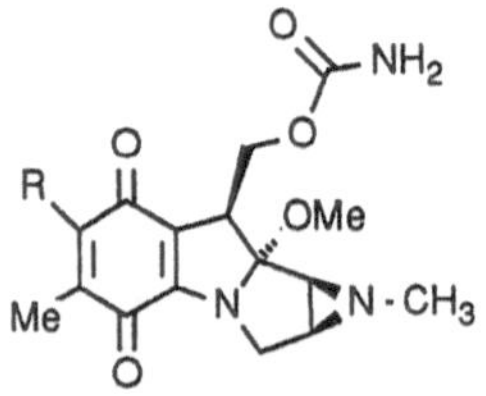

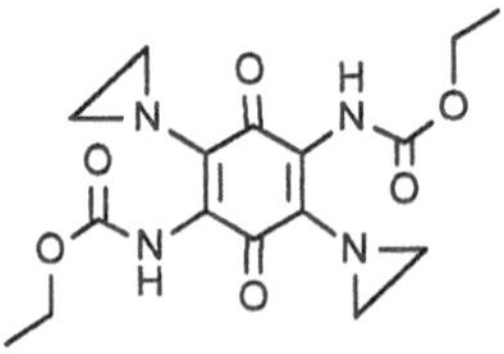

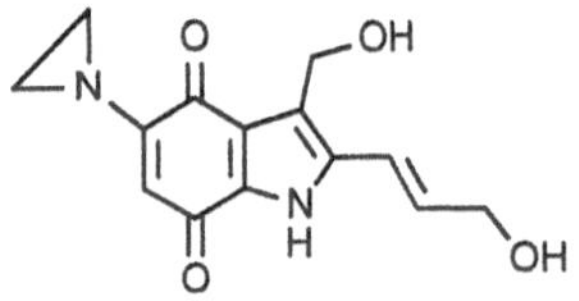

28a : R = NH$_2$: porfiromycin

28b : R = 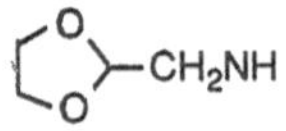 (BMY-42355) structure —CH$_2$NH

29 : diaziquone

30 : EO9

AROMATIC N-OXIDES

In the course of studies of non-nitro hypoxic cell radiosensitizers, the benzo-triazine di-N-oxide SR 4233 (**31**) was found to be a highly selective HSC with cytotoxicity 20–200-fold greater under hypoxic than under aerobic conditions in culture[229]. This compound also enhances killing by X-rays in SCCVII tumours[229], probably mainly through its action as an HSC[51], and is thus an important new lead compound. SR 4233 has been shown to be a bioreductive agent, with oxygen-inhibited reduction to the fluorescent triazine-1-oxide, SR 4317 (**33**, Scheme VII), as the major metabolite in hypoxic cells[230]. It thus represents the paradigm for HSC based on a third oxygen-inhibitable biotransformation, the reduction of an N-oxide.

Laderoute *et al.*[231] demonstrated the 1-electron reduction product to be an oxidizing radical, probably the carbon-centred radical **32**, capable of generating DNA breaks by hydrogen abstraction. This model is consistent with the unusual

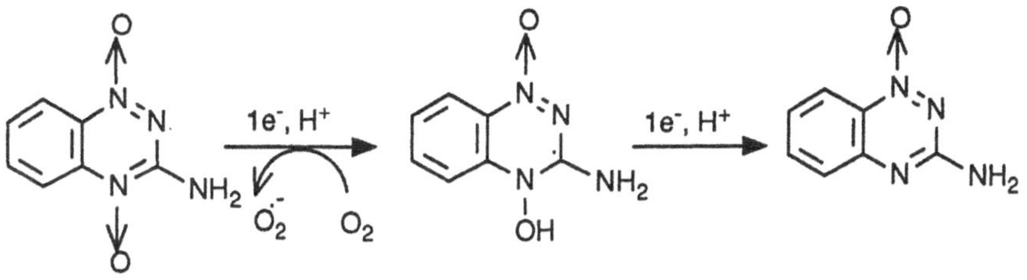

31 : SR 4233   32   33 : SR 4137

Scheme VII

stoichiometry of the radiolytic reduction of SR 4233 in formate (approximately 0.5 electrons per molecule of SR 4233 consumed)[232] if **32** can oxidize formate to the reducing CO_2 radical to provide a reducing chain reaction. The rate of oxidation of the 1-electron reduction product by oxygen was similar to that for the 2- and 5-nitroimidazoles, suggesting that the hypoxic selective of SR 4233 is due to removal of the oxidizing radical by this route in oxygenated cells. Baker *et al.*[230] provided further support for this model by showing that the two- and four-electron reduction products were non-toxic, and providing evidence for an oxygen-sensitive oxidizing radical in cells. Cytochrome P450[233] and NADPH:cytochrome P450 reductase[234] have been variously proposed as the major enzyme responsible for SR 4233 reduction.

The cytotoxicity of SR 4233 appears to depend on induction of double-strand DNA breaks[235], but it is not clear how these arise with such efficiency[236] from the action of a monofunctional radical. One possibility is that a relatively immobile reductase with a high turnover number, situated near the DNA, could generate a cluster of oxidizing radicals and thereby form lesions of a type similar to the multiply damaged sites responsible for the cytotoxicity of ionizing radiation.

The very high selectivity of SR 4233 for hypoxic cells, coupled with its demonstrated efficacy against murine tumours in combination with fractionated irradiation[51], make it a key bioreductive agent. The outcome of a recently commenced clinical trial (M. J. Brown, personal communication) will be awaited with great interest.

ALIPHATIC N-OXIDES

A variety of enzyme systems are known to catalyse the reduction of aliphatic (tertiary) amine N-oxides and to be inhibited by oxygen, although the substrate specificities of these enzyme systems are unclear. Liver cytochrome P450s can reduce[237] imipramine N-oxide (**34**) and other tertiary amine N-oxides with 50% inhibition at $4 \mu mol/L$ O_2. NADPH-cytochrome P450 reductase, although an important nitroreductase, fails to reduce indicine N-oxide[238] and does not appear to have been investigated in relation to other aliphatic N-oxides. Aldehyde oxidase is well characterized as an oxygen-sensitive N-oxide reductase[239]. Rat liver contains a cytosolic N-oxide reductase with characteristics similar to those of horseradish peroxidase[240]. Fe(II) and enzymatically reduced cytochrome c can both reduce indicine N-oxide[238,240]. The latter is also reduced by denatured, but not by native, haemoglobin, with approximately 50% inhibition by oxygen[238]. In contrast, imipramine N-oxide has been reported to be reduced rapidly by native haemoglobin[241] with formation of methaemoglobin[242]. Extensive reduction of Ro 31-0313 (**35**), the piperidinyl-N-oxide metabolite of pimonidazole, has been observed in mice and in isolated whole blood[243] although it is not known whether this reduction is oxygen sensitive or what enzyme systems are involved.

34 : imipramine N-oxide   **35** : Ro 31-0313

While the reduction of aliphatic N-oxides is facile, there is no evidence for reactive or toxic intermediates analogous to those generated during reduction of nitro compounds, quinones, or aromatic N-oxides. In the absence of any mechanism leading to increased toxicity on reduction, aliphatic N-oxides would not, therefore, be expected to give rise to hypoxia-selective cytotoxicity. There is thus a need to link reduction of the N-oxide to the enhancement of cytotoxic potency. Two examples in the recent literature point to interesting possibilities.

(1) Use of N-oxide reduction to activate a nitrogen mustard. White *et al.*[244] have shown that the N-oxide of mechlorethamine, nitromin (**36**), is reduced selectively under hypoxic conditions to form the more reactive des-N-oxide nitrogen mustard. Nitromin is selectively toxic in Walker cell cultures under hypoxic conditions, but with a modest selectivity of only about 4-fold.

36 : nitromin   **37** : nitracrine N-oxide

(2) Use of N-oxide reduction to enhance binding affinity of a DNA intercalator. Wilson *et al.*[245] showed that the aliphatic N-oxide of nitracrine, 1-NC-N-oxide (37), is a weaker DNA binder than nitracrine itself, but is reduced to nitracrine in AA8 cells by a pathway which is strongly inhibited by oxygen. The hypoxic cytotoxicity of both compounds is similar, but the N-oxide has dramatically lower aerobic toxicity, suggesting that the more weakly DNA-binding N-oxide is, in effect, a less toxic prodrug of nitracrine. 1-NC-N-oxide has a hypoxic differential of about 1000-fold in this system, making it the most selective HSC reported to date. Its remarkable selectivity was suggested[245] to reflect a requirement for oxygen-inhibitable reduction at two independent centres (the N-oxide and nitro groups), the requirement for bis-bioreduction imposing exquisite oxygen sensitivity.

TRANSITION METALS

Although metals are important redox centres in biological systems, little work has been done to explore their possible application in the context of HSC. Pt(II) complexes with nitroimidazoles are known to be selectively toxic to hypoxic cells[246], but the active redox centre is the nitroaromatic ligand rather than the metal itself. Ware *et al.*[122,247] suggested that co-ordination of alkylating agents, such as aziridine and nitrogen mustards, to Co(III) through the nitrogen lone pair would provide complexes in which the alkylating moiety is deactivated, but which could release reactive alkylating agents on reduction to Co(II) (Scheme VIII).

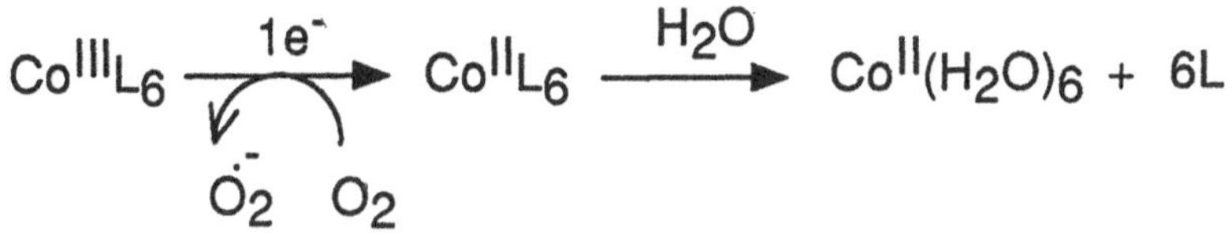

$$Co^{III}L_6 \xrightarrow{1e^-} Co^{II}L_6 \xrightarrow{H_2O} Co^{II}(H_2O)_6 + 6L$$
$$\dot{O}_2^- \quad O_2$$

Scheme VIII

Reduction of Co(III) complexes with monodentate alkylating agents appears not to be inhibited by oxygen[247,248], presumably because rapid loss of ligands from the very labile Co(II) complex[249] precludes reoxidation by oxygen. However, Co(III) complexes with bidentate nitrogen mustards, such as SN 24771 (38), are expected to provide more stable Co(II) complexes[250].

SN 24771 is approximately 5-fold more toxic under hypoxic than under aerobic conditions[122] and provides a first example of a bioreductive agent whose toxicity is triggered by reduction of a metal centre. Thus the reversible Co(III)/Co(II) redox system may be exploitable for the release of cytotoxins under hypoxic conditions.

38 : SN 24771

THE PATH AHEAD: PROBLEMS AND CHALLENGES FOR THE FURTHER DEVELOPMENT OF BIOREDUCTIVE AGENTS

Four bioreductive agents (SR 4233, RB 6145, porfiromycin and EO9) representing three chemical classes have recently entered clinical trial or are expected to do so in the near future. These compounds represent the first generation of agents to be developed as HSCs, although predecessor compounds (such as misonidazole and MMC), not optimized for HSC activity, have been evaluated clinically. While these compounds should be adequate to determine whether there is a role for bioreductive agents in radiotherapy and chemo-therapy, they are unlikely to exploit fully the potential of this class of agent. Some of the challenges for further development of bioreductive drugs are addressed here.

Tissue distribution of reductases

The therapeutic utility of bioreductive drugs depends on higher rates of activation in hypoxic tumour microenvironments than in normal tissues. A high activity of reductases in some normal tissues relative to tumours could compromise this selectivity by countering the advantage offered by oxygenation differences. Rates of reduction of the 2-nitroimidazole benznidazole are much higher in liver that in KHT or RIF-1 tumours in mice, and the V_{max} for anaerobic NADPH-dependent reduction in liver homogenates is 6–10-fold higher than for KHT tumour homogenates[129]. Reductive activation of nitracrine is much faster in liver, kidney, spleen and lung than in Lewis lung tumours[188], and rates of SR 4233 reduction are much higher in hepatocytes than in tumour cells[251].

Even in tumours derived from tissues with a high capacity for xenobiotic metabolism, there is evidence that levels of reductive enzymes are often lower than in the tissue of origin. For example, the activity of xanthine dehydrogenase, a known nitroreductase[134], is 5–6-fold lower in the moderately well-differ-entiated rat hepatocellular carcinoma, HC-252, than in normal liver[252]. Amounts of this enzyme, determined by immunoprecipitation, were only 33 and 2% of that in normal rat liver for hepatomas 20 and 3924A respectively[253]. There is an

114

urgent need for information on activities of reductive enzymes in human tumours.

The problem of expression of nitroreductases extends to the use of continuously passaged tumour cell lines as *in vitro* models for drug development. It is well known that culture of hepatocytes leads to a dramatic decrease in cytochrome P450[254–256], and a less-marked but substantial decrease in cytochrome P450 reductase has also been reported[254,255]. It is not yet clear whether the capacity of tumour cells for reductive bioactivation shows similar marked alterations on adaptation to culture, although it might be expected that enzyme loss due to dedifferentiation and proliferation in culture would be less pronounced with neoplastic cells. It should be of continuing concern that bioreductive drug discovery relies largely on (rodent) tumour cell lines which may not reflect the bioreductive potential of tumours in patients.

Bioactivation under aerobic conditions and K-curve matching

High levels of reductase expression in normal tissue would not be of concern if activation of bioreductive agents were fully inhibited at physiological oxygen concentrations (i.e. by 5% oxygen at most[257]). Unfortunately, this condition does not appear to be met by most available bioreductive drugs. Costa et al.[251] have shown that SR 4233 is rapidly metabolized by rat hepatocytes at 4% oxygen, and is an order of magnitude more toxic to these cells at 4% than at 20% oxygen. The ratios of 2–20-fold between 20% oxygen and anoxia shown by most bioreductive agents are probably inadequate. The need for large differentials is made even more pressing by other factors in tumours which may compromise selectivity. This problem is illustrated by a study of cytotoxicity of RSU 1069 against 9L rat tumours[258] showing a differential of 50-fold in 9L cell cultures between 0 and 2% O_2 but a differential *in vivo* between clamped (fully anoxic) and unclamped (about 2% O_2) tumours of only 5-fold. The authors concluded that factors other than oxygen, such as pH, nutrients and thiol content, modify the effective differential.

As well as the prevention of bioactivation of drugs under normal conditions of oxygen tension, it is important to consider the relationship between 'K-curves' (oxygen dependence of cell killing) for HSCs and radiation. The half value ('K-value') for the latter is approximately 0.5% O_2, while for mitomycin C[212], diaziquone[224] and misonidazole[259] the K-value is in the order of 0.01% O_2. Thus, a population of cells in tumours at oxygen tensions intermediate between the K-value of the HSC and radiation may be spared during their combined use[260]. Ideally then, the K-value should be at least as high as that for radiation, with as large a differential as possible between 0 and 1–5 % O_2.

There is a need to understand in more detail the determinants of the oxic/hypoxic differential of existing agents so that more selective HSCs can be designed. In some cases, large differences are seen within a congeneric series, as for the 5-nitroquinolines where ratios range from 1 to 60-fold (0 vs 20% O_2)[192,193] for reasons that are not yet understood. In general terms, at least two phenomena are known to limit hypoxic selectivity in certain situations.

Oxygen-insensitive reductases

As noted above, aerobic reductive activation of quinoidal HSCs can proceed by two-electron reduction catalysed by DT diaphorase, which bypasses the oxygen-sensitive intermediate formed during one-electron reduction. A directly analogous problem can occur with nitro(hetero)arenes. The existence of oxygen-insensitive two-electron nitroreductases in bacteria ('type I nitroreductases') is well known[261], but several mammalian reductases can also act as oxygen-insensitive nitroreductases. DT diaphorase itself is the best known, catalysing oxygen-insensitive reduction of CB 1954[138], 4-nitroquinoline N-oxide[139] and 1,6-dinitropyrene[140]. It may not always, however, act as an obligate two-electron donor since it also catalyses *cis-trans* isomerization of nitrofuran derivatives[262], a reaction which is considered to be mediated via the nitro radical anion[262].

Several other mammalian nitroreductases are also inefficiently inhibited by oxygen although, again, it is not clear to what extent this reflects obligate two-electron reduction. Rat liver xanthine dehydrogenase can reduce the 5-nitro-furan, nitrofurazone, and is less sensitive to inhibition by oxygen than is xanthine oxidase from the same source[134]. The nitroreductase activity of aldehyde oxidase appears to be less sensitive to oxygen that either xanthine oxidase or the microsomal systems[130]. It has been suggested that oxygen may compete more efficiently with nitro compounds as an electron acceptor for the internal electron transport chain of xanthine oxidase than aldehyde oxidase[130]. Differences in oxygen competition at the substrate level are an interesting possible reason for differences in oxygen sensitivity of nitroreduction which warrant further investigation.

Given these differences in sensitivity to oxygen, it is obviously of key importance to design HSCs which will not be substrates for oxygen-insensitive reductases. An interesting example is provided by SN 23862 (**22**), an analogue of CB 1954 which has lost the sensitivity of the latter to reduction by the Walker adenocarcinoma DT diaphorase[199]. SN 23862 has a hypoxic selectivity of 70-fold against UV4 cells, compared with 3–4-fold for CB 1954 in the same system[199]. SN 23862 also shows hypoxic selectivity much superior to that of CB 1954 in the Walker, FME and EMT6 cell lines (unpublished results). It is likely that the superiority of the mustard analogue of CB 1954 is a consequence of its insensitivity to DT diaphorases.

Kinetic (oxygen competition) problems

Even under circumstances where reductive activation is exclusively by a one-electron mechanism, sensitivity to oxygen can be compromised by inefficient back-oxidation of the one-electron adduct. An interesting example is provided by the much greater sensitivity to oxygen of metronidazole[48] than misonidazole[259]. Rauth *et al.*[263] provided an elegant explanation for this by demonstrating a parallel difference in oxygen sensitivity of radiolytic reduction of metronidazole and 2-nitroimidazoles, and showing that this could be accounted for kinetically by a difference in the stability of 2- and 5-nitroimidazole radical anions. Wardman[144] subsequently confirmed this hypothesis through a pulse radiolysis study, demonstrating a first-order decay of 2-nitroimidazole radicals to unknown products. This decay was sufficiently rapid for its rate to be comparable to that for back-oxidation at approximately $2 \mu mol/L$ O_2, while removal of 5-nitroimidazoles was only by bimolecular disproportionation at a rate which would equal that due to re-oxidation at about $5 nmol/L$ O_2. The difference in radical stability thus appears to account for the relative oxygen insensitivity of 2-nitroimidazole cytotoxicity. The only unsatisfactory aspect of this explanation is that it requires the observed first-order decay to lead to cytotoxic products, and there is currently no indication as to what these could be. Once the nature of such first-order radical decay processes is understood more fully, it may be possible to exercise some control over radical stability, and K-values, at the level of drug design.

Enhancing hypoxic selectivity: bis-bioreductive agents

An interesting strategy for enhancing hypoxic selectivity, when this is limited by either of the above two mechanisms, is to design agents with two reducible centres ($I_{ox}II_{ox}$) which require two independent oxygen-sensitive biotransformations to achieve full activation. Thus, in Scheme IX, if each reduction is moderately inhibited by oxygen, the overall formation of the bis-reduced species ($I_{red}II_{red}$) should be much more sensitively inhibited.

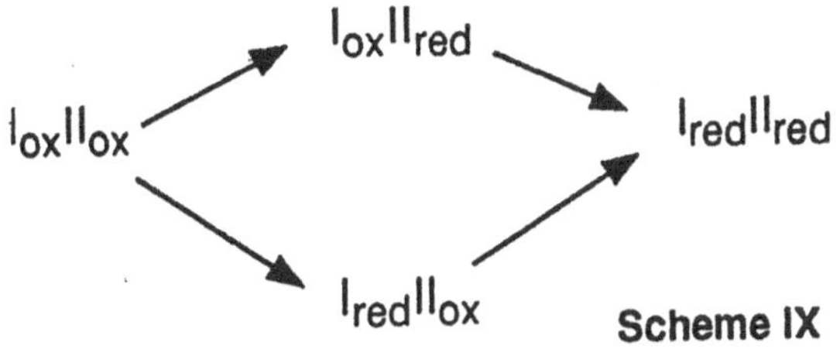

Scheme IX

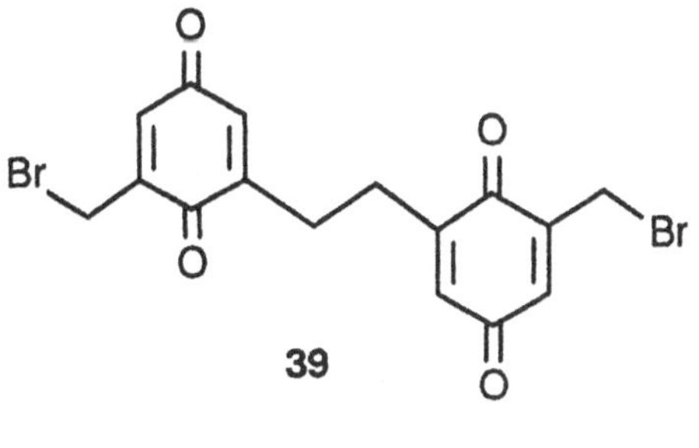

39

Wilson et al.[245] have suggested that reduction of nitracrine N-oxide (**37**) can fulfil these criteria (see above), with the reduction of the N-oxide enhancing toxicity through the resultant increase in DNA binding, and the reduction of the nitro group forming a cytotoxic reactive product. The remarkable hypoxic selectivity of this compound (approximately 1000-fold) suggests that other bis-bioreductive agents should be investigated. Earlier, Witiak et al.[264] linked two quinones to form bis-bioreductive alkylating agents (e.g. **39**) capable of quinone methide formation. Structure **39** was shown to have activity against the D98/HR1 xenograft, but his compound appears not to have been tested for selective toxicity under hypoxia.

Diffusible cytotoxins from bioreductive agents

The problem of K-curve matching noted above will make it difficult to develop bioreductive agents which complement exactly the deficiencies of radiation or other treatment modalities. An obvious solution is to seek drugs which will, on reduction in hypoxic cells, release diffusible cytotoxins capable of killing surrounding cells at higher oxygen tensions. The other major advantage of this approach, as noted above, is that it offers possibilities for exploiting tumour hypoxia so that tumour cell killing by bioreductive agents is not restricted to the hypoxic fraction.

Most classes of bioreductive drugs currently under consideration are probably not well suited to meeting this objective since their active cytotoxic species are transient radicals or highly reactive electrophiles, such as nitrenium or carbonium ions. Diffusion ranges of $100-200\,\mu m$ in a tumour will require compounds with halflives of at least 1 minute (assuming a diffusion coefficient in tissue of the order of $10^{-6}-10^{-5}cm^2s^{-1}$). Halflives considerably longer than this may be appropriate since a dilution on release into the systemic circulation would tend to protect normal tissues. There is a need to devise activation schemes which will provide well-defined active species to enable specific design of the latter to optimize drug diffusion.

Aliphatic or activated aromatic nitrogen mustards have properties which make them appropriate for consideration as the diffusible species. They are potent cytotoxins with reactivities in an appropriate range, and, as a bonus, often have antitumour activity in their own right. Several current approaches to HSC development (see compounds **22, 25, 36** and **38**) are based on the production of diffusible activated nitrogen mustards. As these new compounds enter evaluation against murine tumours, it will be of great interest to test whether killing of normally oxygenated cells can result from metabolic activation in hypoxic microenvironments.

The approach suggested here is an extension of an emerging concept in cancer treatment in which a targeting system is used to provide tumour selectivity, but with a coupled effector which is less well localized. The great advantage of such systems is that the problems presented by intratumour heterogeneity can be minimized. Not all tumour cells need express the characteristic (antigen, hypoxia, low pH etc.) employed by the targeting system if a long-range effector can produce a 'bystander effect' in surrounding cells. Radiolabelled anti-bodies[265], antibody-directed enzyme-prodrug therapy (ADEPT)[266] and hyper-thermic release of liposome-encapsulated drugs[267] all represent examples of this strategy. A bystander effect in the present context would also help to guard against drug resistance through mutations resulting in loss of the bioactivation pathway[220].

CONCLUSIONS

The first hypoxia-selective cytotoxins, represented by misonidazole and mitomycin C, lacked respectively the potency and selectivity required to be effective in this role *in vivo*. The second-generation agents, represented by SR 4233, RB 6145, porfiromycin and EO9, have greater activity against hypoxic cells in mouse tumours. It is reasonable to expect that these drugs will, at the very least, establish whether bioreductive drugs have a future in chemotherapy and/or radiotherapy. However, it is unlikely that the available compounds will be ideal, and probably much can and will be done to develop superior bioreductive drugs. In particular, there are exciting possibilities for rational design of new drugs capable not only of eliminating treatment-refractory hypoxic cells but of exploiting this or other microenvironmental features as a basis for tumour selectivity.

There are several factors which suggest that the recent growth in interest in bioreductive drug development is likely to continue for some time:

(1) The proposed basis of selectivity is well grounded in tumour biology, and can be readily modelled in tissue culture. The latter feature is a boon for systematic drug development, and makes bioreductive drugs quite unusual. For most classes of anticancer agents, tissue culture methods are helpful in studying mechanisms of cytotoxicity but contribute little to an understanding of selectivity, which is the real and often-neglected issue. (The culture-based drug discovery experiment currently being undertaken by the National Cancer Institute, USA, is an ambitious and interesting attempt to use differences between tumour cell types as a surrogate for true tumour selectivity[268].)

(2) The mechanism of tumour selectivity (oxygen-inhibited bioactivation) is well understood, at least in principle, at the biochemical/chemical level and offers great scope to the inventive medicinal chemist.

(3) The conditions which make tumours sensitive to bioreductive agents (lack of oxygen, presence of activating enzymes) can be assessed, probably non-invasively, so the potential exists for developing assays which will help predict individual tumour sensitivity. Bioreductive agents are, again, unusual among prodrugs in that bioactivation occurs locally in the tumour, making this approach uniquely advantageous.

(4) Bioreductive agents, if appropriately designed, might provide diffusible cytotoxic products. As such, they have the potential to take their place among an emerging group of novel techniques (localized targeting systems with delocalized effectors) which have potential for overcoming the fundamentally important problem of intratumour heterogeneity.

No bioreductive agent under clinical or advanced preclinical evaluation can yet claim a genuinely *de novo* rational design, but, with well-defined mechanisms for cytotoxicity and selectivity, this field is poised for such approaches. Several mechanism-based bioreductive drug development programmes are now in evidence, and prospects for the development of drugs able to exploit tumour hypoxia fully are good.

Acknowledgements

The author wishes to thank Dr Stephen Cliffe, Dr Brian D. Palmer, Prof. William A. Denny and Dr Richard P. Hill for helpful discussions, and Ms Lynda Robb for assistance with preparation of the manuscript. This work was undertaken with support from the Health Research Council of New Zealand and The National Cancer Institute, USA.

References

1. Woglom, W. H. (1947). In Moulton, F. R. (ed) *General Review of Cancer Therapy*, pp. 1–10. (Washington D.C.: American Association for the Advancement of Science)
2. Moolten, F. L. (1990). Mosaicism induced by gene insertion as a means of improving chemotherapeutic selectivity. *Immunology*, **10**, 203–233
3. Clarkson, B. (1991). Retinoic acid in acute promyelocytic leukemia: The promise and the paradox. *Cancer Cells*, **3**, 211–220
4. Coleman, C. N. (1988). Hypoxia in tumors: a paradigm for the approach to biochemical and physiological heterogeneity. *J. Natl. Cancer Inst.*, **80**, 310–317
5. Tannock, I. F. and Rotin, D. (1989). Acid pH in tumors and its potential for therapeutic exploitation. *Cancer Res.*, **49**, 4373–4384
6. Kennedy, K. A., Teicher, B. A., Rockwell, S. and Sartorelli, A. C. (1980). The hypoxic tumor cell: a target for selective cancer chemotherapy. *Biochem. Pharmacol.*, **26**, 1–8
7. Adams, G. E. and Stratford, I. J. (1986). Hypoxia-mediated nitroheterocyclic drugs in the radio- and chemotherapy of cancer. An overview. *Biochem. Pharmacol.*, **35**, 71–76
8. Sartorelli, A. C. (1988). Therapeutic attack of hypoxic cells of solid tumors: Presidential address. *Cancer Res.*, **48**, 775–778
9. Jenkins, T. C. (1990). Hypoxia-selective agents: radiosensitizers and cytotoxins. In Wilman, D. E. V. (ed.) *Chemistry of Antitumour Agents*, pp. 342–269. (Glasgow and London: Blackie)
10. Kirkpatrick, D. L. (1989). The development of hypoxic tumor cell cytotoxic agents. *Pharmac. Ther.*, **40**, 383–399
11. Adams, G. E., Stratford, I. J., Bremner, J. C. M., Cole, S., Edwards, H. S. and Fielden, E. M. (1991). Nitroheterocyclic compounds as radiation sensitizers and bioreductive drugs. *Radiother. Oncol.*, (Suppl. 20), 85–91
12. Petry, E. (1923). Zur Kenntnis der Bedingungen der biologischen Wirkung der Röntgenstrahlen. *Biochem. Zeitschr.*, **135**, 353
13. Powers, W. E and Tolmach, L. J. (1963). A multicomponent X-ray survival curve for mouse lymphosarcoma cells irradiated *in vivo*. *Nature (London)*, **197**, 710–711
14. Guichard, M., Courdi, A. and Malaise, E. P. (1980). Experimental data on the radiobiology of solid tumors. *J. Eur. Radiother.*, **1**, 171–191
15. Moulder, J. E. and Rockwell, S. (1984). Hypoxic fractions of solid tumours: experimental techniques, methods of analysis and a survey of existing data. *Int. J. Radiat. Oncol. Biol. Phys.*, **10**, 695–712
16. Rockwell, S. and Moulder, J. E. (1990). Hypoxic fractions of human tumors xenografted into mice. A review. *Int. J. Radiat. Oncol. Biol. Phys.*, **19**, 197–202
17. Thomlinson, R. H. and Gray, L. H. (1955). The histological structure of some human lung cancers and the possible implications for radiotherapy. *Br. J. Cancer*, **9**, 539–549
18. Chaplin, D. J., Durand, R. E. and Olive, P. L. (1986). Acute hypoxia in tumors: implications for modifiers of radiation effects. *Int. J. Radiat. Oncol. Biol. Phys.*, **12**, 1279–1282
19. Chaplin, D. J., Olive, P. L. and Durand, R. E. (1987). Intermittent blood flow in a murine tumor: Radiobiological effects. *Cancer Res.*, **47**, 597–601
20. Chapman, J. D., Franko, A. J. and Sharplin, J. (1981). A marker for hypoxic cells in tumours with potential clinical applicability. *Br. J. Cancer*, **43**, 546–550
21. Raleigh, J. A., Miler, G. G., Franko, A. J., Koch, C. J., Fuciarelli, A. F. and Kelly, D. A. (1987). Fluorescence immunohistochemical detection of hypoxic cells in spheroids and tumours. *Br. J. Cancer*, **56**, 395–396

22. Hodgkiss, R. J., Jones, G., Long, A., Parrick, J., Smith, K. A., Stratford, M. R. L. and Wilson, G. D. (1991). Flow cytometric evaluation of hypoxic cells in solid experimental tumours using fluorescence immunodetection. *Br. J. Cancer*, **63**, 119–125

23. Zeman, E. M., Massenburg, G. S., Cline, J. M., Thrall, D. E. and Raleigh, J. A. (1991). Proliferative and oxygenation status in spontaneous canine tumors: an immunocytochemical approach. In Chapman, J. D., Dewey, W. C. and Whitmore, G. F. (eds.) *Radiation Research, a Twentieth-Century Perspective*, Vol 1, p. 251. (Toronto: Academic Press)(abstract)

24. Peters W., Teixeira, M., Intaglietta, M. and Gross, J. F. (1980). Microcirculatory studies in rat mammary carcinoma. I. Transparent chamber method, development of microvasculature, and pressures in tumor vessels. *J. Natl. Cancer. Inst.*, **65**, 631–642

25. Brown, J. M. (1979). Evidence for acute hypoxic cells in mouse tumours and a possible mechanism of reoxygenation. *Br. J. Radio.*, **52**, 650–656

26. Olive, P. L., Chaplin, D. J. and Durand, R. E. (1985). Pharmacokinetics, binding and distribution of Hoechst 33342 in spheroids and murine tumours. *Br. J. Cancer*, **52**, 739–746

27. Minchinton, A. I., Durand, R. E. and Chaplin, D. J. (1990). Intermittent blood flow in the KHT sarcoma – flow cytometry studies using Hoechst 33342. *Br. J. Cancer*, **62**, 195–200

28. Trotter, M. J., Chaplin, D. J. and Olive, P. L. (1989). Use of a carbocyanine dye as a marker of functional vasculature in murine tumours. *Br. J. Cancer*, **59**, 706–709

29. Trotter, M. J., Chaplin, D. J., Durand, R. E. and Olive, P. L. (1989). The use of fluorescent probes to identify regions of transient perfusion in murine tumors. *Int. J. Radiat. Oncol. Biol. Phys.*, **16**, 931–934

30. Boucher, Y., Baxter, L. T. and Jain, R. K. (1990). Interstitial pressure gradients in tissue-isolated and subcutaneous tumor: implications for therapy. *Cancer Res.*, **50**, 4478–4484

31. Brown, J. M. and Koong, A. (1991). Therapeutic advantage of hypoxic cells in tumors: A theoretical study. *J. Natl. Cancer Inst.*, **83**, 178–185

32. Vaupel, P., Kallinowski, F. and Okunieff, P. (1989). Blood flow, oxygen and nutrient supply, and metabolic microenvironment of human tumors: a review. *Cancer Res.*, **49**, 6449–6465

33. Chapman, J. D. (1991). Measurement of tumor hypoxia by invasive and non-invasive procedures: a review of recent clinical studies. *Radiother. Oncol.*, (Suppl. 20), 13–19

34. Henk, J. M., Kunkler, P. B. and Smith, C. W. (1977). Radiotherapy and hyperbaric oxygen in head and neck cancer. *Lancet*, 101–103

35. Overgaard, J., Hansen, H. S., Andersen, A. P., Hjelm-Hansen, M., Jorgensen, K., Sandberg, E., Bertelsen, A., Hammer, R. and Petersen, M. (1989). Misonidazole combined with split course radiotherapy in treatment of invasive carcinoma of larynx and pharynx: report from the DAHANCA 2 study. *Int. J. Radiat. Oncol. Biol. Phys.*, **16**, 1065–1068

36. Bush, R. S., Jenkin, R. D. T., Allt, W. E. C., Beale, F. A., Bean, H., Dembo, A. J. and Pringle, J. F. (1978). Definitive evidence for hypoxic cells influencing cure in cancer therapy. *Br. J. Cancer*, **37** (Suppl. III), 302–306

37. Gatenby, R. A., Kessler, H. B., Rosenblum, J. S., Coia, L. R., Moldofsky, P. J., Hartz, W. H. and Brodler, G. J. (1988). Oxygen distribution in squamous cell carcinoma metastases and its relationship to outcome of radiotherapy. *Int. J. Radiat. Oncol. Biol. Phys.*, **14**, 831–838

38. Wardman, P. (1977). The use of nitroaromatic compounds as hypoxic cell radiosensitizers. *Curr. Top. Radiat. Res. Q.*, **11**, 347–398

39. Wardman, P. (1987). The mechanism of radiosensitization by electron-affinic compounds. *Radiat. Phys. Chem.*, **30**, 423–432

40. Kappen, L. S., Lee, R. R., Yang, C. and Goldberg, I. H. (1989). Oxygen transfer from a nitro group of a nitroaromatic radiosensitizer to a DNA sugar damage product. *Biochemistry*, **28**, 4540–4542

41. Phillips, T. C., Wassermann, T. H., Johnson, R. J., Levin, V. A. and Van Raalte, G. (1981). Final report on the United States Phase I Clinical Trial of the hypoxic cell radiosensitizer, misonidazole (Ro 07-0582, NSC #261037). *Cancer*, **48**, 1697–1704

42. Brown, J. M. (1989). Keynote address: hypoxic cell sensitizers: where next? *Int. J. Radiat. Oncol. Biol. Phys.*, **16**, 987–993

43. Williams, M. V., Denekamp, J., Minchinton, A. I. and Stratford, M. R. L. (1982). *In vivo* assessment of basic 2-nitroimidazole radiosensitizers. *Br. J. Cancer*, **46**, 127–137

44. Brown, J. M. (1981). Radiosensitizers: rationale and potential. *Cancer Treat. Rep.*, **65** (Suppl. 2), 95–102

45. Wong, T. W., Whitmore, G. F. and Gulyas, S. (1978). Studies on the toxicity and radio-sensitizing ability of misonidazole under conditions of prolonged incubation. *Radiat. Res.*, **75**, 541–555

46. Sutherland, R. M. (1974). Selective chemotherapy of noncycling cells in an *in vitro* tumor model. *Cancer Res.*, **34**, 3501–3503

47. Hall, E. J. and Roizin-Towle, L. A. (1975). Hypoxic cell radiosensitizers: radiobiological studies at the cellular level. *Radiology*, **117**, 453–457

48. Mohindra, J. K. and Rauth, A. M. (1976). Increased killing by metronidazole and nitrofurazone of hypoxic compared to aerobic mammalian cells. *Cancer Res.*, **26**, 930–936

49. Moore, B. A., Palcic, B. and Skarsgard, L. D. (1976). Radiosensitizing and toxic effects of the 2-nitroimidazole Ro-07-0582 in hypoxic mammalian cells. *Radiat. Res.*, **67**, 459–473

50. Sridhar, R., Koch, C. and Sutherland, R. M. (1976). Cytotoxicity of two nitroimidazole radiosensitizers in an *in vitro* tumor model. *Int. J. Radiat. Oncol. Biol. Phys.*, **1**, 1133–1137

51. Brown, J. M. and Lemmon, M. J. (1990). Potentiation by the hypoxic cytotoxin SR4233 of cell killing produced by fractionated irradiation of mouse tumors. *Cancer Res.*, **50**, 7745–7749

52. Hill, R. P. (1986). Sensitizers and radiation dose fractionation: results and interpretations. *Int. J. Radiat. Oncol. Biol. Phys.*, **12**, 1049–1054

53. Murray, J. C. and Randhawa, V. S. (1988). Misonidazole reduces blood flow in two experimental tumours. *Br. J. Cancer*, **58**, 128–132

54. Dische, S. (1992). The clinical trial of hypoxic cell radiosensitizers. In Chapman, J. D., Dewey, W. C. and Whitmore, G. F. (eds.) *Radiation Research, a Twentieth-Century Perspective*, Vol 2. (Toronto: Academic Press)

55. Adams, G. E. (1992). Mechanistic studies of different classes of bioreductive drugs: *in vitro* and *in vivo*. In Chapman, J. D., Dewey, W. C. and Whitmore, G. F. (eds) *Radiation Research, a Twentieth-Century Perspective*, Vol. 2. (Toronto: Academic Press)

56. Brown, J. M. (1977). Cytotoxic effects of the hypoxic cell radiosensitizer Ro 7-0582 to tumor cells *in vivo*. *Radiat. Res.*, **72**, 469–486

57. Davies, B. M. A. and Watling, D. C. (1978). An *in vivo* investigation of the radiosensitization of metastases by nitroimidazoles. *Int. J. Radiat. Oncol. Biol. Phys.*, **4**, 809–819

58. Siemann, D. W. and Kochanski, K. (1981). Combinations of radiation and misonidazole in a murine lung tumor model. *Radiat. Res.*, **86**, 387–397

59. Hall. E. J. (1991). Hypoxia revisited. *J. Natl. Cancer Inst.*, **83**, 156

60. Tannock, I. F. and Guttman, P. (1981). Response of Chinese hamster ovary cells to anticancer drugs under aerobic and hypoxic conditions. *Br. J. Cancer*, **43**, 245–248

61. Teicher, B. A., Lazo, J. S. and Sartorelli, A. C. (1981). Classification of antineoplastic agents by their selective toxicities towards oxygenated and hypoxic tumor cells. *Cancer Res.*, **41**, 73–81

62. Kappen, L. S. and Goldberg, I. H. (1984). Nitroaromatic radiation sensitizers substitute for oxygen in neocarzinostatin induced DNA damage. *Proc. Natl. Acad. Sci. USA*, **81**, 3312–3316

63. Lown, J. W. and Kim, S.-K.(1977). The mechanism of bleomycin-induced cleavage of DNA. *Biochem. Biophys. Res. Commun.*, **77**, 1150–1157

64. Teicher, B. A., Lazo, J. S., Merrill, W. W., Filderman, A. E. and Rose, C. M. (1986). Effect of fluosol-DA/O_2 on the antitumor activity and pulmonary toxicity of bleomycin. *Cancer Chemother. Pharmacol.*, **18**, 213–218

65. Tannock, I. F. (1986). The relation between cell proliferation and the vascular system in a transplanted mouse mammary tumour. *Br. J. Cancer*, **22**, 258–273

66. Pallavicini, M. G., Lalande, M. E., Miller, R. G. and Hill, R. P. (1979). Cell cycle distribution of chronically hypoxic cells and determination of the clonogenic potential of cells accumulated in G_2 + M phases after irradiation of a solid tumor *in vivo*. *Cancer Res.*, **39**, 1891–1897

67. Olive, P. L. and Durand, R. E. (1989). Misonidazole binding in SCCVII tumors in relation to the tumor blood supply. *Int. J. Radiat. Oncol. Biol. Phys.*, **16**, 755–761

68. Koch, C. J., Kruuv, J., Frey, H. E. and Snyder, R. A. (1973). Plateau phase in growth induced by hypoxia. *Int. J. Rad. Biol.*, **23**, 67–74

69. Loffler, M. (1980). On the role of dihydro-orotate dehydrogenase in growth cessation of Ehrlich ascites tumor cells cultured under oxygen deficiency. *Eur. J. Biochem.*, **107**, 207–215

70. Shrieve, D. S., Deen, D. F. and Harris, J. W. (1983). Effects of extreme hypoxia on the growth and viability of EMT6/SF mouse tumor cells *in vitro*. *Cancer Res.*, **43**, 3521–3527

71. Spiro, I. J., Rice, G. C., Durand, R. E., Stickler, R. and Ling, C. C. (1984). Cell killing, radiosensitization and cell cycle redistribution induced by chronic hypoxia. *Int. J. Radiat. Oncol. Biol. Phys.*, **10**, 1275–1280

72. Amellem, O. and Pettersen, E. O. (1991). Cell inactivation and cell cycle inhibition as induced by extreme hypoxia: the possible role of cell cycle arrest as a protection against hypoxia-induced lethal damage. *Cell Prolif.*, **24**, 127–141

73. Sutherland, R. M. (1986). Importance of critical metabolites and cellular interactions in the biology of microregions of tumours. *Cancer*, **58**, 1668–1680

74. Tannock, I. (1978). Cell kinetics and chemotherapy: A critical review. *Cancer Treat. Rep.*, **62**, 1117-1133

75. Kerr, D. J. and Kaye, S. B. (1987). Aspects of cytotoxic drug penetration, with particular reference to anthracyclines. *Cancer Chemother. Pharmacol.*, **19**, 1–5

76. Durand R. E. (1989). Distribution and activity of antineoplastic drugs in a tumor model. *J. Natl. Cancer Inst.*, **81**, 146–152

77. Wilson, W. R. and Denny, W. A. (1992). DNA-binding nitroheterocycles as hypoxia-selective cytotoxins. In Chapman, J. D., Dewey, W. C. and Whitmore, G. F. (eds.) *Radiation Research, a Twentieth-Century Perspective*, Vol. 2. (Toronto: Academic Press)

78. Sutherland, R. M., Eddy, H. A., Bareham, B., Reich, K. and Vanantwerp, D. (1979). Resistance to Adriamycin in multicellular spheroids. *Int. J. Radiat. Oncol. Biol. Phys.*, **5**, 1225–1230

79. Wilson, W. R., Whitmore, G. F. and Hill, R. P. (1981). Activity of 4'-(9-acridinyl-amino)methanesulfon-*m*-anisidide against Chinese hamster cells in multicellular spheroids. *Cancer Res.*, **41**, 2817–2822

80. Ozols, R. F., Locker, G. Y., Doroshow, J. H., Grotzinger, K. R., Myers, C. E. and Young, R. C. (1979). Pharmacokinetics of Adriamycin and tissue penetration in murine ovarian cancer. *Cancer Res.*, **39**, 3209–3214

81. Tannock, I. (1982). Response of aerobic and hypoxic cells in a solid tumor to Adriamycin and cyclophosphamide and the interaction of the drugs with radiation. *Cancer Res.*, **42**, 4921–4926

82. Durand R. E. (1991). Keynote Address: The influence of microenvironmental factors on the activity of radiation and drugs. *Int. J. Radiat. Oncol. Biol. Phys.*, **20**, 245–258

83. Simpson-Herren, L., Noker, P. E. and Wagoner, S. D. (1988). Variability of tumor response to chemotherapy. II. Contributions of tumor heterogeneity. *Cancer Chemother. Pharmacol.*, **22**, 131–136

84. Denny, W. A. and Wilson, W. R. (1986). Considerations for the design of nitrophenyl mustards as agents with selective toxicity for hypoxic tumour cells. *J. Med. Chem.*, **29**, 879–887

85. Skovsgaard, T. (1977). Transport and binding of daunorubicin, Adriamycin and rubidazole in Ehrlich ascites tumour cells. *Biochem. Pharmacol.*, **26**, 215–222

86. Jahde, E., Glusenkamp, K.-H. and Rajewsky, M. F. (1990). Protection of cultured malignant cells from mitoxantrone cytotoxicity by low extracellular pH: A possible mechanism for chemoresistance *in vivo. Eur. J. Cancer*, **26**, 101–106

87. Kennedy, K. A., McGurl, J. M., Leondaridis, L. and Alabaster, O. (1985). pH dependence of mitomycin C induced cross linking activity in EMT6 tumor cells. *Cancer Res.*, **45**, 3541–3547

88. Keyes, S. R., Rockwell, S., Kennedy, K. A. and Sartorelli, A. C. (1991). Distribution of porfirömycin in EMT6 tumors and normal tissues of BALB/c mice. *J. Natl. Cancer Inst.*, **83**, 632–63789.   Rice, G. C., Hoy, C. and Schimke, P. T. (1986). Transient hypoxia enhances the frequency of dihydrofolate reductase gene amplification in Chinese hamster ovary cells. *Proc. Natl. Acad. Sci. USA*, **83**, 5978–5982

90. Young, S. D., Marshall, R. S. and Hill, R. P. (1988). Hypoxia induces DNA overreplication and enhances metastatic potential of murine tumor cells. *Proc. Natl. Acad. Sci. USA*, **85**, 9533–9537

91. Young, S. D. and Hill, R. P. (1990). Effects of reoxygenation on cells from hypoxic regions of solid tumors: Anticancer drug sensitivity and metastatic potential. *J. Natl. Cancer Inst.*, **82**, 371–380

92. Sciandra, J. J., Subjeck, J. R. and Hughes, C. S. (1984). Induction of glucose regulated proteins during anaerobic exposure and of heat shock proteins after reoxygenation. *Proc. Natl. Acad. Sci., USA*, **81**, 4843–4847

93. Shen, J., Hughes, C., Chao, C., Cai, J., Bartels, C., Gressner, T. and Subjeck, J. (1987). Coinduction of glucose regulated proteins and doxorubicin resistance in Chinese hamster ovary cells. *Proc. Natl. Acad. Sci. USA*, **84**, 3278–3282

94. Roll, D. E., Murphy, B. J., Laderoute, K. R., Sutherland, R. M. and Smith, H. C. (1991). Oxygen regulated 80 kDa protein and glucose regulated 78 kDa protein are identical. *Mol. Cell. Biochem.*, **103**, 141–148

95. Hughes, C. S., Shen, J. W. and Subjeck, J. R. (1989). Resistance to etoposide induced by three glucose-regulated stresses in Chinese hamster ovary cells. *Cancer Res.*, **49**, 4452–4454

96. Shen, J. W., Subjeck, J. R., Lock, R. B. and Ross, W. E. (1990). Depletion of topoisomerase II in isolated nuclei during a glucose-regulated stress response. *Mol. Cell. Biol.*, **9**, 3284–3291

97. Finlay, G. J., Wilson, W. R. and Baguley, B. C. (1987). Cytokinetic factors in drug resistance of Lewis lung carcinoma: Comparison of cells freshly isolated from tumours with cells from exponential and plateau-phase cultures. *Br. J. Cancer*, **56**, 755–762

98. Teicher, B. A., Holden, S. A., Al-Achi, A. and Herman, T. S. (1990). Classification of antineoplastic treatments by their differential toxicity towards putative oxygenated and hypoxic tumor subpopulations *in vivo* in the FSaIIC murine fibrosarcoma. *Cancer Res.*, **50**, 3339–3344

99. Tannock, I. F. (1987). Toxicity of 5-fluorouracil for aerobic and hypoxic cells in two murine tumours. *Cancer Chemother. Pharmacol.*, **19**, 53–56

100. Tannock, I. F., Guttman, P. and Rauth, A. M. (1983). Failure of 2-deoxy-D-glucose and 5-thio-D-glucose to kill hypoxic cells of two murine tumors. *Cancer Res.*, **43**, 980–983

101. Rauth, A. M. and Mohindra, J. K. (1981). Selective toxicity of 5-(3,3-dimethyl-1-triazeno) imidazole-4-carboxamide toward hypoxic mammalian cells. *Cancer Res.*, **41**, 4900–4905

102. Hill, R. P. and Stanley, J. A. (1975). The response of hypoxic B16 melanoma cells to *in vivo* treatment with chemotherapeutic agents. *Cancer Res.*, **35**, 1147–1153

103. Brophy, G. T. and Sladek, N. E. (1983). Influence of pH on the cytotoxic activity of chlorambucil. *Biochem. Pharmacol.*, **32**, 79–84

104. Mikkelson, R. B., Asher, C. and Hicks, T. (1985). Extracellular pH, transmembrane distribution and cytotoxicity of chlorambucil. *Biochem. Pharmacol.*, **34**, 2531–2534

105. Minchinton, A. I. and Chaplin, D. J. (1991). Spatial characterization of glutathione depletion in the KHT sarcoma using flow cytometry. *Int. J. Radiat. Biol.*, **59**, 1425–1433

106. Chen, M. and Whistler, R. L. (1957). Action of 5-thio-D-glucose and its 1-phosphate with hexokinase and phosphoglucomutase. *Arch. Biochem. Biophys.*, **169**, 392–396

107. Wick, N. R., Drury, R., Naxada, H. L. and Wolf, J. B. (1957). Localization of the primary metabolic block produced by 2-DG. *J. Biol. Chem.*, **244**, 963–969

108. Song, C. W., Clement, J. J. and Levitt, S. H. (1976). Preferential cytotoxicity of 5-thio-D-glucose against hypoxic tumor cells. *J. Natl. Cancer Inst.*, **57** (Suppl. III), 603–605

109. Song, C. W., Sung, J. H., Clement, J. J. and Levitt, S. H. (1978). Cytotoxic effect of 5-thio-D-glucose on chronically hypoxic cells in multicellular spheroids. *Br. J. Cancer*, **32**, 136–140

110. Tannock, I. (1983). Toxicity of aziridinylbenzoquinone for aerobic and hypoxic cells of a transplanted mouse mammary tumour and interaction of the drug with radiation and Adriamycin. *Cancer Res.*, **43**, 2059–2062

111. Rockwell, S. and Schultz, R. J. (1984). Failure of 5-thio-D-glucose to alter cell survival in irradiated or unirradiated EMT6 tumors. *Radiat. Res.*, **100**, 527–535

112. Aw, T. Y. (1991). Postnatal changes in pyridine nucleotides in rat hepatocytes: composition and O_2 dependence. *Pediatr. Res.*, **30**, 112–117

113. Costa, A. K., Heffel, D. F., Schieble, T. M. and Trudell, J. R. (1987). Toxicity of t-butylhydroperoxide in hepatocyte monolayers exposed to hypoxia and reoxygenation. *In Vitro Cell. Dev. Biol.*, **23**, 501–506

114. Tribble, D. L., Jones, D. P. and Edmondson, D. E. (1988). Effect of hypoxia on *tert*-butylhydroperoxide-induced oxidative injury in isolated hepatocytes. *Mol. Pharmacol.*, **34**, 413–420

115. Tribble, D. L. and Jones, D. P. (1990). Oxygen dependence of oxidative stress. Rate of NADPH supply for maintaining the GSH pool during hypoxia. *Biochem. Pharmacol.*, **39**, 729–736

116. Sarkar, A., Ho, J. T., Marton, L. J. and Deen, D. F. (1990). Effect of hypoxia on 1,3-bis(2-chloroethyl)-1-nitrosourea cytotoxicity in 9L cells. *Cancer Res.*, **50**, 2719–2723

117. Palmer, B. D., Wilson, W. R., Pullen, S. M. and Denny, W. A. (1989). Hypoxia-selective antitumor agents. 3. Relationships between structure and cytotoxicity against cultured tumour cells for substituted N,N-bis-(2-chloroethyl)anilines. *J. Med. Chem.*, **33**, 112–121

118. Chaplin, D. J., Acker, M. D. and Olive, P. L. (1989). Potentiation of the tumor cytotoxicity of melphalan by vasodilating agents. *Int. J. Radiat. Oncol. Biol. Phys.*, **16**, 1131–1135

119. Begg, A. C., Shrieve, D. C., Smith, K. A. and Terry, N. H. A. (1985). Effects of hypoxia, pH and growth stage on cell killing in Chinese hamster V79 cells *in vitro* by activated cyclophosphamide. *Cancer Res.*, **45**, 3454–3459

120. Grau, C., Bentzen, S. M. and Overgaard, J. (1990). Cytotoxic effect of misonidazole and cyclophosphamide on aerobic and hypoxic cells in a C_3H mammary carcinoma. *Br. J. Cancer*, **61**, 61–64

121. Lin, A. J., Cosby, L. A., Shansky, C. W. and Sartorelli, A. C. (1972). Potential bioreductive alkylating agents. I. Benzoquinone derivatives. *J. Med. Chem.*, **15**, 1247–1254

122. Ware, D. W., Wilson, W. R., Denny, W. A. and Rickard, C. E. F. (1991). Design and synthesis of cobalt(III) nitrogen mustard complexes as hypoxia selective cytotoxins. The X-ray crystal structure of bis(3-chloro-2,4-pentanedioato)(RS-N,N'-bis(2-chloroethyl)-ethylene-diamine) cobalt(III) perchlorate, $[Co(Clacac)_2(BCE)]ClO_4$. *J. Chem. Soc. Chem. Commun.*, **17**, 1171–1173

123. Mason, R. P. and Holtzman, J. L. (1975). The role of catalytic superoxide formation in the O_2 inhibition of nitroreductase. *Biochem. Biophys. Res. Commun.*, **67**, 1267–1275

124. Wardman, P. and Clarke, E. D. (1976). Oxygen inhibition of nitroreductase: electron transfer from nitro radical-anions to oxygen. *Biochem. Biophys. Res. Commun.*, **69**, 942–949

125. Biaglow, J. E., Nygaard, O. F. and Greenstock, C. L. (1975). Electron transfer in Ehrlich ascites tumor cells in the presence of nitrofurans. *Biochem. Pharmacol.*, 25, 393–398

126. Biaglow, J., Varnes, M., Roizen-Towle, L., Clarke, E., Epp, E., Astor, M. and Hall, E. (1986). Biochemistry of reduction of nitroheterocycles. *Biochem. Pharmacol.*, **35**, 77–90

127. Grisham, M. B., Volkmer, C., Tso, P. and Yamada, T. (1991). Metabolism of trinitrobenzene sulfonic acid by the rat colon produced reactive oxygen species. *Gastroenterology*, **101**, 540–547

128. Feller, D. R., Morita, M. and Gillette, J. R. (1971). Reduction of heterocyclic nitro compounds in the rat liver (35594). *Proc. Soc. Exp. Biol. Med.*, **137**, 433–437

129. Walton, M. I. and Workman, P. (1987). Nitroimidazole bioreductive metabolism. Quantitation and characterisation of mouse tissue benznidazole nitroreductases *in vivo* and *in vitro*. *Biochem. Pharmacol.*, **36**, 887–896

130. Wolpert, M. K., Althans, J. R. and Jones, D. C. (1973). Nitroreductase activity of mammalian liver aldehyde oxidase. *J. Pharmacol. Exp. Ther.*, **185**, 202–213

131. Morita, M., Feller, D. R. and Gillette, J. R. (1971). Reduction of niridazole by rat liver xanthine oxidase. *Biochem. Pharmacol.*, **20**, 217–226

132. Gillette, J. R., Kamm, J. J. and Sasame, H. A. (1968). Mechanisms of *p*-nitrobenzoate reduction in liver. The possible role of cytochrome P-450 in liver microsomes. *Mol. Pharmacol.*, **4**, 541–548

133. Feller, D. R., Morita, M. and Gillette, J. R. (1971). Enzymatic reduction of niridazole by rat liver microsomes. *Biochem. Pharmacol.*, **20**, 203–215

134. Kutcher, W. W. and McCalla, D. R. (1984). Aerobic reduction of 5-nitro-2-furaldehyde semicarbazone by rat liver xanthine dehydrogenase. *Biochem. Pharmacol.*, **33**, 799–805

135. Robertson, J. A., Chen, H.-C. and Nebert, D. W. (1986). NAD(P)H:menadione oxidoreductase. *J. Biol. Chem.*, **261**, 15794–15799

136. Jaiswal, A. K., Burnett, P., Adesnik, M. and Wesley McBride, O. (1990). Nucleotide and deduced amino acid sequence of a human cDNA (NQO₂) corresponding to a second member of the NAD(P)H:quinone oxidoreductase gene family. Extensive polymorphism at the NQO_2 gene locus on chromosome 6. *Biochemistry*, **29**, 1899–1906

137. Lind, C., Cadenas, E., Hochstein, P. and Ernster, L. (1990). DT-diaphorase: purification, properties and function. *Meth. Enzymol.*, **186**, 287–301

138. Knox, R. J., Boland, M. P., Friedlos, F., Coles, B., Southan, C. and Roberts, J. J. (1988). The nitroreductase enzyme in Walker cells that activates 5-(aziridin-1-yl)-2,4-dinitrobenzamide (CB 1954) is a form of NAD(P)H dehydrogenase (quinone)(EC 1.6.99.2). *Biochem. Pharmacol.*, **37**, 4671–4677

139. De Flora, S., Bennicelli, C., Camoirano, A., Serra, D. and Hochstein, P. (1988). Influence of DT diaphorase on the mutagenicity of organic and inorganic compounds. *Carcinogenesis*, **9**, 611–617

140. Hajos, A. K. D. and Winston, G. W. (1991). Dinitropyrene nitroreductase activity of purified NAD(P)H:quinone oxidoreductase: role in rat liver cytosol and induction by Aroclor-1254 pretreatment. *Carcinogenesis*, **12**, 697–702

141. Westfall, B. B. (1943). The reduction of symmetrical trinitrotoluene by a succinic dehydrogenase preparation. *J. Pharmacol. Exp. Ther.*, **79**, 23–26
142. Beuding, E. and Jolliffe, N. (1946). Metabolism of trinitrotoluene (TNT) *in vitro*. *J. Pharmacol. Exp. Ther.*, **88**, 300–312
143. Boon, P. J., Cullis. P. M., Symons, M. C. R. and Wren, B. W. (1985). Effects of ionising radiation on deoxyribonucleic acid. Part 2. The influence of nitroimidazole drugs on the course of radiation damage to aqueous deoxyribonucleic acid. *J. Chem. Soc. Perkin Trans.*, **2**, 1057–1061
144. Wardman, P. (1985). Lifetimes of the radical-anions of medically-important nitroaryl compounds in aqueous solution. *Life Chem. Rep.*, **3**, 22–28
145. Polnaszek, C. F., Peterson, F. J., Holtzman, J. L. and Mason, R. P. (1984). No detectable reaction of the anion radical metabolite of nitrofurans with reduced glutathione or macromolecules. *Chem.–Biol. Interactions*, **51**, 263–271
146. Noss, M. B., Panicucci, R., McClelland, R. A. and Rauth, A. M. (1988). Preparation, toxicity and mutagenicity of 1-methyl-2-nitrosoimidazole: a toxic 2-nitroimidazole reduction product. *Biochem. Pharmacol.*, **37**, 2585–2593
147. Noss, M. B., Panicucci, R., McClelland, R. A. and Rauth, A. M. (1989). 1-Methyl-2-nitrosoimidazole: cytotoxic and glutathione depleting capabilities. *Int. J. Radiat. Oncol. Biol. Phys.*, **16**, 1015–1019
148. Ehlhardt, W. J., Beaulieu Jr, B. B. and Goldman, P. (1988). Nitrosoimidazoles: highly bactericidal analogues of 5-nitroimidazole drugs. *J. Med. Chem.*, **31**, 323–329
149. Beland, F. A., Ribovich, M., Howard, P. C., Heflich, R. H., Kurian, P. and Milo, G. E. (1986). Cytotoxicity, cellular transformation and DNA adducts in normal human diploid fibroblasts exposed to 1-nitrosopyrene, a reduced derivative of the environmental contaminant 1-nitropyrene. *Carcinogenesis*, **7**, 1279–1283
150. Lafi, A, and Parry. J. M. (1987). Chromosome aberrations induced by nitro-, nitroso- and amino-pyrenes in cultured Chinese hamster cells. *Mutagenesis*, **2**, 23–26
151. Heflich, R. H., Fifer, E. K., Djuric, Z. and Beland, F. A. (1985). DNA adduct formation and mutation induction by nitropyrenes in *Salmonella* and Chinese hamster ovary cells: relationship with nitroreduction and acetylation. *Environ. Health Perspect.*, **62**, 135–143
152. Miller, J. A. (1970). Carcinogenesis by chemicals: An overview – G. H. A. Clowes Memorial Lecture. *Cancer Res.*, **30**, 559–576
153. Rosencrantz, H. S. and Mermelstein, R. (1983). Mutagenicity and genotoxicity of nitroarenes – all nitro-containing chemicals were not created equal. *Mutat. Res.*, **114**, 217–267
154. Wild, D. (1990). A novel pathway to the ultimate mutagens of aromatic amino and nitro compounds. *Envir. Health Perspect.*, **88**, 27–31
155. Tada, M. and Tada, M. (1975). Seryl-tRNA synthetase and activation of the carcinogen, 4-hydroxylaminoquinoline-1-oxide. *Nature (London)*, **255**, 510–512
156. Miller, E. C. (1978). Some current perspectives on chemical carcinogenesis in humans and experimental animals: Presidential address. *Cancer Res.*, **38**, 1479–1496
157. Djuric, Z., Fifer, E. K. and Beland, F. A. (1985). Acetyl coenzyme A-dependent binding of carcinogenic and mutagenic dinitropyrenes to DNA. *Carcinogenesis*, **6**, 941–944
158. Djuric, Z., Potter, D. W., Heflich, R. H. and Beland, F. A. (1986). Aerobic and anaerobic reduction of nitrated pyrenes *in vitro*. *Chem.–Biol. Interactions*, **59**, 309–324
159. Tee, L. B. G., Minchin, R. F. and Ilett, K. F. (1988). Metabolism of 1,8-dinitropyrene by rabbit lung. *Carcinogenesis*, **9**, 1869–1874
160. Pfau, W., Schmeiser, H. H. and Wiessler, M. (1990). Aristolochic acid binds covalently to the exocyclic amino group of purine nucleotides in DNA. *Carcinogenesis*, **11**, 313–319
161. Whillans, D. W. and Whitmore, G. F. (1981). The radiation reduction of misonidazole. *Radiat. Res.*, **86**, 311–324
162. McClelland, R. A., Fuller, J. R., Seaman, N. E., Rauth, A. M. and Battistella, R. (1984). 2-Hydroxylaminoimidazoles – unstable intermediates in the reduction of 2-nitroimidazoles. *Biochem. Pharmacol.*, **33**, 303–309
163. Varghese, A. J. (1983). Glutathione conjugates of misonidazole. *Biochem. Biophys. Res. Commun.*, **112**, 1013–1020
164. Heimbrook, D. C. and Sartorelli, A. C. (1986). Biochemistry of misonidazole reduction by NADPH-cytochrome c(P-450) reductase. *Mol. Pharmacol.*, **29**, 168–172
165. Varghese, A. J. and Whitmore, G. F. (1983). Modification of guanine derivatives by reduced 2-nitroimidazoles. *Cancer Res.*, **43**, 78–82

166. Varghese, A. J. and Whitmore, G. F. (1980). Binding to cellular macromolecules as a possible mechanism for the cytotoxicity of misonidazole. *Cancer Res.*, **40**, 1265–1269

167. Middlestadt, M. V. and Rauth, A. M. (1982). The effects of reduction products of misonidazole on Chinese hamster ovary cells. *Int. J. Radiat. Oncol. Biol. Phys.*, **8**, 709–712

168. Ehlhardt, W. J., Beaulieu B. B. Jr. and Goldman, P. (1987). Chemical and biological properties of acetyl derivatives of the hydroxylamino reduction products of metronidazole and dimetridazole. *Biochem. Pharmacol.*, **36**, 931–935

169. Symons, M. C. R., Bowman, W. R. and Taylor, P. F. (1990). Radical anions of nitro-soimidazoles: Putative intermediates in the mechanism of action of nitroimidazole antibiotics. *Tetrahedron Lett.*, **31**, 3221–3224

170. Rauth, A. M., Paciga, J. E. and Mohindra, J. K. (1980). *In vivo* studies of the cytotoxicity of hypoxic cell radiosensitizers. In Brady, L. W. (ed.) *Radiation Sensitizers. Their Use in the Clinical Management of Cancer,* pp. 207–214. (New York: Masson Publishing USA, Inc.)

171. Adams, G. E., Stratford, I. J., Wallace, R. G., Wardman, P. and Watts, M. E. (1980). Toxicity of nitro compounds towards hypoxic mammalian cells *in vitro*: dependence on reduction potential. *J. Natl. Cancer Inst.*, **64**, 555–560

172. Clarke, E. D., Goulding, K. H. and Wardman, P. (1982). Nitroimidazoles as anaerobic electron acceptors for xanthine oxidase. *Biochem. Pharmacol.*, **31**, 3237–3242

173. Battelli, M. G., Della Corte, E. and Stirpe, F. (1972). Xanthine oxidase type D (dehydrogenase) in the intestine and other organs of the rat. *Biochem. J.*, **126**, 747–749

174. McKelvey, T. G., Hollwarth, M. E., Granger, D. N., Engerson, T. D., Landler, U. and Jones, H. P. (1988). Mechanisms of conversion of xanthine dehydrogenase to xanthine oxidase in ischemic rat liver and kidney. *Am. J. Physiol.*, **254**, G753–G760

175. O'Connor, C. J., McLennan, D. J., Sutton, B. M., Denny, W. A. and Wilson, W. R. (1991). Effect of reduction potential on the rate of reduction of nitroacridines by xanthine oxidase and by dihydro-flavin mononucleotide. *J. Chem. Soc. Perkin Trans.*, **2**, 951–954

176. Stratford, I. J., O'Neill, P., Sheldon, P. W., Silver, A. R. J., Walling, J. M. and Adams, G. E. (1986). RSU-1069, a nitroimidazole containing an aziridine group. *Biochem. Pharmacol.*, **35**, 105–109

177. Adams, G. E., Ahmed, I., Sheldon, P. W. and Stratford, I. J. (1984). Radiation sensitization and chemopotentiation: RSU-1069 a compound more efficient than misonidazole *in vitro* and *in vivo*. *Br. J. Cancer*, **40**, 571–577

178. Hill, R. P., Gulyas, S. and Whitmore, G. F. (1986). Studies on the *in vivo* and *in vitro* cytotoxicity of the drug RSU-1069. *Br. J. Cancer*, **53**, 743–751

179. O'Neill, P., McNeil, S. S. and Jenkins, T. C. (1987). Induction of DNA crosslinks *in vitro* upon reduction of the nitroimidazole-aziridines RSU-1069 and RSU-1131. *Biochem. Pharmacol.*, **36**, 1787–1792

180. Whitmore, G. F. and Gulyas, S. (1986). Studies on the toxicity of RSU-1069. *Int. J. Radiat. Oncol. Biol. Phys.*, **12**, 1219–1222

181. Fielden, E. M., Adams, G. E., Cole, S., Naylor. M. A., O'Neil, P., Stephens, M. A. and Stratford, I. J. (1992). Assessment of a range of novel nitro-aromatic radiosensitizers and bioreductive drugs. *Int. J. Radiat. Oncol. Biol. Phys.* **22**, 707–711

182. Cole, S., Stratford, I. J., Adams, G. E., Fielden, E. M. and Jenkins, T. C. (1990). Dual function 2-nitroimidazoles as hypoxic cell radiosensitizers and bioreductive cytotoxins: *in vivo* evaluation in KHT murine sarcomas. *Radiat. Res.*, **124**, S38–S44

183. Horwich, A., Holliday, S. B., Deacon, J. M. and Peckham, M. J. (1986). A toxicity and pharmacokinetic study in man of the hypoxic cell radiosensitizer RSU-1069. *Br. J. Radiol*, **59**, 1238–1243

184. Hesketh, P. J. and Gandara, D. R. (1991). Serotonin antagonists: a new class of antiemetic agents. *J. Natl. Cancer Inst.*, **9**, 613–620

185. Cole, S., Stratford, I. J., Bowler, J., Nolan, J., Wright, E. G., Lorimore, S. A. and Adams, G. E. (1991). Oral (po) dosing with RSU 1069 or RB 6145 maintains their potency as hypoxic cell radiosensitizers and cytotoxins but reduces systemic toxicity compared with parenteral (ip) administration in mice. *Int. J. Radiat. Oncol. Biol. Phys.*, **21**, 387–395

186. Gniazdowski, M., Filipski, J. and Chorzay, M. (1978). Nitracrine. In Hahn (ed.) *Antibiotics V/Part 2*, pp. 275. (Berlin: Springer-Verlag)

187. Wilson, W. R., Denny, W. A., Twigden, S. J., Baguley, B. C. and Probert, J. C. (1984). Selective toxicity of nitracrine to hypoxic mammalian cells. *Br. J. Cancer*, **49**, 215–223

188. Wilson, W. R., Denny, W. A., Stewart, G. M., Fenn, A. and Probert, J. C. (1986). Reductive metabolism and hypoxia-selective toxicity of nitracrine. *Int. J. Radiat. Oncol. Biol. Phys.*, **12**, 1235–1238

189. Wilson, W. R., Anderson, R. F. and Denny, W. A. (1989). Hypoxia-selective antitumor agents. 1. Relationships between structure, redox properties and hypoxia-selective cytotoxicity for 4-substituted derivatives of nitracrine. *J. Med. Chem.*, **32**, 23–30

190. Wilson, W. R., Thompson, L. H., Anderson, R. F. and Denny, W. A. (1989). Hypoxia-selective antitumor agents. 2. Electronic effects of 4-substituents on the mechanisms of cytotoxicity and metabolic stability of nitracrine derivatives. *J. Med. Chem.*, **32**, 31–38

191. Wilson, W. R., Siim, B. G., Denny, W. A., van Zijl, P., Taylor, M. L., Chambers, D. M. and Roberts, P. B. (1992). *S*-Nitro-4-(*N*,*N*-dimethylaminopropylamino)quinoline (5-nitraquine), a new DNA affinic hypoxic cell radiosensitizer and bioreductive agent: Comparison with nitracrine. *Radiat. Res.*, (in press)

192. Denny, W. A., Wilson, W. R., Atwell, G. J., Boyd, M., Pullen, S. M. and Anderson, R. F. (1990). Nitroacridines and nitroquinolines as DNA-affinic hypoxia-selective cytotoxins. In Adams, G. E., Breccia, A., Fielden, E. M. and Wardman, P. (eds.) *Selective Activation of Drugs by Redox Processes*, pp. 149–158. (New York and London: Plenum)

193. Denny, W. A., Atwell, G. J., Roberts, P. B., Anderson, R. F., Boyd, M., Lock, C. J. L. and Wilson, W. R. (1992). Hypoxia-selective agents. 6. 4-Alkylaminonitroquinolines: a new class of hypoxia-selective cytotoxins. *J. Med. Chem.*, submitted

194. Sebolt, J. S., Scavone, S. V., Pinter, C. D., Hamelehle, K. L., Von Hoff, D. D. and Jackson, R. C. (1987). Pyrazoloacridines, a new class of intercalating agents with selectivity against solid tumors *in vitro*. *Cancer Res.*, **47**, 4299–4304

195. Cowan, D. M. S., Panicucci, R., McClelland, R. A. and Rauth, R. M. (1991). Targeting radiosensitizers to DNA by attachment of an intercalating group: Nitroimidazole-linked phenanthridines. *Radiat. Res.*, **127**, 81–89

196. Denny, W. A., Roberts, P. B., Anderson, R. F., Brown, J. M. and Wilson, W. R. (1992). NLA-1: A 2-nitroimidazole radiosensitizer targeted to DNA by intercalation. *Int. J. Radiat. Oncol. Biol. Phys.* **22**, 553–556

197. Teicher, B. A. and Sartorelli, A. C. (1980). Nitrobenzyl halides and carbamates as prototype bioreductive alkylating agents. *J. Med. Chem.*, **23**, 955–960

198. Palmer, B. D., Wilson, W. R. and Denny, W. A. (1990). Nitro analogues of chlorambucil as potential hypoxia-selective antitumour drugs. *Anticancer Drug Design*, **5**, 337–349

199. Palmer, B. D., Wilson, W. R., Cliffe, S. and Denny, W. A. (1992). Hypoxia-selective antitumor agents. 5. Synthesis of water-soluble nitroaniline mustards with selective toxicity for hypoxic mammalian cells. *J. Med. Chem.*, (in press)

200. Roberts, J. J., Friedlos, F. and Knox, R. J. (1986). CB 1954 (2,4-dinitro-5-aziridinyl benzamide) becomes a DNA interstrand crosslinking agent in Walker tumour cells. *Biochem. Biophys. Res. Commun.*, **140**, 1073–1078

201. Knox, J. J., Friedlos, F., Jarman, M. and Roberts, J. J. (1988). A new cytotoxic, DNA interstrand crosslinking agent, 5-(aziridin-1-yl)-4-hydroxylamino-2-nitrobenzamide, is formed from 5-(aziridin-1-yl)-2,4-dinitrobenzamide (CB 1954) by a nitroreductase enzyme in Walker carcinoma cells. *Biochem. Pharmacol.*, **37**, 4661–4669

202. Lewis, D. F. V. (1989). Molecular orbital calculations on tumour-inhibitory phenyl aziridines: QSARs. *Xenobiotica*, **19**, 341–356

203. Wong, K.-H., King, B. T. and Agrawal, K. C. (1986). The mechanism of action of 3-ethoxy-3-(2-nitroimidazol-1-yl)-1-propene (NBK-50), a bioreductive cytotoxic agent. *Proc. Am. Assoc. Cancer Res.*, **27**, 1120

204. Firestone, A., Mulcahy, T. and Borch, R. F. (1991). Nitroheterocycle reduction as a paradigm for intramolecular catalysis of drug delivery to hypoxic cells. *J. Med. Chem.*, **34**, 2933–2935

205. Mulcahy, R. T., Gipp, J. J., Schmidt, J. and Borch, R. F. (1991). Preferential hypoxic toxicity of a bioreductively-activated phosphorodiamidate mustard (JSD-231). In Chapman, J. D., Dewey, W. C. and Whitmore, G. F. (eds.) *Radiation Research, a Twentieth-Century Perspective*, Vol. 1, p. 348. (Toronto: Academic Press) (abstract)

206. Siegel, D., Gibson, N. W., Preusch, P. C. and Ross, D. (1990). Metabolism of mitomycin C by DT-diaphorase: Role in mitomycin C-induced DNA damage and cytotoxicity in human colon carcinoma cells. *Cancer Res.*, **50**, 7483–7489

207. Bachur, N. R., Gordon, S. L. and Gee, M. V. (1978). A general mechanism for microsomal activation of quinone anticancer agents to free radicals. *Cancer Res.*, **38**, 1745–1750

208. Moore, H. W. and Czerniak, R. (1981). Naturally occurring quinones as potential bioreductive alkylating agents. *Med. Res. Rev.*, **1**, 249–280
209. Wilson, I., Wardman, P., Lin, T.-S. and Sartorelli, A. C. (1987). Reactivity of thiols towards derivatives of 2- and 6-methyl-1,4-naphthoquinone bioreductive alkylating agents. *Chem.–Biol. Interactions.*, **61**, 229–240
210. Kennedy, K. A., Rockwell, W. and Sartorelli, A. C. (1980). Preferential activation of mitomycin C cytotoxic metabolites by hypoxic tumor cells. *Cancer Res.*, **40**, 2356–2361
211. Ludwig, C. U., Peng, Y. M., Beaudry, J. N. and Salmon, S. E. (1984). Cytotoxicity of mitomycin C on clonogenic human carcinoma cells is not enhanced to hypoxia. *Cancer Chemother. Pharmacol.*, **12**, 146–150
212. Marshall, R. S. and Rauth, A. M. (1986). Modification of the cytotoxic activity of mitomycin C by oxygen and ascorbic acid in Chinese hamster ovary cells and in a repair deficient mutant. *Cancer Res.*, **46**, 2709–2713
213. Rauth, A. M., Mohindra, J. K. and Tannock, I. F. (1983). Activity of mitomycin C for aerobic and hypoxic cells *in vitro* and *in vivo*. *Cancer Res.*, **43**, 4154–4158
214. Weissberg, J. B., Son, Y. H., Papac, R. J., Sasaki, C., Fischer, D. B., Lawrence, R., Rockwell, S., Sartorelli, A. C. and Fischer, J. J. (1989). Randomized clinical trial of mitomycin C as an adjunct to radiotherapy in head and neck cancer. *Int. J. Radiat. Oncol. Biol. Phys.*, **17**, 3–9
215. Keyes, S. R., Rockwell, S. and Sartorelli, A. C. (1985). Porfiromycin as a bioreductive alkylating agent with selective toxicity to hypoxic EMT6 tumor cells *in vivo* and *in vitro*. *Cancer Res.*, **45**, 3642–3645
216. Rockwell, S., Keyes, S. R. and Sartorelli, A. C. (1988). Modulation of the cytotoxicity of mitomycin C to EMT6 mouse mammary tumor cells by dicoumarol *in vitro*. *Cancer Res.*, **48**, 5471–5474
217. Dulhanty, A. M. and Whitmore, G. F. (1991). Chinese hamster ovary cell lines resistant to mitomycin C under aerobic but not hypoxic conditions are deficient in DT diaphorase. *Cancer Res.*, **51**, 1860–1865
218. Marshall, R. S., Paterson, M. C. and Rauth, A. M. (1991). Studies on the mechanism of resistance to mitomycin C and porfiromycin in a human cell strain derived from a cancer prone individual. *Biochem. Pharmacol.*, **41**, 1351–1360
219. Rockwell, S., Keyes, S. R. and Sartorelli, A. C. (1989). Modulation of the antineoplastic efficacy of mitomycin C by dicoumarol *in vivo*. *Cancer Chemother. Pharmacol.*, **24**, 349–353
220. Hoban, P. R., Walton, M. I., Robson, C. N., Godden, J., Stratford, I. J., Workman, P., Harris, A. L. and Hickson, I. D. (1990). Decreased NADPH:cytochrome P-450 reductase activity and impaired drug activation in a mammalian cell line resistant to mitomycin C under aerobic but not hypoxic conditions. *Cancer Res.*, **50**, 4692–4697
221. Siegel, D., Gibson, N. W., Preusch, P. C. and Ross, D. (1990). Metabolism of mitomycin C by DT-diaphorase: role in mitomycin C-induced DNA damage and cytotoxicity in human colon carcinoma cells. *Cancer Res.*, **50**, 7483–7489
222. Gold, L. G., Foley, H. T. and Shnider, B. I. (1965). A preliminary study with porfiromycin. *Proc. Am. Assoc. Cancer Res.*, **6**, 22 (abstract)
223. Rockwell, S., Keyes, S. R., Loomis, R., Kelley, M., Vyas, D. M., Wong, H., Doyle, T. W. and Sartorelli, A. C. (1991). Activity of C-7 substituted cyclic acetal derivatives of mitomycin C and porfiromycin against hypoxic and oxygenated EMT6 carcinoma cells *in vitro* and *in vivo*. *Cancer Commun.*, **3**, 191–198
224. O'Brien, P. J., Kaul, H. K. and Rauth, A. M. (1990). Differential cytotoxicity of diaziquone toward Chinese hamster ovary cells under hypoxic and aerobic exposure conditions. *Cancer Res.*, **50**, 1516–1520
225. Siegel, D., Gibson, N. W., Preusch, P. C. and Ross, D. (1990). Metabolism of diaziquone by NAD(P)H: (Quinone acceptor) oxidoreductase (DT-diaphorase): Role in diaziquone-induced DNA damage and cytotoxicity in human colon carcinoma cells. *Cancer Res.*, **50**, 7293–7300
226. Oostveen, E. A. and Speckamp, W. N. (1987). Mitomyc... C analogues. 1. Indoloquinones as potential bisalkylating agents. *Tetrahedron*, **43**, 255–262
227. Workman, P., Binger, M. and Kooistra, K. L. (1992). Pharmacokinetics, distribution and metabolism of the novel bioreductive alkylating indoloquinone EO9 in rodents. *Int. J. Radiat. Oncol. Biol. Phys.* **22**, 713–716

228. Walton, M. I., Smith, P. J. and Workman, P. (1991) The role of NAD(P)H:quinone reductase (EC 1.6.99.2, DT-diaphorase) in the reductive bioactivation of the novel indoloquinone antitumor agent EO9. *Cancer Commun.*, **3**, 199–206

229. Zeman, E. M., Brown, J. M., Lemmon, M. J., Hirst, V. K. and Lee, W. W. (1986). SR 4233, a new bioreductive agent with high selective toxicity for hypoxic mammalian cells. *Int. J. Radiat. Oncol. Biol. Phys.*, **12**, 1239–1242

230. Baker, M. A., Zeman, E. M., Hirst, V. K. and Brown, J. M. (1988). Metabolism of SR 4233 by CHO cells: Basis for selective hypoxic cytotoxicity. *Cancer Res.*, **48**, 5947–5952

231. Laderoute, K., Wardman, P. and Rauth, A. M. (1988). Molecular mechanisms for the hypoxia-dependent activation of 3-amino-1,2,4-benzotriazine-1,4-dioxide (SR 4233). *Biochem. Pharmacol.*, **37.**, 1487–1495

232. Laderoute, K. R. and Rauth, M. A. (1986). Identification of two major reduction products of the hypoxic cell toxin 3-amino-1,2,4-benzotriazine-1,4-dioxide. *Biochem. Pharmacol.*, **35**, 3417–3420

233. Walton, M. I. and Workman, P. (1989). Enzymology of the reductive bioactivation of SR 4233 – a novel benzotriazine di-n-oxide hypoxic cell cytotoxin. *Biochem. Pharmacol.*, **39**, 1735–1742

234. Cahill, A. and White, I. N. H. (1990). Reductive metabolism of 3-amino-1,2,4-benzotriazine-1,4-dioxide (SR 4233) and the induction of unscheduled DNA synthesis in rat and human derived cell lines. *Carcinogenesis*, **11**, 1407–1411

235. Biedermann, K. A., Wang, J., Graham, R. P. and Brown, J. M. (1991). SR 4233 cytotoxicity and metabolism in DNA repair-competent and repair-deficient cell cultures. *Br. J. Cancer*, **63**, 358–361

236. Wang, J., Evans, J. W., Biederman, K. A. and Brown, J. M. (1991). The mechanism of cell killings by SR 4233 under hypoxic conditions. In Chapman, J. D., Dewey, W. C. and Whitmore, G. F. (eds.) *Radiation Research, a Twentieth-Century Perspective*, Vol 1, p. 349. (Toronto: Academic Press) (abstract)

237. Sugiura, M., Iwasaki, K. and Kato, R. (1977). Reduced nicotinamide adenine dinucleotide-dependent reduction of tertiary amine N-oxide by liver microsomal cytochrome P-450. *Biochem. Pharmacol.*, **26**, 489–495

238. Powis, G. and DeGraw, C. L. (1980). N-oxide reduction by hemoglobin, cytochrome C and ferrous ions. *Res. Commun. Chem. Pathol. Pharmacol.*, **30**, 143–150

239. Kitamura, S. and Tatsumi, K. (1984). Reduction of tertiary amine N-oxides by liver preparations: function of aldehyde oxidase as a major N-oxide reductase. *Biochem. Biophys. Res. Commun.*, **121**, 749–754

240. Gillespie, S. G. and Duffel, M. W. (1989). Peroxidase as a model for reduction of tertiary amine oxides catalysed by rat hepatic supernatant and microsomal fractions. *Biochem. Pharmacol.*, **38**, 573–579

241. Bickel, M. H., Weder, H. J. and Aebi, H. (1968). Metabolic interconversions between imipramine, its N-oxide and its desmethyl derivative in rat tissues *in vitro. Biochem. Biophys. Res. Commun.*, **33**, 1012–1018

242. Bickel, M. H. (1969). The pharmacology and biochemistry of N-oxides. *Pharmacol. Rev.*, **21**, 325–355

243. Walton, M. I., Bleehan, N. M. and Workman, P. (1985). The reversible N-oxidation of the nitroimidazole radiosensitizer Ro 03-8799. *Biochem. Pharmacol.*, **34**, 3939–3940

244. White, I. N. H., Suzanger, M., Mattocks. A. R., Bailey, E., Farmer, P. B. and Connors, T. A. (1989). Reduction of nitromin to nitrogen mustard: unscheduled DNA synthesis in aerobic or anaerobic rat hepatocytes, JB1, BL8 and Walker carcinoma cell lines. *Carcinogenesis*, **10**, 2113–2118

245. Wilson, W. R., van Zijl, P. and Denny, W. A. (1992). Bis-bioreductive agents as hypoxia-selective cytotoxins: Nitracrine N-oxide. *Int. J. Radiat. Oncol. Biol. Phys.*, **22**, 693–696

246. Skov K. A., Adomat, H., Chaplin, D. J. and Farrell, N. P. (1990). Toxicity of [PtCl₂(NH₃)L] in hypoxia; L = misonidazole or metronidazole. *Anticancer Drug Design*, **5**, 121–128

247. Ware, D. W., Siim, B. G., Robinson, K. G., Denny, W. A., Brothers, P. J. and Clark, G. R. (1991). Synthesis and characterization of aziridine complexes of cobalt(III) and chromium(III) designed as hypoxia-selective cytotoxins. X-ray crystal structure of *trans*[Co(Az)₂(NO₂)₂] Br₂.2H₂O.LiBr. *Inorg. Chem.*, **30**, 3750–3757

248. Teicher, B. A., Abrams, M. J., Rosbe, K. W. and Herman, T. S. (1990). Cytotoxicity, radiosensitization, antitumor activity, and interaction with hyperthermia of a Co(III) mustard complex. *Cancer Res.*, **50**, 6971–6975
249. Simic, M. and Lilie, J. (1974). Kinetics of ammonia detachment from reduced Cobalt(III) complexes based on conductometric pulse radiolysis. *J. Am. Chem. Soc.*, **96**, 291–292
250. Shinohara, N., Lilie, J. and Simic, M. G. (1977). Kinetics and mechanism of ligand dissociation of cobalt(II)-polyamine complexes in aqueous solution. *Inorg. Chem.*, **16**, 2809–2813
251. Costa, A. K., Baker, M. A., Brown, J. M. and Trudell, J. R. (1989). *In vitro* hepatotoxicity of SR 4233 (3-amino-1,2,4-benzotriazine-1,4-dioxide), a hypoxic cytotoxin and potential antitumor agent. *Cancer Res.*, **49**, 925–929
252. Sun. A. S. and Cederbaum, A. I. (1980). Oxidoreductase activities in normal rat liver, tumor-bearing rat liver, and hepatoma HC-252. *Cancer Res.*, **40**, 4677–4681
253. Ikegami, T., Natsumeda, Y. and Weber, G. (1986). Decreased concentration of xanthine dehydrogenase (EC 1.1.1.204) in rat hepatomas. *Cancer Res.*, **46**, 3838–3841
254. Guzelian, P. S., Bissel, D. M. and Meyer, U. A. (1977). Drug metabolism in adult rat hepatocytes in primary monolayer culture. *Gastroenterology*, **72**, 1232–1239
255. Fahl, W. E., Michalopoulos, G., Sattler, G. L., Jefcoate, C. R. and Pitot, H. C. (1979). Characteristics of microsomal enzyme controls in primary cultures of rat hepatocytes. *Arch. Biochem. Biophys.*, **192**, 61–72
256. Sirica, A. E. and Pitot. H. C. (1980). Drug metabolism and effects of carcinogens in cultured hepatic cells. *Pharmacol. Rev.*, **31**, 205–228
257. Vanderkooi, J. M., Erecinska, M. and Silver, I. A. (1991). Oxygen in mammalian tissue: methods of measurement and affinities of various reactions. *Am. J. Physiol.*, **29**, C1131–C1150
258. Wong, K.-H., Koch, C. J., Wallen, C. A. and Wheeler, K. T. (1991). Pharmacokinetics and cytotoxicity of RSU-1069 in subcutaneous 9L tumours under oxic and hypoxic conditions. *Br. J. Cancer*, **63**, 484–488
259. Taylor, Y. C. and Rauth, A. M. (1982). Oxygen tension, cellular respiration and redox state as variables influencing the cytotoxicity of the radiosensitizer misonidazole. *Radiat. Res.*, **91**, 104–123
260. Marshall, R. S. and Rauth, A. M. (1988). Oxygen and exposure kinetics as factors influencing the cytotoxity of Porfiromycin, a Mitomycin C analogue, in Chinese hamster ovary cells. *Cancer Res.*, **48**, 5655–5659
261. Kedderis, G. and Miwa, G. (1988). The metabolic activation of nitroheterocyclic therapeutic drugs. *Drug Metab. Rev.*, **19**, 33–62
262. Tatsumi, K., Koga, N., Kitamura, S., Yoshimura, H., Wardman, P. and Kato, Y. (1979). Enzymic *cis-trans* isomerization of nitrofuran derivative. Isomerizing activity of xanthine oxidase, lipoyl dehydrogenase, DT-diaphorase and liver microsomes. *Biochim. Biophys. Acta*, **567**, 75–87
263. Rauth, A. M., McClelland, R. A., Michaels, H. B. and Battistella, R. (1984). The oxygen dependence of the reduction of nitroimidazoles in a radiolytic model system. *Int. J. Radiat. Oncol. Biol. Phys.*, **10**, 1323–1326
264. Witiak, D. T., Kamat, P. L., Allison, D. L., Leibowitz, S. M., Glaser, R., Holliday, J. E., Moeschberger, M. L. and Schaller, J. P. (1983). Bis(bioreductive) alkylating agents: synthesis and biological activity in a nude mouse human carcinoma model. *J. Med. Chem.*, **26**, 1679–1686
265. Wessels, B. W. (1990). Current status of animal radioimmunotherapy. *Cancer Res. (Suppl.)*, **50**, 970s–973s
266. Bagshawe, K. D. (1990). Antibody-directed enzyme/prodrug therapy (ADEPT). *Biochem. Soc. Transact.*, **18**, 750–752
267. Nishimura Y., Ono, K., Hiraoka, M., Masunaga, S., Jo, S., Shibamoto, Y., Sasai, K., Abe. M., Iga, K. and Ogawa, Y. (1990). Treatment of murine SCCVII tumors with localized hyperthermia and temperature-sensitive liposomes containing cisplatin. *Radiat. Res.*, **122**, 161–167
268. Skehan, P., Storeng, R., Scuderio, D., Monks, A., McMahon, J., Vistica, D., Warren, J. T., Bokesch, H., Kenney, S. and Boyd, M. R. (1990). A new colorimetric cytotoxicity assay for anticancer-drug screening. *J. Natl. Cancer Inst.*, **82**, 1107–1112

5
Computer modelling and drug design

S. NEIDLE AND C. A. LAUGHTON

INTRODUCTION

Our understanding of biological processes at the molecular level is, in large part, a direct consequence of knowledge obtained over the past three decades on the three-dimensional structures of biological molecules. Thus, the determination of the double-helical structure of DNA by Crick, Franklin, Watson and Wilkins led directly to the rationalization of much of genetics, and ultimately to the ability to manipulate and dissect genes at the molecular level. The knowledge that specific cellular genes, when activated by, for example, point mutations or translocations, can give rise to tumorigenic events provides for the first time the possibility of a totally specific target for chemotherapy. In order to exploit this information, it will be necessary to design drugs which interact with DNA with complete sequence-specificity; this, in turn, will require an understanding of the detailed three-dimensional structure and dynamics of these oncogene targets. This chapter describes the role of molecular modelling in the elucidation of the three-dimensional structure of biomolecules, in the analysis of the relationship between structure and function, and in the evaluation and design of drugs that can interact with DNA, proteins or enzymes.

One can define molecular structure in general terms as the mutual arrangement of atoms in a molecule, held together by chemical bonds. The shape of a complex molecule is largely defined by the relatively weak forces between its non-bonded atoms – these may be steric, electrostatic, hydrogen-bonding or hydrophobic. These forces are also responsible for intermolecular recognition. Hydrogen bonding is the most specific, involving discrete donor and acceptor atoms, and is highly directional. The other weak forces tend to be non-directional, and, for example, can be mapped on a molecular surface where they play a major role in non-specific recognition between molecules and in shape recognition generally. Hydrogen bonding is thus the primary contributor to specificity in drug action, as well as in more general intermolecular interactions. In molecular modelling, we can use existing knowledge of these bonding and non-bonding interactions to predict the structure of biomolecules and their complexes, or, conversely, to use knowledge of the three-dimensional structure to analyse the importance and role of different inter- and intramolecular forces. Modelling of the molecular interactions of a drug with its receptor provides understanding of its mode of action, and, crucially, enables the rational design of analogues that will interact with their target in distinct defined ways in order to elicit a distinct biological response.

THE MOLECULAR STRUCTURAL TOOLS OF DRUG DESIGN

The most detailed level of information on the atomic environment surrounding a bound ligand comes from X-ray crystallographic analysis. Of especial interest are intermolecular distances signifying: (1) non-bonded attractive interactions, for example between oppositely charged groups; (2) hydrogen bonds; and (3) hydrophobic interactions involving van der Waals contacts between, for example, methyl and phenyl groups. Two-dimensional NMR techniques are increasingly useful as a complement to such X-ray results, since they can also provide short-range distance data, albeit for averaged dynamic structures of molecular weight less than about 20 000. However, at the present time, they do not provide an equivalent degree of atomic resolution; nor is it readily possible to assess quantitatively the quality of an NMR-derived model whereas this is standard for X-ray-derived ones. It is common to quote the overall agreement between observed and calculated X-ray models in terms of a 'reliability' factor, R, which is considered to be < 0.20 for a well-defined structure. No such factor is in use for NMR-derived structural data. An important factor in the consideration of structures from X-ray crystallography is the resolution limit of the experimental data itself, which is a major factor in defining the degree of precision of the final structure. A low resolution analysis (> 3 Å) means that fine detail of the structure cannot be observed in the electron-density maps. The level of detail required for reliable side-chain definition is only obtained with a resolution of < 2 Å. Otherwise, the refinement procedures used provide best-fits with a degree of ambiguity related to the resolution limit. Thus, X-ray crystallographic analysis of proteins and nucleic acids is essentially a molecular-modelling process, albeit with experimental data against which the model(s) can be compared.

Three-dimensional structural data detailing the interactions between an anti-cancer drug and its target macromolecule are available at present in very few cases. These are for:

Adenosine deaminase
Dihydrofolate reductase and the antifolate, methotrexate
Thymidylate synthase and CB3717
Doxorubicin/daunomycin, actinomycin, *cis*-platinum and
ellipticine with various short DNA sequences

This paucity of experimental data has necessitated theoretical molecular modelling approaches in order to attempt to define likely modes of interaction for analogues of these drugs as well as others, such as amsacrine, mitoxantrone and bleomycin. Modelling of protein targets where only the primary sequence is established is most powerful when there is homology with proteins of established structure. As yet, such studies have not yielded model structures for major targets, such as oncogene proteins (apart from p21 RAS), protein kinase C or

DNA topoisomerase II, and certainly not at the < 1 Å level of accuracy in atomic positions needed for drug design. Some 400 protein crystal structures have been determined to date[29]; there is currently a rapid increase in the rate of analysis due in part to the advent of fast X-ray data acquisition methods and relatively inexpensive supercomputer power. The other major factor is the increasing ability to obtain hitherto inaccessible proteins in large quantities ($> 10\,mg$) by expression of recombinant genes, even though this is technically more difficult for eukaryotic proteins.

Even when knowledge of DNA structure was limited to the simplistic classic Watson-Crick model, drug–DNA complexes were perceived to be accessible to study by molecular modelling methods. Initially, these were restricted to crude considerations of physical space-filling models. These have now been superseded by various methods of computer-aided molecular design[1–3].

MOLECULAR MODELLING METHODS

Molecular graphics

Interactive high-performance computer graphics were originally exploited by protein crystallographers for fitting and analysing electron density to putative protein structures. The power of the method to visualize molecules in three dimensions has resulted in its widespread application to molecular modelling and drug design. In addition, the economic cost of the hardware required has decreased in real terms by an order of magnitude over the past ten years, so that molecular modelling facilities are now available in the majority of molecular biology and medicinal chemistry research laboratories. Molecules can be shown and manipulated as stick-like figures. Surface characteristics of both large and small molecules can be represented in a variety of ways, depending on the properties being highlighted. Visualization of the solvent-accessible surface of a macromolecule[4] is often useful when locating binding sites in that macromolecule. This can be combined with information on surface charge distribution[5], which utilizes calculated molecular electrostatic potentials (see, for example, reference 6 for definitive results on B-DNA). Colour visualization of this property is informative when locating reactive regions on macromolecule or drug for, say, attack by a charged species. Surface representation of hydrophobic properties is a newer development which is likely to be particularly powerful when combined with these others.

Empirical energy calculations

In addition to manipulative operations on complete molecules, molecular design requires the ability to analyse the intramolecular forces in a molecule that determine its shape, and the intermolecular forces that determine how one molecule, e.g. a protein or nucleic acid, interacts with another, e.g. a drug. In general, at equilibrium, a molecule or complex of molecules will adopt a conformation in which all the forces balance to give the minimum total energy – the global minimum conformation. An important part of molecular modelling is concerned with attempts to identify this conformation by computing the relationship between structure and energy through molecular mechanics. This is done by assigning parameters to different structural features. These parameters describe equilibrium bond-lengths, angles and torsions, together with their deformation energies/energetic barriers to bond rotation. Other parameters describe non-bonding interactions, such as van der Waals and electrostatic forces. A self-consistent set of such parameters is described as a force field. There are many of these in the literature, some designed for use with proteins and nucleic acids[7–9] and others for small molecules. Their usage together when, for example, drug–macromolecule interaction energies are calculated, must be undertaken with caution, as individual parameters are not always readily transferable from one force field to another. Typically, each force field is packaged with a set of computer programs for implementing it: three examples which have been extensively validated for macromolecular studies are AMBER – Assisted Model Building with Energy Refinement[10]; CHARM – Chemistry at Harvard Macromolecular Mechanics[7]; and GROMOS – Groningen Molecular Simulation Program[11].

The potential energy calculated by molecular mechanics methods[7,10] is an estimate of the internal energy of the system, and is not to be confused with the thermodynamic free energy measured experimentally

$$\Delta G_0 = RT \ln K$$

where K is the equilibrium constant for an interaction between molecules. ΔG_0 is the correct descriptor of the energetic driving force for reactions between molecules; the energy obtained from calculations as described above is equivalent to the enthalpy, ΔH, which requires a knowledge of the change in entropy of the system in order to be related to ΔG_0.

In general, the application of molecular mechanics to systems of macromolecular complexity does not lead directly to the identification of the global minimum energy conformation, but to one of maybe many local minimum energy conformations. Various techniques have been developed for systematic conformational searching of relatively simple molecules and drug–receptor complexes in order to find global minimum structures (for example, references 12 and 13), but they are not extendible to molecules of even moderate complexity because of the enormous computational expense involved. In order to screen initially for likely candidates, methods have been developed[14] to examine the interaction of a probe group with a macromolecule surface at a large number of grid points. Combining the results of searches with different probes representing different characteristics of the relevant ligand is a powerful method of locating both known and unknown binding clefts, especially on protein surfaces. However, these approaches take no account of possible conformational change in either drug or receptor during binding.

The development of molecular dynamics methods[15–18] by which molecular motions can be simulated over a course of time through application of classical equations of motion has enabled much more extensive explorations of complex intra- and intermolecular interactions to be made, and provides a more realistic simulation of a real biological system than the static snapshot provided by the molecular mechanics approach. The methods are extremely expensive in computer time, although the increasing availability of supercomputers is ensuring their widening use. Even so, simulations of drug–receptor complexes are at present restricted to a maximum of a few hundred picoseconds, which is a far shorter timescale than most biological events. In particular, the simulation with atomic resolution of large-scale events, such as protein folding, is many orders of magnitude beyond the capabilities of the current generation of computers.

Treatment of solvent in energy calculations

Most processes of biological interest take place in aqueous solution, and the treatment of solvent effects in simulations is a major consideration. Interaction of a macromolecule with a ligand may require displacement of bound water at the binding site, and solvent can shield electrostatic interactions between components. Explicit inclusion of solvent can be made by means of the 'Monte-Carlo technique' by which water molecules are added to a structure, initially at random, and are then allowed to equilibrate to a physically acceptable arrangement[16,19]. But, to include explicit solvent in a molecular simulation can be computationally very expensive, as it greatly increases the number of atoms, and so the number of interactions, which must be evaluated. The electrostatic shielding factor is generally assumed to be the most important one[20], and so, in many simulations, explicit solvent is not used but alterations are made to the force field to simulate this shielding effect. This greatly increases the speed of the calculations, or, in the case of molecular dynamics the possible duration of the simulation, but the approximations introduced may be excessive, particularly where electrostatic or solvation factors are major contributions to the interaction, as they often are in drug–DNA simulations.

Free-energy calculations

The above discussions have indicated some of the inadequacies of current molecular modelling methodologies in reproducing and ultimately predicting experimental findings. Provided the structures of both drug and receptor are known, current approaches will yield reliable qualitative pictures for modes of interaction. Calculations of the energetics of interactions are, in general, less reliable for the reasons indicated above. However, the more recently developed methods of free-energy perturbation analysis[21,22] are providing much-improved estimates of changes in free energies as opposed to the enthalpy-related quantities determined by molecular mechanics. The new approach combines molecular dynamics calculations with statistical thermodynamics. As yet, relatively few ligand–receptor complexes have been studied by it, in view of the enormous computer resources required. In the test case of the benzamidine–trypsin complex[23], agreement between predicted and experimental free energy is remarkably good. In general, a well-determined high-resolution X-ray structure of the macromolecule involved constitutes an indispensable starting point for an analysis of drug–receptor energetics.

Free-energy perturbation methods have been applied with considerable success to several small-molecule systems of special relevance to cancer chemotherapy. Following a suggestion that two-electron bioreductive compounds might have tumour cell selectivity by virtue of differences in hypoxic properties[24], free-energy methods have been successfully used to calculate redox potential values for simple benzoquinones[25,26] which are good models for compounds of promising utility in this approach. The power of the methods is illustrated by its application to the calculation of free-energy differences for simple alcohols in water compared with carbon tetrachloride[27]. This simulation is, in effect, an estimation of partition coefficients – the calculated log P values are within 0.06 units of experiment. It therefore provides, in principle, a predictive methodology for transport properties of drugs.

Other drug design methods

This section would be incomplete without at least some mention of the important methodologies required when no structural data on the macromolecular target are available, the common situation in drug design.

The Cambridge crystallographic database contains X-ray structural data on over 70 000 organic compounds[28], and is an indispensable tool in these circumstances. Molecular shape analysis and quantitative structure–activity relation (QSAR) methods have been extensively employed[1,3], often in conjunction with the database. A typical approach would use energy minimization (and perhaps dynamic simulation) on several related molecules of varying biological activities, followed by matching ('receptor mapping') of the resulting low-energy features. This technique has been used in a study of phorbol ester tumour promoters (protein kinase C activators) which has identified critical structural features and possible roles for particular chemical groups[30]. Molecular volume considerations have been included, together with molecular mechanics minimizations in studies of steroid hormone-like inhibitors of the cytochrome P450 enzymes, aromatase and lyase[31,32]. A recent extension of shape analysis has been the development of combinatorial methods for computing steric and electrostatic fields – this has been applied with some success to steroids involved in binding to carrier proteins[33].

MOLECULAR MODELLING OF DNA-BINDING DRUGS

These are, in terms of numbers, the most important category of current anticancer drugs. Molecular structural and modelling studies on them have been extensive. In general, ligands can interact with DNA in two distinct ways:

(1) Covalently: with bases, sugars or phosphate groups. The established DNA cross-linking antitumour drugs, such as the nitrogen mustards and *cis*-platinum, all react with nucleophilic atoms of the bases, most commonly guanine or adenine. Access to the bases is via either major or minor grooves of the double helix (Figure 5.1).

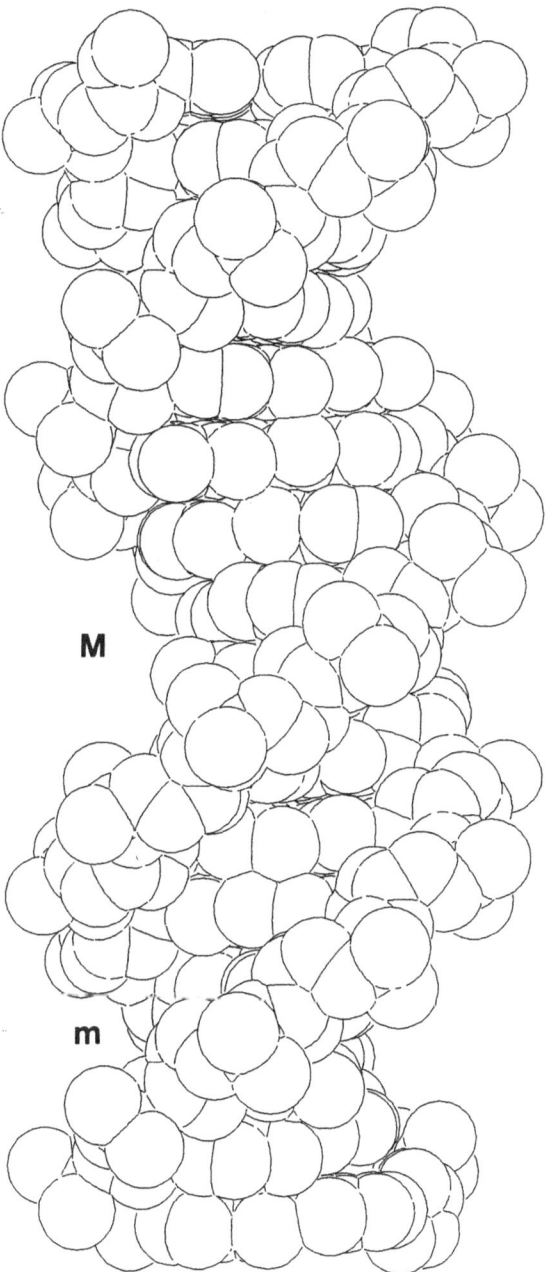

Figure 5.1 The molecular structure of the B form of double-helical DNA. The major and minor grooves are marked M and m, respectively

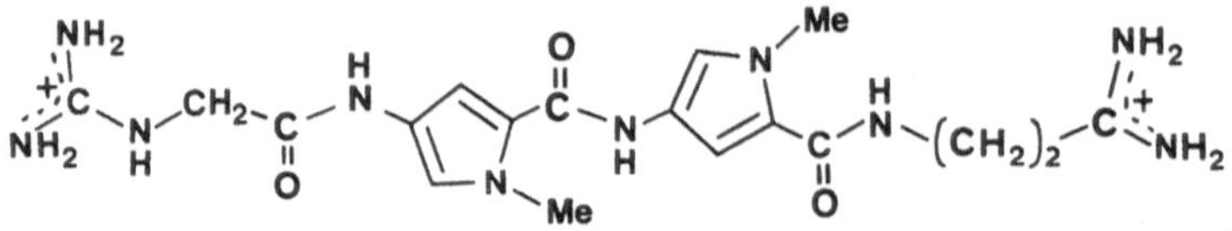

Netropsin

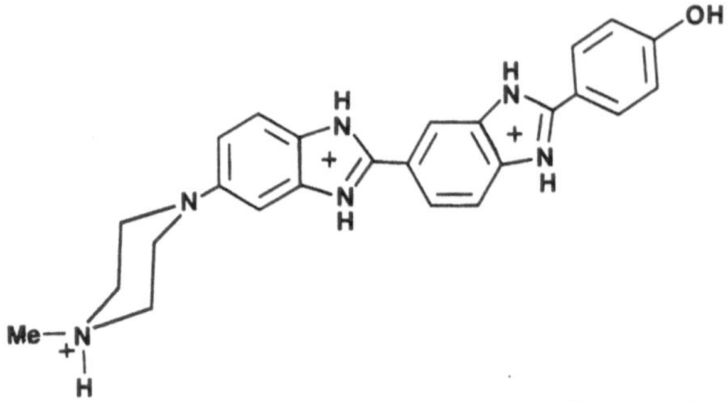

Hoechst 33258

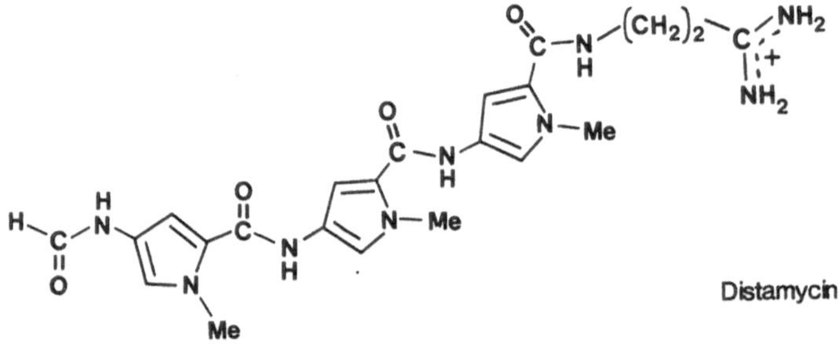

Distamycin

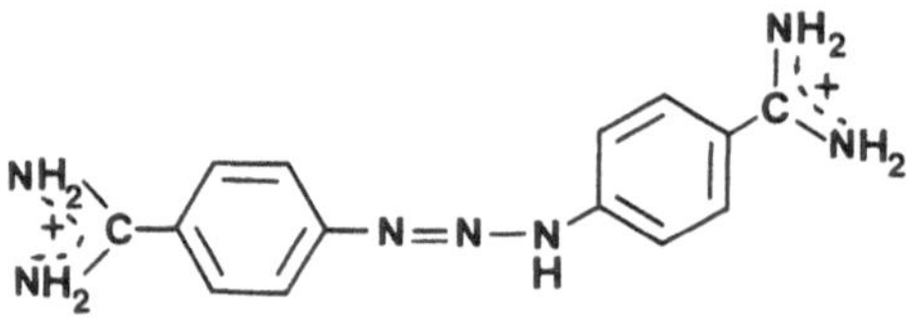

Berenil

Figure 5.2 Structural formulae for some non-covalent groove-binding drugs

(2) Non-covalently: interactions involve hydrogen-bonding, electrostatic and hydrophobic forces. Binding modes can be categorized as:

   (a) Intercalative interaction between base pairs, as shown by Adriamycin, actinomycin and amsacrine (Figure 5.2).

140

(b) Binding in the grooves of a DNA double helix. Non-covalent minor-groove binding has been established for molecules, such as netropsin, Hoechst 33258, distamycin and berenil (Figure 5.2), none of which show significant cytotoxic or antitumour activity. Many in this series have significant antiviral activity.

(c) Generalized external binding to phosphate groups of DNA by electro-static interaction. Polyamines, such as spermine, bind in this manner. It is unlikely that this mode is, by itself, of significance for anticancer drug action on account of its inherent non-selectivity.

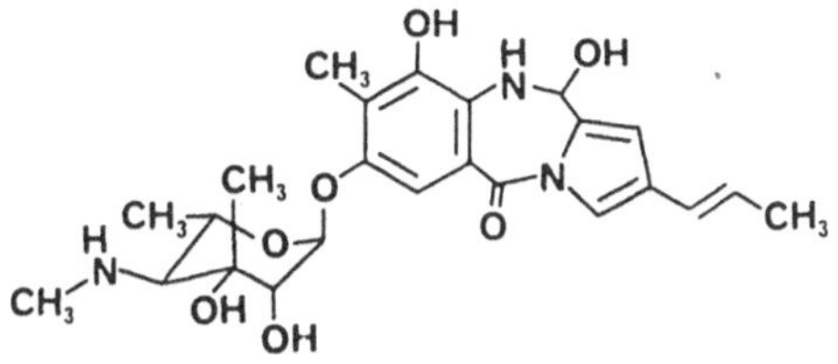

anthramycin

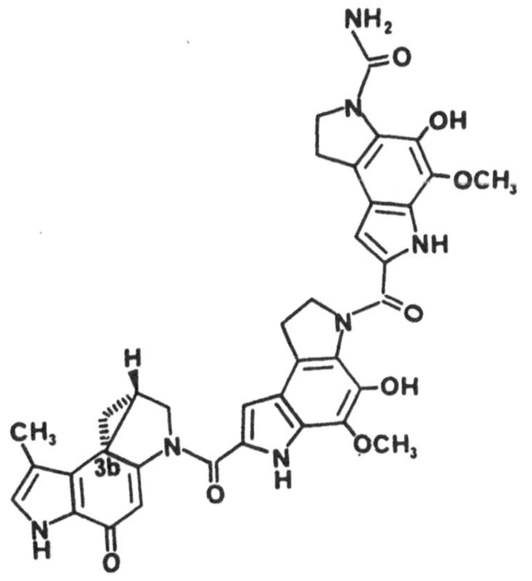

CC-1065

Figure 5.3 Structural formulae for some covalent groove-binding drugs

141

In reality, many small molecules bind to DNA by a combination of these factors[34]. Thus, the potent antitumour agents of the anthramycin series (Figure 5.3) are minor-groove binders, forming covalent bonds to the N2 atoms of guanine residues. Intercalating molecules with attached groups, such as alkyl chains (mitoxantrone), peptide groups (actinomycin, echinomycin) or sugars (the anthracyclines), leave these groups residing in one or other groove where they are stabilized by non-bonded attractive interactions. Sometimes these are specific for particular sequences, with actinomycin and its requirement for a 5′-position guanine being a well-studied example[35].

In general, the necessary (though by themselves insufficient) requirements for antitumour activity are apparently simple: either covalent binding to one of several base sites, possibly with inter/intra-strand cross-linking, or non-covalent intercalative interaction with the intercalating chromophore having an appended side chain or substituent group. This might suggest (erroneously) that the active clinically useful compounds would be non-specific in their interaction with genomic DNA and hence inherently incapable of having a discriminating effect on cancer vs normal cell regulation at the DNA level. Lack of understanding of the molecular basis for the antitumour action shown by DNA-interactive anti-tumour drugs in general, has, until recently, ensured a relatively empirical approach to the development of new drugs. It is now clear that the field is on the threshold of rapid advances based on knowledge of the underlying cell and molecular biology of antitumour action[36], allied with the large body of experimental and theoretical data on drug–DNA complexes *in vitro*.

Molecular modelling of intercalation

The class of intercalators includes some of the currently most clinically effective antitumour drugs, with the anthracyclines, such as Adriamycin, showing broad-spectrum activity. It is now established that DNA sequence selectivity is shown by several members of the class[37,38]. However, this effect appears to be only for a few base pairs at a time, and is thus not, by itself, a critical factor in anticancer terms. The relationship between level of DNA affinity and activity *in vitro* or *in vivo* is complex[39]. Studies indicate that, although there is unsurprisingly no general linear relationship between interaction with DNA and ultimate biological effect, intercalation is a necessary prerequisite (though not by itself sufficient) for anticancer activity[40,41]. Nonetheless, it is well established that, in some individual series of compounds, the relationship can be approximately linear[35]. The critical finding for the understanding of the anticancer activity of many intercalators has been that only those that can stabilize a ternary complex with DNA and the enzyme DNA topoisomerase II, which produces lethal double-strand breaks *in vivo* (this has been termed a 'cleavable complex'[42,43]), have a significant level of antitumour activity. However, as yet there is no structural information at all on this large enzyme, and hence none on the ternary complexes.

Instead, modelling studies have focused on the simpler drug–DNA systems themselves, in the hope that these will provide useful insights into structure–activity relationships, bearing in mind the key importance of the intercalative recognition step in the overall antitumour response.

There are no X-ray or NMR structural data on a drug molecule embedded within a long DNA sequence. The structures available are all, therefore, to be considered as first-order models for biological DNA. The majority are of dinucleoside monophosphate duplexes (for example, references 44, 45 (with ellipticine) and 46). A number, involving daunomycin and related anthracyclines, are with hexanucleotides (see below); in these, the drug is intercalated at the ends of the short hexamer double helix and thus is still not representative of a true intercalation conformation. In the cases of the dinucleoside models, the nucleotide conformations are not dependent on the nature of the bound drug molecule[47] and have been utilized as an approximate model for use in molecular design studies of new intercalators[48]. A number of more general, non-experimentally-based DNA intercalation models have been developed for longer stretches of helix, although few have been energy-refined with an all-atom force field[49-51] or have been derived from molecular dynamics simulations[52,53].

The likely active conformation of the daunomycin and Adriamycin molecules was established by X-ray and conformational analyses on the parent drug[54,55]. The X-ray structure of a daunomycin–hexanucleotide complex with the sequence d(CGTACG)$_2$ shows the drug chromophore intercalating at the CG sites and the daunosamine lying in the minor groove[56,57]. This has been confirmed by subsequent X-ray analyses[58-60] of daunomycin and Adriamycin and several of their derivatives complexed with the sequence d(CGATCG)$_2$ and d(CGTACG)$_2$. The results of these structure determinations show the importance of a number of substituents on the daunomycin molecule, both in terms of DNA binding *in vitro* and in relation to antitumour activity. For example, the essential substituents at C9 are strongly hydrogen bonded to the CG base pairs at the intercalation site. Thus, alterations at C9, even in stereochemistry, would diminish these interactions. Similar arguments can be advanced for the daunosamine substituents. These structural results are fully consistent with DNA-binding characteristics observed in solution for the more recently developed anthracycline analogues, such as the 4' epimer (epirubicin), which have activities comparable to Adriamycin but with improved toxicity profiles[61]. These structural studies show that there is no significant difference between daunomycin and Adriamycin in terms of DNA interaction; however, marked differences in solvent structure surrounding the bound drugs were observed[59], which may relate to differing abilities to form ternary complexes, and hence to their differing anticancer profiles.

Theoretical molecular modelling has correctly predicted the observed DNA sequence-selectivity of the anthracyclines[62]. Calculations of binding energies for several daunomycin derivatives substituted at the 4-position and epimerized at the 7- and 9-positions are in good general agreement with experimental DNA-binding data[63]. This correlation has also been found for analogues, such as the 9-deoxy derivative[64], although it is not biologically active. As with the amsacrine family of compounds, differences in DNA topoisomerase II cleavable complex formation are probably important factors in the manifestation of activity[65].

The acridine compound *m*-AMSA (amsacrine) is used in the clinic in the treatment of acute leukaemia. Many hundreds of derivatives have been synthesized in the search for drugs active, in particular, against solid tumours[66].

There are good correlations for well-defined subclasses of compounds in the series between antitumour activity and DNA binding[67–69], although correlation between subclasses is not always possible. In general, the correlations lend further support to the theory that intercalation is a fundamental determinant of cytotoxicity for acridines, when taken together with other factors. There is no X–ray structure of an acridine drug–oligonucleotide complex, but, instead, a number of molecular modelling studies are available[70–72]. All indicate that the parent drug is a minor-groove intercalator (Figure 5.4). These studies confirm the experimental finding of equivalent DNA-affinity for the biologically inactive *ortho* isomer[69]. Molecular modelling has not, as yet, defined any detailed structural differences between DNA complexes of *ortho* and *meta* isomers, although presumably DNA topoisomerase is able to do so.

Carboxamide derivatives of amsacrine have been found to have high activity *in vivo* against solid tumour models, such as the Lewis lung tumour[73,74], with the structural requirement of heterocyclic chromophore planarity[75]. It is likely that distribution properties are of particular importance for their antitumour activity, although the evidence from molecular modelling[76,77] is that major-groove intercalation is preferred, which may be suggestive of more fundamental differences compared with amsacrine compounds. The 'minimal intercalator' concept has been developed from these studies for carboxamides in general[73], favouring compounds that have lower DNA affinities on account of small chromophore size and, hence, improved distribution properties in solid tumours. Molecular modelling studies[78] on a series of phenyl-substituted phenyl quinoline carboxamides has shown that it is possible to optimize DNA affinity rationally within this series and has related it to improved activity.

The development of the anthraquinone-based compound, mitoxantrone, as a synthetic anthracycline-like drug has been paralleled by molecular modelling studies on it and analogues, including the anthrapyrazoles[48,79–81]. These have shown that mitoxantrone is a DNA major-groove intercalator and that structure–activity data are strongly suggestive of a relationship between DNA affinity and activity *in vitro*. Activity *in vivo* is much less well indicated by quantitative modelling predictions, suggestive of a role for topoisomerase and/or pharmacokinetic factors. Molecular modelling has nonetheless been able to predict the structural features required for a minimal level of activity, such as the need to have side chains with a two-carbon atom link and terminating in a protonated amino group in order to produce effective electrostatic interactions with phosphate groups or bases on the DNA.

Actinomycin is one of the best-studied intercalators with clinically useful activity against Wilms' tumour and gestational choriocarcinoma. It is an inhibitor of transcription and has a near-absolute requirement for guanine at the 3' end of its DNA binding site. Crystal structures of complexes with deoxyguanosine[82] and the dinucleoside phosphate d(GpC)[83] have shown a hydrogen bond between the N2 of guanine and the carbonyl oxygen atom of a threonine residue in the peptide moiety of the drug. However, neither structure shows actinomycin–DNA intercalation directly. A detailed modelling study[49] has provided further support for this explanation of actinomycin sequence selectivity. It is, perhaps, a consequence of the relatively narrow spectrum of antitumour activity shown by this drug that no rational drug design studies

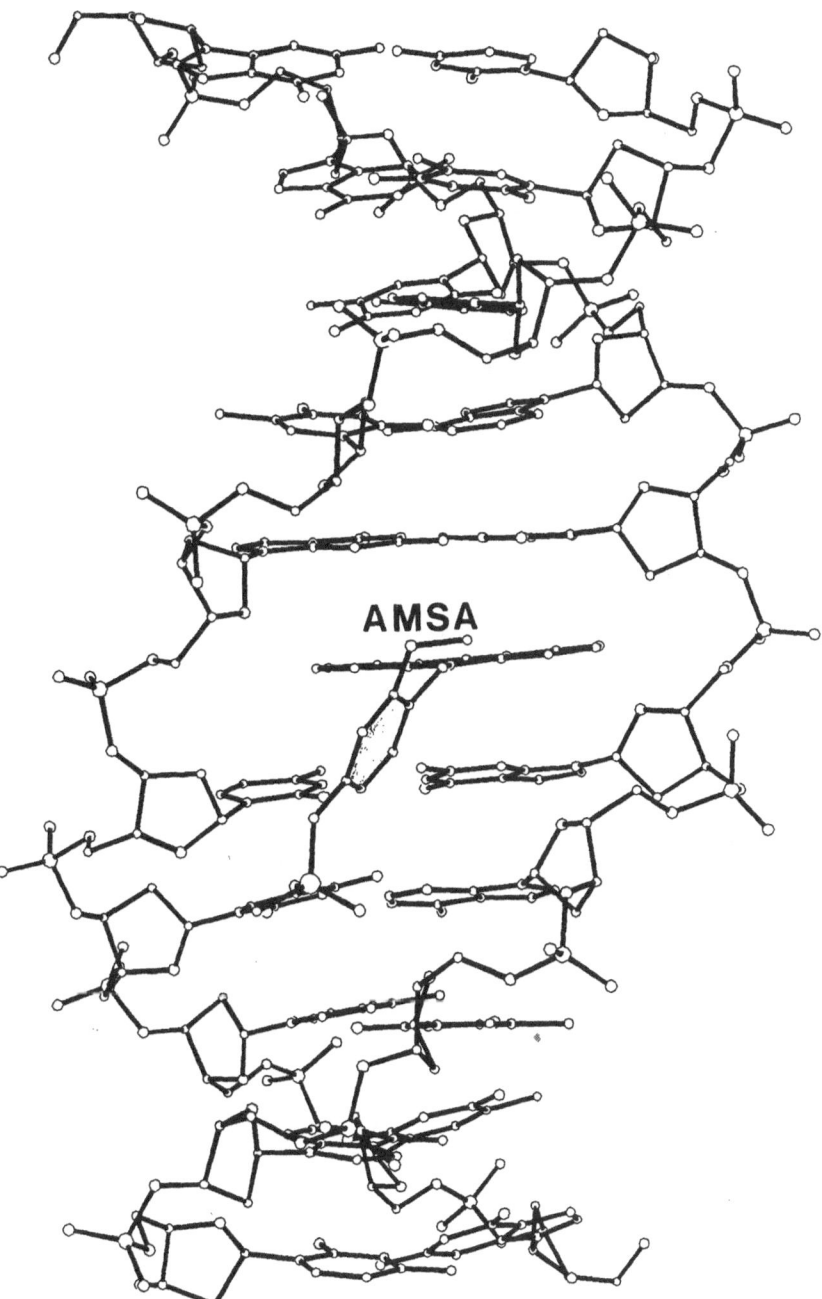

Figure 5.4 Molecular model for amsacrine intercalated into a DNA sequence. The phenyl ring of the drug molecule is shown shaded; it is lying in the minor groove, as indicated by energy calculations[71]

seeking new analogues have been reported, in spite of the exceptionally detailed view of its mode of action on DNA that is now available.

Groove-binding drugs

The antibiotics, netropsin and distamycin, are representative of a large class of natural and synthetic molecules that bind to B-DNA double helices at AT-rich sequences[84]. These drugs are generally only mildly cytotoxic but often have pronounced antiviral activity[85]. Interest in these compounds has increased in recent years with their exploitation as starting points for the rational development of sequence-specific ligands. An often-stated major goal is eventually to recognize selectively a run of 14–16 contiguous base pairs, which is approximately the length of a statistically unique sequence in the human genome of ca 2.5 billion base pairs[86]. Such totally selective recognition could be used to regulate the expression of particular genes, and to compete with regulatory proteins. The binding constraints required to achieve this are of the order of $10^{12}M^{-1}$, which is easily achievable, even with current types of synthetic gene regulators. The stringent recognition requirement of 14–16 nucleotides need not be adhered to in practical terms if one is targeting one of a relatively small number of strongly expressed oncogenes, such as the P53 locus. X-ray crystallographic studies have defined the molecular basis for the interaction of the drugs, netropsin, Hoechst 33258 and berenil, with the dodecanucleotide sequence d(CGCGAATTCGCG)[87–90] and with several related sequences (for example distamycin with d(CGCAAATTTGCG)[91]). All show a drug molecule bound in the minor groove at the AT region, with hydrogen-bond contacts to the bases, especially to atom N3 of adenine or O2 of thymine (Figure 5.5). Theoretical modelling has indicated that minor-groove non-covalent binding has components of hydrogen-bonding (to provide specific directional base recognition), electrostatic and hydrophobic forces[92–94]. A crucial factor governing AT binding in general is that an AT sequence has a smooth minor-groove inner surface, thus enabling an isohelical fit of ligands that have a concave shape into the groove[95]. Attempts have been made to alter systematically the structure of netropsin and distamycin molecules in order to recognize GC sequences as well as AT ones, by the introduction of appropriately positioned hydrogen-bond acceptors that can, in principle, interact with the exocyclic N2 group of a guanine[96,97]. These molecules, termed lexitropsins, are, as yet, only partially successful in being able to switch recognition to GC base pairs. However, they do indicate that the underlying molecular design premise is well founded. A molecular modelling study of berenil interactions with a 60-base-pair DNA sequence has indicated that differences in flexibility between AT and GC regions are important factors in determining selectivity[98].

Covalent binding

There are various sites of covalent attack on DNA bases; guanine is the most susceptible one, with atoms N2, N3 and N7 being preferred. The N3 of adenine

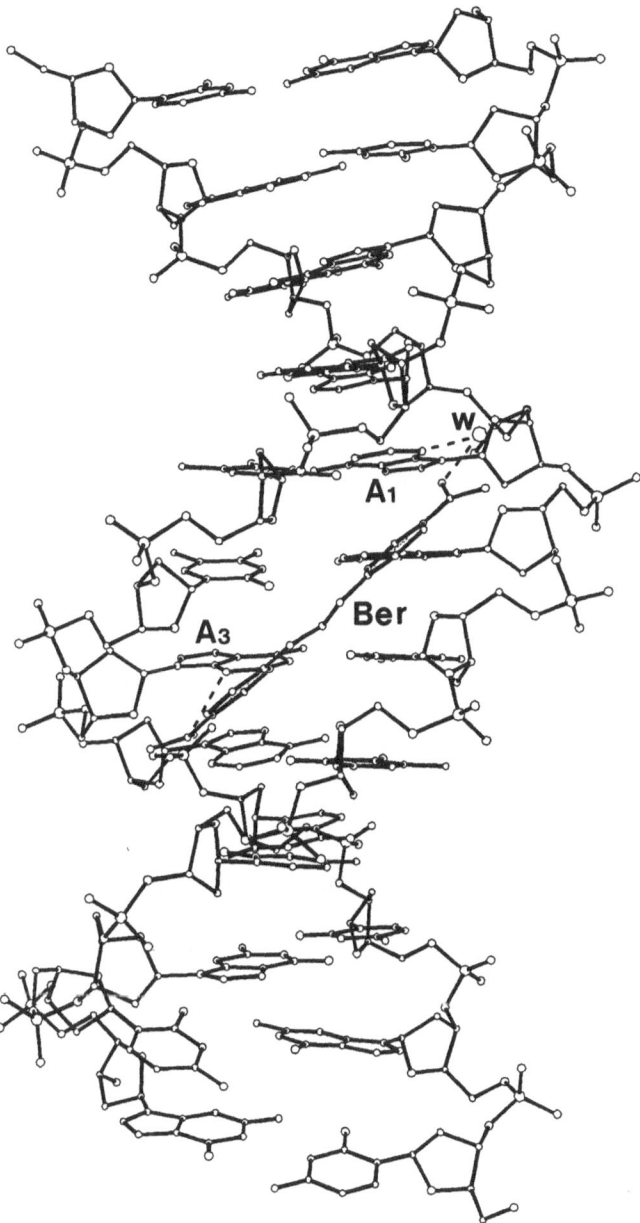

Figure 5.5 The molecular structure of the berenil-d(CGCGAATTCGCG)$_2$ complex, with the drug shown lying in the minor groove of the double helix. The phenyl rings of the drug molecule lie almost in the plane of view. Dashed lines indicate hydrogen bonds between the amidinium groups of the drug and N3 atoms of the adenine bases A1 and A3. In the case of A1, the interaction is indirect, via a water molecule (w). The structure is described further in reference 90

is also a common target. Intra- and/or interstrand cross-linking is possible with bifunctional agents, such as melphalan. There are, as yet, no X-ray structural data on these systems. The minor-groove covalent binders generally produce relatively small-scale perturbations to B-form DNA structure. This has meant that computer modelling studies have had a plausible starting point compared with, for example, *cis*-platinum major-groove cross-linking, which results in major structural changes to B-DNA that are not yet well understood. This difference in the effect on DNA structure between minor- and major-groove binders has an important biological consequence; the lesions produced by a minor-groove-binding drug, such as CC1065, are highly resistant to the action of DNA repair enzymes. It is tempting to speculate that this relates to the extraordinarily high cytotoxicity and antitumour potency of some minor-groove alkylators.

Anthramycin (Figure 5.3) is the best-studied member of the pyrrolo[1,4]benzodiazepine class of antitumour antibiotics[99]. Interaction with double-stranded DNA is at N2 of guanine and shows a preference for purine–guanine–purine sequences. Several molecular modelling studies[100–102] have rationalized much of the fine detail of sequence and orientation preferences. The antibiotic, CC-1065, with three benzodipyrrole subunits (Figure 5.3), is one of the most potent anticancer compounds known[103]. It alkylates adenine at the N3 position and has stringent sequence-specificity requirements, for 5'-AAAAA or 5'-PuNTTA. These may be biologically important sequences for certain regulatory proteins. In part, these preferences may be due to the need for isohelicity, as with the non-covalent groove binders, but, surprisingly, it is now apparent that the major contributor to the sequence effect is a more subtle combination of sequence-induced reactivity and sequence-dependent nucleotide deformability[104,105]. The covalent bonding is largely responsible for the antitumour effects.

A synthetic alkylating derivative of distamycin, N-deformyl-N(4-N,N-bis, (2-chloroethylamino)benzoyl)distamycin, has very high experimental anti-tumour activity[106] and also probably alkylates at the N3 position of adenine. It thus appears that the manifestation of minor-groove sequence selectivity, even at levels much less than 14–16 base pairs, is sufficient for a highly potent antitumour effect. It may well be that this is in part related to the ability of minor-groove-binding drugs to inhibit transcription factor–DNA binding[107], as well as to the lack of repairability of the resulting drug–DNA complex.

Modelling of DNA triple helices

It has been known for some time that, under the right conditions, a DNA duplex can associate with a third polynucleotide strand through the formation of a triple-stranded helix[108]. However, only recently has this phenomenon been exploited as an approach to sequence-specific DNA recognition (for a review, see reference 109). Although there are known to be several types of DNA triple helix, the one that has received the most attention is that resulting from the association of a second polypyrimidine strand with a homopurine/homopyrimidine sequence in a length of duplex DNA. This form may be of importance biologically[110]. Details of the structure of this type of triplex have been elucidated from fibre-diffraction[111,112] and NMR[113–115] data.

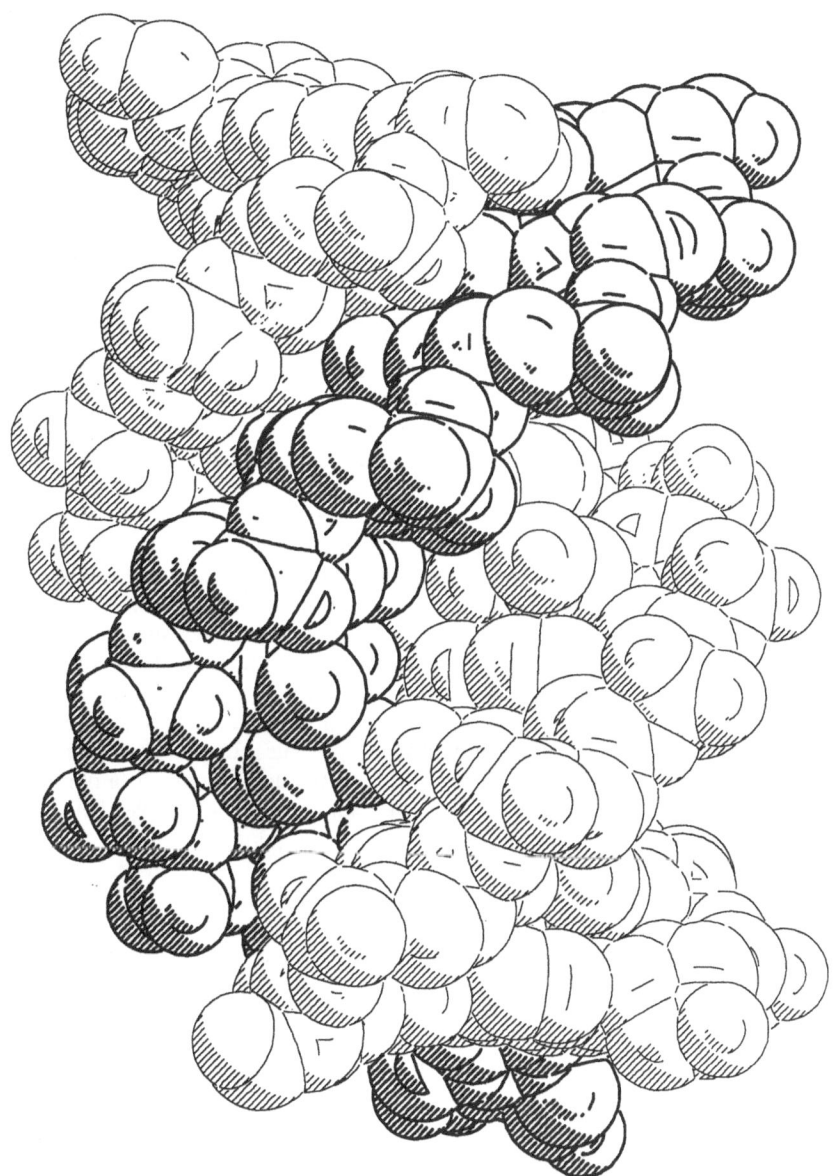

Figure 5.6 The molecular structure of a DNA triple helix, with the Hoogsteen-binding pyrimidine strand in bold

The interaction is basically one of groove binding; the recognition poly-nucleotide strand winds into the major groove of the DNA duplex, interacting with it through the formation of Hoogsteen hydrogen bonds (Figure 5.6). This mode of binding means that, like the anti-sense approach (Chapter 10), triple helix formation has the conceptual advantage over other sequence recognition methods of a one-to-one correspondence between the basic building blocks of the recognition element and those of the target, greatly simplifying the process of designing a ligand for a given DNA sequence. It has the advantage over the anti-sense approach that the target is one of a few copies of a DNA sequence per cell, rather than a large number of mRNA transcripts. Its principal disadvantage at the present time is that effective triple helix formation is restricted to homopurine/homopyrimidine sequences.

Overcoming this limitation is a major goal of much experimental and theoretical work[116,117]. But, even with this limitation, the triple-strand, or 'anti-gene', approach has been used with success to produce artificial repressors[118,119] and restriction enzymes[120], and to direct the attack on DNA of photocross-linkers[121], intercalators[122] and alkylators[123].

Attempts to increase the range of sequences for which triple strand formation can be achieved have been hampered by a lack of detailed structural information. To date, there are no single-crystal X-ray structures of triple helices, and NMR studies have concentrated on a small number of short symmetrical sequences which, in any case, yield only a limited amount of structural data. In such circumstances, the utility of a molecular modelling approach to the study of triple helix structure is evident.

Molecular mechanics has been used to study the effect of 'mismatches' between the duplex sequence and the recognition strand on the stability of the resultant triple helix[124]. The same question has been investigated using molecular dynamics[125]. NMR evidence of perturbations from the fibre diffraction-based model for triplex structure, particularly with regard to sugar puckers, has been supported by other dynamic studies[126,127]. The former of these two studies also examined the effect of substituting methylphosphonates for phosphates on triplex stability. The latter study also related various structural features to a number of experimental observations, including the stabilization of triple helices by polyvalent cations[119] and cationic ligands, such as spermine[128], and interactions between triplexes and groove-binding ligands, such as a distamycin analogue[115].

All these results help to increase our understanding of the forces that hold the triple helix structure together, and how structural modifications might be made to the recognition element in order to overcome the homopurine/homo-pyrimidine sequence limitation, and potentiate binding generally.

ENZYMES AND PROTEINS AS ANTICANCER DRUG TARGETS

Dihydrofolate reductase (DHFR) with the anticancer drug, methotrexate, bound in the folate active site is by far the best-studied of all drug–receptor systems at the atomic level. This enzyme is important in the biosynthetic pathway to thymidine, and, hence, its inhibition can have cytotoxic consequences. The crystal structures of several bacterial DHFRs have been solved, as binary and ternary complexes as well as in ligand-free form[129–131]. Mammalian DHFRs have significant sequence differences compared with the bacterial enzymes – this is shown by the much weaker binding of the antibacterial drug, trimethoprim, to chicken DHFR. These differences have been elucidated by X-ray analysis of the chicken enzyme complex[130] which shows a loss of a drug–valine hydrogen bond and a general movement of active-site residues compared with the bacterial complex. The crystal structure of a human DHFR–folate complex has been reported, with and without bound methotrexate[132]. The drug is bound in the active site quite differently from the structure observed in the complex with enzyme from mouse L1210 cells[133], which may reflect distinct conformational states for the enzyme. In view of this large amount of structural information, many molecular modelling studies have been reported, especially with methotrexate and trimethoprim analogues. Molecular shape analysis has been used in the design of benzylpyrimidine inhibitors[134]. A combination of computer graphics modelling and structure–activity relationship (QSAR) analysis has been used to good effect in order to show that predicted and observed enzyme affinities have a high degree of correlation[135,136]. New analogues of trimethoprim have been designed by graphics modelling whose predicted binding mode has been subsequently verified in detail by crystallographic analysis, although this non-quantitative modelling approach was not able to rationalize the experimental binding affinities[137].

The related enzyme, thymidylate synthase, plays an even more central role in DNA synthesis and has long been established as the major target for 5-fluorouracil. More recently, it has been exploited as a target for new antifolate drugs[138]. Structural studies on the enzyme are at an early stage compared with DHFR and no new drugs have yet been reported that are derived from molecular modelling/crystallographic studies. The determination of the crystal structure of *Lactobacillus casei* thymidylate synthase in the form of its dUMP complex[139] is undoubtedly being followed by homology modelling studies in order to define the three-dimensional structure of the human enzyme (which has high sequence homology with the bacterial one) and thereby circumvent a separate X-ray analysis of the human enzyme. However, the conflicting results on human and murine dihydrofolate reductase[132,133] suggest that this approach requires considerable caution: several crystallographic analyses of thymidylate synthase ternary complexes have been reported. The *Escherichia coli* enzyme has been co-crystallized with 5-fluoro-2'-deoxyuridylate and the antifolate drug, CB3717 (10-propargyl-5,8-dideazafolate)[140,141]; this shows a large conformational change around the active site compared with the dUMP complex of the *L. casei* enzyme. The roles played by conserved residues in these changes present another layer of complexity that must be understood before successful detailed modelling can be undertaken with a view to designing superior new inhibitors of the human enzyme.

The X-ray analyses of the p21 *ras* oncogene protein[142,143] provide the first results on a macromolecule directly involved in human tumours, and are thus of major significance for the future development of highly selective anti-*ras* agents. Changes in the protein on going from inactive (GDP-bound) to active (GTP-bound) states are found in the effector region[143,144]. The structural differences between normal and transforming mutants have also been explored[145] although it is not clear at present how such differences, which tend to change the GTPase activity of p21 and keep it in the 'on' signal state[143,145], can be exploited in chemotherapeutic terms. Cellular and mutant proteins have almost identical structures, with most differences being located in the vicinity of the phosphate. It is likely that knowledge of p21 interactions with its effector molecule will be required in order to understand fully the oncogenic events which it triggers, and eventually exploit the information for rational drug design.

The cytochrome P450 superfamily contains two broad groups of enzymes which are interesting targets for cancer chemotherapy for quite different reasons. Firstly, there is a group of enzymes involved with the oxygenation of (principally aromatic) compounds which are responsible for the metabolic activation of some of the most powerful carcinogens[146,147]. Secondly, there is the group of enzymes involved with steroid biosynthesis which are potential targets in the treatment of hormone-dependent cancers, particularly of the breast and prostate[148].

Because of the varied and vital roles played by the P450 enzymes, it is important to maximize selectivity in the design of inhibitors for these particular targets. The rational design of such inhibitors will require a detailed knowledge of the three-dimensional structures of the relevant enzymes, but, at present, this knowledge is lacking. There is only one enzyme in the P450 superfamily whose crystal structure has been determined, the camphor-binding $P450_{cam}$ from *Pseudomonas putida*. Molecular modelling has been extensively employed in attempts to predict the tertiary structures of other P450 enzymes from this starting point. The bacterial enzymes are soluble, while the eukaryotic ones are membrane bound; however, sequence analysis suggests[149–152] that the membrane-binding region is largely restricted to an N-terminal domain and that the remaining eukaryotic enzymes share a similar tertiary fold to $P450_{cam}$. Molecular modelling has therefore been employed to help predict what effect amino-acid sequence differences between different P450 enzymes will have on the details of this common general fold.

The procedure falls into three general stages. Firstly, the sequence of interest is aligned with that of $P450_{cam}$. Residues that can be equivalenced in this way form the 'core' of the structure. Backbone coordinates for these residues are transferred directly from the $P450_{cam}$ structure. Secondly, the backbone coordinates of the remaining residues, those around insertions and deletions – the 'loops' – are modelled, typically via a database search of known loop structures (for example, reference 153). This step may be skipped if all the residues of interest, e.g. those around the active site, are found in the core. The third step consists of structural refinement in which the positions of the protein backbone atoms and the orientation of the amino-acid side chains are optimized. This, again, may make use of database techniques (see, for example, reference 154) as well as molecular mechanics and dynamics calculations[155].

For cytochrome P450IA1, which has been implicated in the metabolic activation of a number of carcinogens, molecular modelling has led to the prediction of the structure of all but the N-terminal region of the human enzyme[156]. Because of the low overall homology between $P450_{cam}$ and P450IA1 (15% sequence identity), it was necessary to enhance the sequence-alignment method through the use of simultaneous multiple alignments and secondary structure predictions.

The same approach has been applied to the prediction of the structure of the 17α-hydroxylase/C_{17-20} enzyme[157], which catalyses the last step in the biosynthesis of the androgen steroid hormones. The enzyme is predicted to contain an interesting bilobal active site cavity, whose structure may be the key to the dual functionality of this enzyme (Figure 5.7).

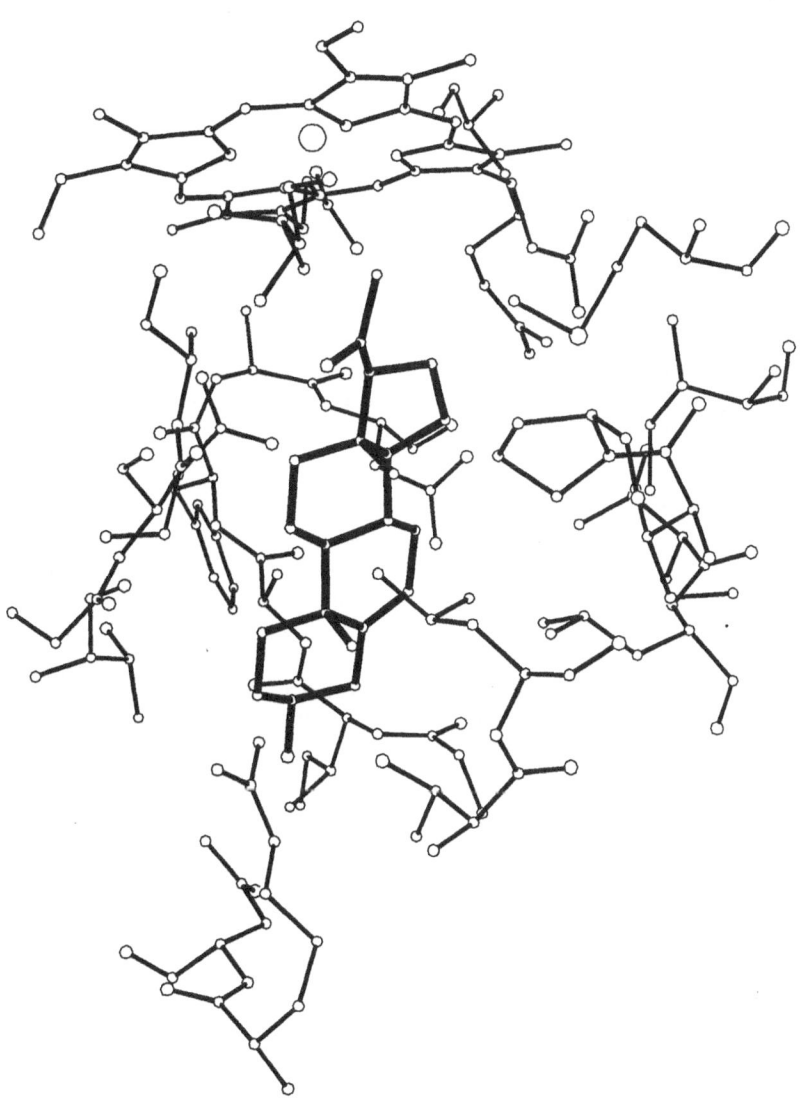

Figure 5.7 Molecular model for the interaction of pregnenolone (in bold) with the predicted structure of the active site of the enzyme 17α-hydroxylase/$C_{17,20}$ lyase. The heme group is visible at the top of the picture

Gene-regulatory proteins – potential future targets

As yet, there is relatively little detailed three-dimensional structural data pertinent to the recognition of DNA sequences by eukaryotic proteins, and consequently scant information on the molecular basis of eukaryotic gene regulation. There is some precise information on bacterial repressor–operator systems, which may be relevant to the future design of synthetic gene regulators, although it is unclear to what extent the principles observed in them are utilized by higher organisms. It has long been presumed that specific DNA base reading is, in general, controlled by the different hydrogen-bonding patterns presented in the major and minor grooves of B-DNA by G.C, C.G, A.T or T.A base pairs (Figure 5.1), with the major groove being sterically preferred. The crystal structures of several repressor-protein–operator complexes from, for example, bacteriophage λ[158] show a common helix-turn-helix structural motif for the protein, with the α-helices fitting into the major groove of the B-DNA recognition sequence. This general pattern has also been observed for the *Eco RI* restriction nuclease–DNA complex[159]. The homeodomain is a DNA-binding motif frequently found in eukaryotic gene regulatory proteins, especially those involved in transcriptional regulation. The crystal structure of its DNA complex shows that its helix-turn-helix structural elements interact with DNA bases and grooves in a manner that is quite distinct in detail from that observed in the bacterial systems[160]. Of particular interest is the minor-groove binding of the N-terminus arm, which may be relevant to the observed inhibitory action of some minor-groove-binding drugs on the binding of transcription factors to DNA[107]. Details of specific amino acid–nucleotide base hydrogen-bond contacts have been surprisingly difficult to generalize to a recognition code since they appear to vary from one complex to another. Indeed, the tryptophan repressor/operator complex[161] does not appear to have any direct amino acid–base hydrogen bonding at all. Instead, recognition seems to involve primarily sequence-dependent structural changes at the sugar–phosphate backbone. This underlines the central importance of understanding the most subtle features of DNA structure, as outlined earlier in this chapter. The other major structural motifs in eukaryotic DNA-regulatory proteins from a wide range of organisms appear to be the 'zinc finger' and the 'leucine zipper'. The former has a pattern of four zinc-binding residues per finger that is folded around the metal ion. There are some structural data on single- and two-finger domains[162–164] from NMR experiments, but no detail for their side-chain orientations. An individual finger almost certainly comprises an α-helix near the C-terminus and an anti-parallel β sheet near the N-terminus arranged around the hydrophobic core. Fingers appear to be modular with little interaction between them. A recent crystal structure of a three-zinc-finger polypeptide complexed with its consensus DNA recognition sequence[165] has shown that each finger resides in the major groove of the DNA double helix, with residues from the N-terminal portion of each α-helix contacting base pairs. Each finger makes similar contacts; however, it is premature to generalize these into a recognition code. The 'leucine zipper' motif comprises a periodic repeat of leucine residues at every seventh position in a region of ca 30 residues. It occurs in a number of transcriptional activator proteins. NMR studies[166] have shown that the unit is α-

helical, with two forming a stable dimer. Knowledge of regulation at the molecular level for oncogenes or drug-resistance genes may well be exploitable in the future, and may lead to highly specific drug therapies, either at the protein or at the DNA level.

CONCLUSIONS

The rational design of new anticancer drugs at the molecular level by computer modelling and X-ray crystallography offers the promise of being able to exploit the increases in our understanding of oncogenic events in molecular and cellular terms, and of eventually leading to highly selective drugs for the treatment of human cancers. In addition, these technologies are now able to provide rationally developed improvements for many existing drugs in terms of optimizing their molecular features responsible for biological activity. The underlying simplistic picture of DNA–drug interaction, whilst not fully explaining the undoubted tumour selectivity of drugs such as Adriamycin and amsacrine, is remarkably effective in providing the basis for the successful application of this rational design. However, the clear limitations of relatively non-specific small molecules (even though the involvement of DNA topoisomerase II in rapidly proliferating tumour cells does enhance their utility beyond earlier expectations) suggest that a future focus of rational drug design on inherently more-selective targets will eventually be more fruitful for effective tumour therapy. X-ray studies on families of oncogenic proteins will provide the basis for computer modelling of specific inhibitors, probably highly disease-type specific. As yet, we do not know whether tumour cells will develop defensive responses to such agents, but it may well be that targeting the genes of such proteins with anti-sense or anti-gene oligonucleotides would circumvent them. Thus, we see that the competing claims of nucleic acids versus their gene products as the better targets for chemotherapy still present an unresolved argument.

References

1. Hopfinger, A. J. (1985). Computer-assisted drug design. *J. Med. Chem.*, **28**, 1133
2. Kollman, P. (1987). Molecular modelling. *Ann. Rev. Phys. Chem.*, **38**, 303
3. Marshall, G. R. (1987). Computer-aided drug design. *Ann. Rev. Pharmacol. Toxicol.*, **27**, 1934.
4. Connolly, M. (1983). Solvent-accessible surfaces of proteins and nucleic acids. *Science*, **221**, 709
5. Weiner, P. K., Langridge, R., Blaney, J. M., Schaefer, R. and Kollman, P. A. (1982). Electrostatic potential molecular surfaces. *Proc. Natl. Acad. Sci. USA*, **79**, 3754
6. Lavery, R. and Pullman, B. (1981). Molecular electrostatic potential on the surface envelopes of macromolecules: B-DNA. *Int. J. Quantum Chem.*, **20**, 259
7. Brooks, B. R., Bruccoleri, R. E., Olafson, H. D., States, D. J., Swaminathan, S. and Karplus, M. (1983). CHARM: a program for macromolecular energy, minimization, and dynamics calculations. *J. Comp. Chem.*, **4**, 187
8. Weiner, S. J., Kollman, P. A., Case, D. A., Singh, U. C., Ghio, C., Alagona, G., Profeta, S. and Weiner, P. (1984). A new force field for molecular mechanical simulation of nucleic acids and proteins. *J. Am. Chem. Soc.*, **106**, 765

9. Weiner, S. J., Kollman, P. A., Nguyen, D. T. and Case, D. A. (1986). An all atom force field for simulations of proteins and nucleic acids. *J. Comput. Chem.*, **7**, 230
10. Weiner, P. K. and Kollman, P. A. (1981). AMBER: assisted model building with energy refinement. A general program for modelling molecules and their interactions. *J. Comput. Chem.*, **2**, 287
11. Van Gunsteren, W. F., Berendsen, H. J. C., Hermans, J., Hol, W. G. J. and Postma, J. P. M. (1983). Computer simulation of the dynamics of hydrated protein crystals and its comparison with X-ray data. *Proc. Natl. Acad. Sci. USA*, **80**. 4315
12. Howard, A. E. and Kollman, P. A. (1988). An analysis of current methodologies for conformational search of complex molecules. *J. Med. Chem.*, **31**, 1669
13. Pearl, L. H. and Neidle, S. (1986). Origins of stereospecificity in DNA damage by anti-benzo[a]pyrene diol-epoxides. *FEBS Lett.*, **209**, 269
14. Goodford, P. J. (1985). A computational procedure for determining energetically favourable binding sites on biologically important macromolecules. *J. Med. Chem.*, **28**. 849
15. Dean, P. M. (1987). *Molecular Foundation of Drug-receptor Interaction*. (Cambridge: Cambridge University Press)
16. McCammon, A. J. and Harvey, S. C. (1987). *Dynamics of Proteins and Nucleic Acids*. (Cambridge: Cambridge University Press)
17. van Gunsteren, W. F. and Berendsen, H. J. C. (1990). Computer simulation of molecular dynamics: methodology, applications and perspectives in chemistry. *Angew. Chem. Int. Ed.*, **29**, 992
18. Brünger, A. T. and Karplus, M. (1991). Molecular dynamics simulations with experimental restraints. *Acc. Chem. Res.*, **24**, 54
19. Richards, W. G., King, P. M. and Reynolds, C. A. (1989). Solvation effects. *Protein Eng.*, **2**, 319
20. Harvey, S. C. (1989). Treatment of electrostatic effects in macromolecular modelling. *Proteins*, **5**, 78
21. Bash, P. A., Singh, U. C., Langridge, R. and Kollman, P. A. (1987). Free energy calculations by computer simulation. *Science*, **236**, 564
22. McCammon, A. J. (1987). Computer-aided molecular design. *Science*, **238**, 486
23. Wong, C. F. and McCammon, J. A. (1986). Dynamics and design of enzymes and inhibitors. *J. Am. Chem. Soc.*, **108**, 3830
24. Reynolds, C. A., Richards, W. G. and Goodford, P. J. (1987). Introducing selectivity into dihydrofolate reductase inhibitors. *Anti-Cancer Drug Design*, **1**, 291
25. Reynolds, C. A., King, P. M. and Richards, W. G. (1988). Accurate redox potentials from theoretical calculations: methyl-substituted benzoquinones. *J. Chem. Soc. Commun.*, 1434
26. Reynolds, C. A., King, P. M. and Richards, W. G. (1988). Computed redox potentials and the design of bioreductive agents. *Nature (London)*, **334**, 80
27. Essex, J. W., Reynolds, C. A. and Richards, W. G. (1989). Relative partition coefficients from partition functions: a theoretical approach to drug transport. *J. Chem. Soc. Chem. Commun.*, 1152
28. Allen, F. H., Bellard, S., Brice, M. D., Cartwright, B. A., Doubleday, A., Higgs, H., Hummelink, T., Hummelink-Peters, B. G., Kennard, O., Motherwell, W. D. S., Rogers, J. R. and Watson, D. G. (1979). The Cambridge Crystallographic Data Centre: computer-based search, retrieval, analysis and display of information. *Acta Crystallogr.* **B35**, 2311
29. Bernstein, F. C., Koetzle, T. F., Williams, G. J. B., Meyer, E. F., Rogers, J. R., Kennard, O., Simanouchi, T. and Tatsumi, M. (1977). The Protein Data Bank: A computer-based archival file for macromolecular structure. *J. Mol. Biol.*, **112**, 535
30. Jeffrey, A. M. and Liskamp, R. M. J. (1986). Computer-assisted molecular modelling of tumour promoters: Rationale for the activity of phorbol esters, telecidin B, and aplysiatoxin. *Proc. Natl. Acad. Sci. USA*, **84**, 241
31. Laughton, C. A., McKenna, R., Neidle, S., Jarman, M., McCague, R. and Rowlands, M. G. (1990). Crystallographic and molecular modelling studies on 3-ethyl-3-(4-pyridyl)piperidine-2,6-dione and its butyl analogue, inhibitors of mammalian aromatase. Comparison with natural substrates: Prediction of enantioselectivity for N-alkyl derivatives. *J. Med. Chem.*, **33**, 2673
32. Laughton, C. A. and Neidle, S. (1990). Inhibitors of the P450 enzymes aromatase and lyase. Crystallographic and molecular modelling studies suggest structural features of pyridyl acetic derivatives responsible for differences in enzyme inhibitory activity. *J. Med. Chem.*, **33**, 3055
33. Cramer, R. D. III, Patterson, E. D. and Bunce, J. D. (1988). Comparative molecular field analysis (CoMFA). 1. Effect of shape on binding of steroids to carrier proteins. *J. Am. Chem. Soc.*, **110**, 5959

34. Waring, M. J. (1981). DNA modification and cancer. *Ann. Rev. Biochem.*, **50**, 159
35. Neidle, S. (1979). The molecular basis for the action of some DNA-binding drugs. *Prog. Med. Chem.*, **16**, 151
36. Hurley, L. H. (1989). DNA and associated targets for drug design. *J. Med. Chem.*, **32**, 2027
37. Phillips, D. R. and Crothers, D. M. (1986). Kinetics and sequence specificity of drug–DNA interactions: an *in vitro* transcription assay. *Biochemistry*, **25**, 7355
38. Chaires, J. B., Fox, K. R., Herrera, J. E., Britt, M. and Waring, M. J. (1987). Site and sequence specificity of daunomycin–DNA interaction. *Biochemistry*, **26**, 8227
39. Wilson, W. R. and Jones, R. L. (1981). Intercalation drugs: DNA binding and molecular pharmacology. *Adv. Pharmacol. Chemother.*, **18**, 177
40. Denny, W. A. (1989). DNA-intercalating ligands as anti-cancer drugs: Prospects for future design. *Anti-Cancer Drug Design*, **4**, 241
41. Baguley, B. C., Denny, W. A., Atwell, G. J. and Cain, B. F. (1981). Potential antitumour agents. 35. Quantitative relationships between antitumour (L1210) potency and DNA binding for 4'-(9-acridinylamino)-methanesulfon-m-anisidide analogues. *J. Med. Chem.*, **24**, 520
42. Nelson, E. M., Tewey, K. M. and Liu, L. F. (1984). Mechanism of antitumour drug action: Poisoning of mammalian DNA topoisomerase II on DNA by 4'-(9-acridinylamino) methanesulfon-m-anisidide. *Proc. Natl. Acad. Sci. USA*, **81**, 1361
43. Pommier, Y., Schwartz, R. E., Zwelling, L. A. and Kohn, K. W. (1985). Effects of DNA intercalating agents on topoisomerase II induced DNA strand cleavage in isolated mammalian cell nuclei. *Biochemistry*, **24**, 6406
44. Neidle, S., Achari, A., Taylor, G. L., Berman, H. M., Carrell, H. L., Glusker, J. P. and Stallings, W. C. (1977). Structure of a dinucleoside phosphate–drug complex as model for nucleic-acid interaction. *Nature (London)*, **269**, 304
45. Jain, S. C., Bhandary, K. K. and Sobell, H. M. (1979). Visualization of drug–nucleic acid interactions at atomic resolution. *J. Mol. Biol.*, **135**, 813
46. Shieh, H. S., Berman, H. M., Dabrow, M. and Neidle, S. (1980). The structure of drug–deoxydinucleoside phosphate complex: generalized conformational behaviour of intercalation complexes with RNA and DNA fragments. *Nucleic Acids Res.*, **8**, 85
47. Berman, H. M., Neidle, S. and Stodola, R. K. (1978). Drug–nucleic acid interactions: Conformational flexibility at the intercalation site. *Proc. Natl. Acad. Sci. USA*, **75**, 828
48. Islam, S. A., Neidle, S., Gandecha, B. M., Partridge, M., Patterson, L. H. and Brown, J. R. (1985). Comparative computer graphics and solution of the DNA interaction of substituted anthraquinones based on doxorubicin and mitoxantrone. *J. Med. Chem.*, **28**, 857
49. Lybrand, T. P., Brown, S. C., Creighton, S., Shafer, R. H. and Kollman, P. A. (1986). Computer modelling of actinomycin D interactions with double-helical DNA. *J. Mol. Biol.*, **191**, 495
50. Neidle, S., Pearl, L. H., Herzyk, P. and Berman, H. M. (1988). A molecular model for proflavine–DNA intercalation. *Nucleic Acids Res.*, **16**, 8999
51. Pullman, B. (1989). Molecular mechanisms of specificity in DNA–antitumour drug interactions. *Adv. Drug Res.*, **18**, 1
52. Prabhakaran, M. and Harvey, S. C. (1985). Molecular dynamics anneals large-scale deformations of model macromolecules: stretching the DNA double helix to form an intercalation site. *J. Phys. Chem.*, **89**, 5767
53. Prabhakaran, M. and Harvey, S. C. (1988). Molecular dynamics of structural transitions and intercalation in DNA. *Biopolymers*, **27**, 1239
54. Neidle, S. and Taylor, G. (1977). Nucleic acid binding drugs. Part IV. The crystal structure of the anti-cancer agent daunomycin. *Biochim. Biophys. Acta*, **479**, 450
55. Islam, S. A. and Neidle, S. (1983). Nucleic acid binding drugs. VII. Molecular mechanics studies on the conformational properties of the anti-cancer drug daunomycin: Some observations of the use of differing potential-energy functions. *Acta Crystallogr.*, **B39**, 114
56. Quigley, G. J., Wang, A. H.-J., Ughetto, G., van der Marel, G., van Boom, J. H. and Rich, A. (1980). Molecular structure of an anticancer drug–DNA complex: Daunomycin plus d(CpGpTpApCpGp). *Proc. Natl. Acad. Sci. USA*, **77**, 7204
57. Wang, A. H.-J., Ughetto, G., Quigley, G. J. and Rich, A. (1987). Interactions between an anthracycline antibiotic and DNA: molecular structure of daunomycin complexed to d(CpGpTpApCpGp) at 1.2-Å resolution. *Biochemistry*, **26**, 1152
58. Moore, M. H., Hunter, W. N., Langlois-D'Estaintot, B. and Kennard, O. (1989). DNA–drug interactions. The crystal structure of d(CGATCG) complexed with daunomycin. *J. Mol. Biol.*, **206**, 693

59. Frederick, C. A., Williams. L. D., Ughetto, G., van der Marel, G. A., van Boom, J. H., Rich, A. and Wang, A. H.-J. (1990). Structural comparison of anticancer drug–DNA complexes: Adriamycin and daunomycin. *Biochemistry*, **29**, 2538

60. Williams, L. D., Frederick, C. A., Ughetto, G. and Rich, A. (1990). Ternary interactions of spermine with DNA: 4'-epi-adriamycin and other DNA:anthracycline complexes. *Nucleic Acids Res.*, **18**, 5533

61. Bonfante, V., Ferrari, L., Brambilla, C., Rossi, A., Villani, F., Crippa, F., Valagussa, P. and Bonadonna, G. (1986). New anthracycline analogs in advanced breast cancer. *Eur. J. Cancer Clin. Oncol.*, **22**, 1379

62. Chen, K.-X., Gresh, N. and Pullman, B. (1986). A theoretical investigation on the sequence selective binding of Adriamycin to double-stranded polynucleotides. *Nucleic Acids Res.*, **14**, 5, 2251

63. Chen, K.-X., Gresh, N. and Pullman, B. (1986). A theoretical study of the comparative binding affinities of daunomycin derivatives to a double-stranded oligomeric DNA. Proposals of new high affinity derivatives. *Mol. Pharmacol.*, **30**, 279

64. Gresh, N., Pullman, B., Arcamone, F., Menozzi, M. and Tonani, R. (1989). Joint experimental and theoretical investigation of the comparative DNA binding affinities of intercalating anthracycline derivatives. *Mol. Pharmacol.*, **35**, 251

65. Zunino, F. and Capranico, G. (1990). DNA topoisomerase II as the primary target for anti-tumour anthracyclines. *Anti-Cancer Drug Design*, **5**, 307

66. Baguley, B. C. and Finlay, G. J. (1988). Derivatives of amsacrine: Determinants required for high activity against Lewis lung carcinoma. *J. Natl. Cancer Inst.*, **80**, 195

67. Baguley, B. C., Denny, W. A., Atwell, G. J. and Cain, B. F. (1981). Potential antitumour agents. 35. Quantitative relationships between antitumour (L1210) potency and DNA binding for 4'-(9-acridinylamino)-methanesulfon-m-anisidide analogues. *J. Med. Chem.*, **24**, 520

68. Baguley, B. C., Denny, W. A., Atwell, G. J. and Cain, B. F. (1981). Potential antitumour agents. 34. Quantitative relationships between DNA binding and molecular structure for 9-anilinoacridines substituted in the anilino ring. *J. Med. Chem.*, **24**, 170

69. Wilson, W. R., Baguley, B. C., Wakelin, L. P. G. and Waring, M. J. (1981). Interaction of the antitumour drug 4'-(9-acridinylamino)methanesulfon-m-anisidide and related acridines with nucleic acids. *Mol. Pharmacol.*, **20**, 404

70. Neidle, S., Abraham, Z. H. L., Collier, D. A. and Islam, S. A. (1987). Application of computer-assisted modelling to structure–activity studies with intercalating drugs. In Harrap, K. R. and Connors, T. A. (eds.) *New Avenues in Developmental Cancer Chemotherapy*. (Florida: Academic Press)

71. Abraham, Z. H. L., Agbandje, M., Neidle, S. and Acheson, R. M. (1988). Experimental DNA-binding and computer modelling studies on an analogue of the anti-tumour drug amsacrine. *J. Biomol. Struct. Dynamics*, **6**, 471

72. Chen, K. X., Gresh, N. and Pullman, B. (1988). Energetics and stereochemistry of DNA complexation with the antitumour AT specific intercalators tilorone and m-AMSA. *Nucleic Acids Res.*, **16**, 3061

73. Atwell, G. J., Box, C. D., Baguley, B. C. and Denny, W. A. (1988). Potential antitumour agents. 56. "Minimal" DNA-intercalating ligands as antitumour drugs: Phenylquinoline-8-carboxamides. *J. Med. Chem.*, **31**, 1048

74. Denny, W. A., Atwell, G. J., Rewcastle. G. W. and Baguley, B. C. (1987). Potential antitumour agents. 49. 5-substituted derivatives of N-[2-dimethylamino)ethyl]-9-aminoacridine-4-carboxamide with *in vivo* solid-tumour activity. *J. Med. Chem.*, **30**, 658

75. Palmer, B. D., Rewcastle, G. W., Atwell, G. J., Baguley, B. C. and Denny, W. A. (1988). Potential antitumour agents. 54. Chromophore requirements for *in vivo* antitumour activity among the general class of linear tricyclic carboxamides. *J. Med. Chem.*, **31**, 707

76. Hudson, B. D., Kuroda, R., Denny, W. A. and Neidle, S. (1987). Crystallographic and molecular mechanics calculations on the anti-tumour drugs N[-(2-dimethylamino)ethyl]- and N-[2-dimethylamino)butyl]-9-aminoacridine-4-carboxamides and their dications: Implications for models of DNA-binding. *J. Biomol. Struct. Dynamics*, **5**, 145

77. Chen, K.-X., Gresh, N. and Pullman, B. (1987). Groove selectivity in the interaction of 9-aminoacridine-4-carboxamide antitumour agents with DNA. *FEBS Lett.*, **224**, 361

78. McKenna, R., Beveridge, A. J., Jenkins, T. C., Neidle, S. and Denny, W. A. (1989). Molecular modelling of DNA–antitumour drug intercalation interactions: correlation of structural and energetic features with biological properties for a series of phenylquinoline-8-carboxamide compounds. *Mol. Pharmacol.*, **35**, 720

79. Chen, K.-X., Gresh, N. and Pullman, B. (1986). A theoretical investigation on the sequence selective binding of mitoxantrone to double-stranded tetranucleotides. *Nucleic Acids Res.*, **9**, 3799

80. Chen, K.-X., Gresh, N. and Pullman, B. (1987). A theoretical study of the intercalative binding of the anti-tumour drug anthrapyrazole to double-stranded oligonucleotides. *Anti-Cancer Drug Design*, **2**, 70

81. Collier, D. A. and Neidle, S. (1988). Synthesis, molecular modelling, DNA binding, and antitumour properties of some substituted amidoanthraquinones. *J. Med. Chem.*, **31**, 847

82. Sobell, H. M. and Jain, S. C. (1972). Stereochemistry of actinomycin binding to DNA II. Detailed molecular model of actinomycin–DNA complex and its implications. *J. Mol. Biol.*, **68**, 21

83. Takusagawa, F., Dabrow, M., Neidle, S. and Berman, H. M. (1982). The structure of a pseudo intercalated complex between actinomycin and the DNA binding sequence d(GpC). *Nature* (*London*), **296**, 466–469

84. Zimmer, C. and Wähnert, U. (1986). Nonintercalating DNA-binding ligands: specificity of the interaction and their use as tools in biophysical, biochemical and biological investigations of the genetic material. *Prog. Biphys. Mol. Biol.*, **47**, 31

85. De Clercq, E. D. and Dann, O. (1980). Diaryl amidine derivatives as oncornaviral DNA polymerase inhibitors. *J. Med. Chem.*, **23**, 787

86. Dervan, P. B. (1986). Design of sequence-specific DNA-binding molecules. *Science*, **232**, 646

87. Kopka, M. L., Yoon, C., Goodsell, D., Pjura, P. and Dickerson, R. E. (1985). Binding of an antitumour drug to DNA. Netropsin and C-G-C-G-A-A-T-T-BrC-G-C-G. *J. Mol. Biol.*, **183**, 553

88. Pjura, P. E., Grzeskowiak, K. and Dickerson, R. E. (1987). Binding of Hoechst 33258 to the minor groove of B-DNA. *J. Mol. Biol.*, **197**, 257

89. Teng, M.-K., Usman, N., Frederick, C. A. and Wang, A. H.-J. (1988). The molecular structure of the complex of Hoechst 33258 and the DNA dodecamer d(CGCGAATTCGCG). *Nucleic Acids Res.*, **16**, 2671

90. Brown, D., Sanderson, M. R., Skelly, J. V., Jenkins, T. C., Brown, T., Garman, E., Stuart, D. I. and Neidle, S. (1990). Crystal structure of a berenil–dodecanucleotide complex: The role of water in sequence-specific ligand binding. *EMBO J.*, **9**. 1329

91. Coll, M., Frederick, C. A., Wang, A. H.-J. and Rich, A. (1987). A bifurcated hydrogen-bonded conformation in the d(A.T) base pairs of the DNA dodecamer d(CGCAAATTTGCG) and its complex with distamycin. *Proc. Natl. Acad. Sci. USA*, **84**, 8385

92. Caldwell, J. and Kollman, P. (1986). A molecular mechanical study of netropsin–DNA interactions. *Biopolymers*, **25**, 249

93. Gago, F., Reynolds, C. A. and Richards, W. G. (1989). The binding of nonintercalative drugs to alternating DNA sequences. *Mol. Pharmacol.*, **35**, 232

94. Pearl, L. H., Skelly, J. V., Hudson, B. D. and Neidle, S. (1987). The crystal structure of the DNA-binding drug berenil: molecular modelling studies of berenil–DNA complexes. *Nucleic Acids Res.*, **15**, 3469

95. Goodsell, D. and Dickerson, R. E. (1986). Isohelical analysis of DNA groove-binding drugs. *J. Med. Chem.*, **29**, 727

96. Lown, J. W. (1988). Lexitropsins: rational design of sequence reading agents as novel anti-cancer agents and potential cellular probes. *Anti-Cancer Drug Design*, **3**, 25

97. Lee, M., Krowicki, K., Hartley, J. A., Pon, R. T. and Lown, J. W. (1988). Molecular recognition between oligopeptides and nucleic acids: influence of van der Waals contacts in determining the 3'-terminus of DNA sequences read by monocationic lexitropsins. *J. Am. Chem. Soc.*, **110**, 3641

98. Laughton, C. A., Jenkins, T. C., Fox, K. R. and Neidle, S. (1990). Interaction of berenil with the *tyrT* DNA sequence studied by footprinting and molecular modelling. Implications for the design of sequence-specific DNA recognition agents. *Nucleic Acids Res.*, **18**. 4479

99. Hurley, L. H., Reck, T., Thurston, D. E. and Langley, D. R. (1988). Pyrrolo[1,4]benzodiazepine antitumour antibiotics: Relationship of DNA alkylation and sequence specificity to the biological activity of natural and synthetic compounds. *Chem. Res. Toxicol.*, **1**, 258

100. Rao, S. N., Chandra Sing, U. and Kollman, P. A. (1986). Molecular mechanics simulations on covalent complexes between anthramycin and B-DNA. *J. Med. Chem.*, **29**, 2484

101. Remers, W. A., Mabilia, M. and Hopfinger, A. J. (1986). Conformations of complexes between pyrrolo[1,4]benzodiazepines and DNA segments. *J. Med. Chem.*, **29**, 2492

102. Zakrzewska, K. and Pullman, B. (1986). A theoretical investigation of the sequence specificity in the binding of the antitumour drug anthramycin to DNA. *J. Biomol. Struct. Dynamics*, **4**, 127

103. Warpehoski, M. A. and Hurley, L. H. (1988). Sequence selectivity of DNA covalent modification. *Chem. Res. Toxicol.*, **1**, 315
104. Hurley, L. H., Lee, C.-S., McGovren, P., Warpehoski, M. A., Mitchell, M. A., Kelly, R. C. and Aristoff, P. A. (1988). Molecular basis for sequence-specific DNA alkylation by CC-1065. *Biochemistry*, **27**, 3886
105. Warpehoski, M. A., Gebhard, I., Kelly, R. C., Krueger, W. C., Li, L. H., McGovren, J. P., Praire, M. D., Wicnienski, N. and Wierenga, W. (1988). Stereoselectivity factors influencing the biological activity of DNA interaction of synthetic antitumour agents modelled on CC-1065. *J. Med. Chem.*, **31**, 590
106. Arcamone, F. M., Animati, F., Barbieri, B., Configliacchi, E. D., Alessio, R., Geroni, C., Giuliani, F. C., Lazzari, E., Menozzi, M., Mongelli, N., Penco, S. and Verini, M. A. (1989). Synthesis, DNA-binding properties and anti-tumour activity of novel distamycin derivatives. *J. Med. Chem.*, **32**, 774
107. Broggini, M., Ponti, M., Ottolenghi, S., D'Incalci, M., Mongelli, N. and Mantovani, R. (1989). Distamycins inhibit the binding of OTF-1 and NFE-1 trans factors to their conserved DNA elements. *Nucleic Acids Res.*, **17**, 1051
108. Felsenfeld, G., Davies, D. R. and Rich, A. (1957). Formation of a three-stranded polynucleotide molecule. *J. Am. Chem. Soc.*, **79**, 2023–2024
109. Moffat, A. A. (1991). Triplex DNA finally comes of age. *Science*, **252**, 1374–1375
110. Wells, R. D., Collier, D. A., Hanvey, J. C., Shimizu, M. and Wohlrab, F. (1988). The chemistry and biology of unusual DNA structures adopted by oligopurine.oligopyrimidine sequences. *FASEB J.*, **2**, 2939–2949
111. Arnott, S., Bond, P. J., Selsing, E. and Smith, P. J. C. (1976). Models of triple-stranded polynucleotides with optimised stereochemistry. *Nucleic Acids Res.*, **11**, 4141–4155
112. Arnott, S. and Selsing, E. (1974). Structures of the polynucleotide complexes poly(dA).poly(dT) and poly(dT).poly(dA).poly(dT). *J. Mol. Biol.*, **88**, 509–521
113. Rajagopal, P. and Feigon, J. (1989). NMR studies of triple-strand formation from the homopurine-homopyrimidine deoxyribonucleotides d(GA)$_4$ and d(TC)$_4$. Biochemistry, **28**, 7859–7870
114. Pilch, D. A., Levenson, C. and Shafer, R. H. (1990). Structural analysis of the (dA)$_{10}$.2(dT)$_{10}$ triple helix. *Proc. Natl. Acad, Sci. USA*, **87**, 1942–1946
115. Umemoto, K., Sarma, M. H., Gupta, G., Luo, J. and Sarma, R. H. (1990). Structure and stability of a DNA triple helix in solution: NMR studies on d(T)$_6$.d(A)$_6$d(T)$_6$ and its complex with a minor groove binding drug. *J. Am. Chem. Soc.*, **112**, 4539–4545
116. Horne, D. A. and Dervan, P. B. (1990). Recognition of mixed-sequence duplex DNA by alternate-strand triple-helix formation. *J. Am. Chem. Soc.*, **112**, 2435–2437
117. Griffin, L. C. and Dervan, P. B. (1989). Recognition of thymine.adenine base pairs by a guanine in a pyrimidine triple helix motif. *Science*, **245**, 967–971
118. Coone, M., Czernuszewicz, G., Postel, E. H., Flint, S. J. and Hogan, M. E. (1988). Site-specific oligonucleotide binding represses transcription of the human *c-myc* gene *in vitro*. *Science*, **241**, 456–459
119. Maher, L. J. III, Wold, B. and Dervan, P. B. (1989). Inhibition of DNA binding proteins by oligonucleotide-directed triple helix formation. *Science*, **245**, 725–730
120. Strobel, S. A. and Dervan, P. B. (1990). Site-specific cleavage of a yeast chromosome by oligonucleotide-directed triple-helix formation. *Science*, **249**, 73–75
121. Praseuth, D., Perrouault, L., Le Doan, T. L., Chassignol, M., Thuong, N. and Helene, C. (1988). Sequence-specific binding and photo-crosslinking of α and β oligodeoxynucleotides to the major groove of DNA via triple-helix formation. *Proc. Natl. Acad. Sci. USA*, **85**, 1349–1353
122. Birg, F., Praseuth, D., Zerial, A., Thuong, N. T., Asseline, U., Le Doan, T. and Helene, C. (1990). Inhibition of Simian virus 40 DNA replication in CV-1 cells by an oligodeoxynucleotide covalently linked to an intercalating agent. *Nucleic Acids Res.*, **18**, 2901–2908
123. Povsic, T. J. and Dervan, P. B. (1990). Sequence-specific alkylation of double-helical DNA by oligonucleotide-directed triple-helix formation. *J. Am. Chem. Soc.*, **112**, 9428–9430
124. Sun, J. S., Mergny, J. L., Lavery, R., Montenay-Garestier, T., and Hélène, C. (1992). Triple helix structures: sequence dependence, flexibility and mismatch effects. *J. Biomol. Struct. Dynamics*, **9**, 411
125. Laughton, C. A. and Neidle, S. (1991). DNA triple helices – a molecular dynamics study. *J. Chim. Phys.* **88**, 2597

126. Hausheer, F. H., Singh, U. C., Saxe, J. D., Colvin, O. M. and T'so, P. O. P. (1990). Can oligonucleotide methylphosphonates form a stable triplet with a double DNA helix? *Anti-Cancer Drug Design*, **5**, 159–167

127. Laughton, C. A. and Neidle, S. (1992). A molecular dynamics simulation of the DNA triplex d(TC)$_5$.d(GA)$_5$.d(C+T)$_5$, *J. Mol. Biol.* **223**, 519

128. Hampel, K. J., Crosson, P. and Lee, J. S. (1991). Polyamines favor DNA triplex formation at neutral pH. *Biochemistry*, **30**, 4455

129. Matthews, D. A., Alden, R. A., Bolin, J. T., Filman, D. J., Freer, S. T., Hamlin, R., Hol, W. G. J., Kisliuk, R. L., Pastore, E. J., Plante, L. T., Xuong, N.-H. and Kraut, J. (1978). Dihydrofolate reductase from lactobacillus casei. *J. Biol. Chem.*, **253**, 6946

130. Matthews, D. A., Bolin, J. T., Burridge, J. M., Filman, D. J., Volz, W. K., Kaufman, B. T., Beddell, C. R., Champness, J. N., Stammers, D. K. and Kraut, J. (1985). Refined crystal structures of Escherichia coli and chicken liver dihydrofolate reductase containing bound trimethoprim. *J. Biol. Chem.*, **260**, 381

131. Filman, D. J., Bolin, J. T., Matthews, D. A. and Kraut, J. (1982). Crystal structures of Escherichia coli and Lactobacillus casei dihydrofolate reductase refined at 1.7 Å resolution. *J. Biol. Chem.*, **257**, 16336

132. Oefner, C., D'Arcy, A. and Winkler, F. K. (1988). Crystal structure of human dihydrofolate reductase complexed with folate. *Eur. J. Biochem.*, **174**, 337

133. Stammers, D. K., Champness, J. N., Beddell, C. R., Dann, J. G., Eliopulos, E., Geddes, A. J., Ogg, D. and North, A. C. T. (1987). The structure of mouse L1210 dihydrofolate reductase–drug complexes and the construction of a model of human enzymes. *FEBS Lett.*, **218**, 178

134. Mabilia, M., Pearlstein, R. A. and Hopfinger, A. J. (1985). Molecular shape analysis and energetics-based intermolecular modelling of benzylpyrimidine dihydrofolate reductase inhibitors. *Eur. J. Med. Chem.*, **20**, 163

135. Hansch, C., Li, R.-L., Blaney, J. M. and Langridge, R. (1982). Comparison of the inhibition of Escherichia coli and Lactobacillus casei dihydrofolate reductase by 2,4-diamino-5-(substituted-benzyl)pyrimidines: Quantitative structure–activitiy relationships, X-ray crystallography, and computer graphics in structure–activity analysis. *J. Med. Chem.*, **25**, 777

136. Selassie, C. D., Fang, Z.-X., Li, R.-L., Hansch, C., Klein, T., Langridge, R. and Kaufman, B. T. (1986). Inhibition of chicken liver dihydrofolate reductase by 5-(substituted benzyl)-2,4diaminopyrimidines. A quantitative structure–activity relationship and graphics analysis. *J. Med. Chem.*, **29**. 621

137. Kuyper, L. F., Roth, B., Baccanari, D. P., Ferone, R., Beddell, C. R., Champness, J. N., Stammers, D. K., Dann, J. G., Norrington, F. E., Baker, D. J. and Goodford, P. J. (1985). Receptor-based design of dihydrofolate reductase inhibitors: comparison of crystallography determined enzyme binding with enzyme affinity in a series of carboxy-substituted trimethoprim analogues. *J. Med. Chem.*, **28**, 303

138. Harrap, K. R., Jackman, A. L., Newell, D. R., Taylor, G. A., Hughes, L. R. and Calvert, A. H. (1989). Thymidylate synthase: a target for anticancer drug design. *Adv. Enzyme Regulation*, **29**, 161

139. Hardy, L. W., Finer-Moore, J. S., Montfort, W. R., Jones, M. O., Santi, D. V. and Stroud, R. M. (1987). Atomic structure of thymidylate synthase: target for rational drug design. *Science*, **235**, 448

140. Matthews, D. A., Appelt, K., Oatley, S. J. and Xuong, N. H. (1990). Crystal structure of *Escherichia coli* thymidylate synthase containing bound 5-fluoro-2'-deoxyuridine and 10-propargyl-5,8-dideazafolate. *J. Mol. Biol.*, **214**, 923

141. Montfort, W. R., Perry, K. M., Fauman, E. B., Finer-Moore, J. S., Maley, G. F., Hardy, L., Maley, F. and Stroud, R. M. (1990). Structure, multiple site binding and segmental accommodation in thymidylate synthase on binding dUMP and an anti-folate. *Biochemistry*, **29**, 6964

142. de Vos, A. M., Tong, L., Milburn, M. V., Matias, P. M., Jancarik, J., Noguchi, S., Nishimura, S., Miura, K., Ohtsuka, E. and Kim, S. H. (1988). Three-dimensional structure of an oncogene protein: catalytic domain of human c-H-ras p21. *Science*, **239**, 888

143. Pai, E. F., Kabsch, W., Krengel, U., Holmes, K. C., John, J. and Wittinghofer, A. (1989). Structure of the guanine-nucleotide-binding domain of the Ha-ras oncogene produce p21 in the triphosphate conformation. *Nature (London)*, **341**, 209

144. Milburn, M. V., Tong, L., de Vos, A. M., Brunger, A., Yamaizumi, Z., Nishimura, S. and Kim, S.-H. (1990). Molecular switch for signal transduction: Structural differences between active and inactive forms of protooncogenic ras proteins. *Science*, **247**, 939

145. Krengel, U., Schlicting, I., Scherer, A., Schumann, R., Frech, M., John, J., Kabsch, W., Pai, E. F. and Wittinghofer, A. (1990). Three-dimensional structures of H-*ras* p21 mutants: molecular basis for their inability to function as signal switch molecules. *Cell*, **62**, 539

146. Wolf, C. R, (1986). Cytochrome P-450s: polymorphic multigene families involved in carcinogen activation. *Trends Genet.*, **2**, 209–214

147. Guengerich, F. P., Umbenhauer, D. R., Ged, C., Martin, M. V., Wilkinson, G. R. and Lloyd, R. S. (1987). In Milners, J., Birkett, D. J., Drew, R. and McManus, M. *Microsomes and Drug Oxidations. Proceedings of the 7th International Symposium*, pp. 195–200 (London: Taylor and Francis)

148. Van Wanwe, J. P. and Janssen, P. A. J. (1989). Is there a case for P-450 inhibitors in cancer treatment? *J. Med. Chem.*, **32**, 2231–2239

149. Poulos, T. L., Finzel, B. C. and Howard, A. J. (1987). High-resolution structure of cytochrome $p450_{cam}$. *J. Mol. Biol.*, **195**, 687–700

150. Nelson, D. R. and Strobel, H. W. (1989). Secondary structure prediction of 52 membrane-bound cytochromes P450 shows a strong structural similarity to $P450_{cam}$. *Biochemistry*, **28**, 656–660

151. Kalb, V. F. and Loper, J. C. (1988). Proteins from eight eukaryotic cytochrome P-450 families share a segmented region of sequence similarity. *Proc. Natl. Acad. Sci. USA*, **85**, 7221–7225

152. Edwards, R. J., Murray, B. P., Boobis, A. R. and Davies, D. S. (1989). Identification and location of α-helices in mammalian cytochromes P450. *Biochemistry*, **28**, 3762–3770

153. Bates, P. A., McGregor, M. J., Islam, S. A., Sattentau, Q. J. and Sternberg, M. J. E. (1989). A predicted three-dimensional structure for the human immunodeficiency binding domains of CD4 antigen. *Protein Eng.*, **3**, 13–21

154. Summers, N. L. and Karplus, M. (1989). Construction of side-chains homology modelling. Application to the C-terminal lobe of rhizopuspepsin. *J. Mol. Biol.*, **3**, 13–21

155. Lee, C. and Subbiah, S. (1991). Prediction of protein side-chain conformation by packing optimisation. *J. Mol. Biol.*, **217**, 373–388

156. Zvelebil, M. J. J. M., Wolf, C. R. and Sternberg, M. J. E. (1991). A predicted three-dimensional structure of human cytochrome P450: implications for substrate specificity. *Prot. Eng.*, **4**, 271–282

157. Laughton, C. A., Neidle, S., Zvelebil, M. J. J. M. and Sternberg, M. J. E. (1990). A molecular model for the enzyme cytochrome P450 a major target for the chemotherapy of prostatic cancer. *Biochem. Biophys. Res. Commun.*, **171**, 1160–1167

158. Jordan, S. R. and Pabo, C. O. (1988). Structure of the Lambda complex at 2.5 Å resolution: details of the repressor–operator interactions. *Science*, **242**, 893

159. McClarin, J. A., Frederick, C. A., Wang, B.-C., Greene, P., Boyer, H. W., Grable, J. and Rosenberg, J. M. (1986). Structure of the DNA-Eco RI endonuclease recognition complex at 3 Å resolution. *Science*, **234**, 1526

160. Kissinger, C. R., Liu, B., Martin-Blanco, E., Kornberg, T. B. and Pabo, C. O. (1990). Crystal structure of an engrailed homeodomain–DNA complex at 2.8 Å resolution: a framework for understanding homeodomain–DNA interactions. *Cell*, **63**, 579

161. Otwinowski, Z., Schevitz, R. W., Zhang, R. G., Lawson, C. L., Joachimiak, A., Marmorstein, R. Q., Luisi, B. and Sigler, P. B. (1988). Crystal structure of trp repressor/operator complex at atomic resolution. *Nature (London)*, **332**, 321

162. Parraga, G., Horvath, S. J., Eisen, A., Taylor, W. E., Hood, L., Young, E. T. and Klevit, R. E. (1988). Zinc-dependent structure of a single-finger domain of yeast ADR1. *Science*, **241**, 1489

163. Lee, M. S., Gippert, G. P., Soman, K. V., Case, D. A. and Wright, P. E. (1989). Three-dimensional solution structure of a single zinc finger DNA-binding domain. *Science*, **245**, 635

164. Neuhaus, D., Nakaseko, Y., Nagai, K. and Klug, A. (1990). Sequence-specific [^{1}H]NMR resonance assignments and secondary structure identification for 1- and 2-zinc finger constructs from SW15. *FEBS Lett.*, **262**, 179

165. Pavletich, N. P. and Pabo, C. O. (1991). Zinc finger–DNA recognition: Crystal structure of a zif 268–DNA complex at 2.1 Å. *Science*, **252**, 809

166. Oas, T. G., McIntosh, L. P., O'Shea, E. K., Dahlquist, F. W. and Kim, P. S. (1990). Secondary structure of a leucine zipper determined by nuclear magnetic resonance spectroscopy. *Biochemistry*, **29**, 2891–2894

6
Differentiation inducers and their potential use in the treatment of acute myelogenous leukaemia

A. TOBLER AND H. P. KOEFFLER

INTRODUCTION

Human acute myelogenous leukaemia (AML) arises from neoplastic trans-formation at the stem cell level. Transformation-related mutations result in an arrest of cellular maturation at an immature stage. Thus, many of the leukaemic cells remain in the proliferative pool and rapidly accumulate. Due to the lack of functional mature peripheral blood cells, leukaemic patients often succumb to haemorrhages and infections. As yet, the therapeutic approach which aims to kill the leukaemic cells by cytotoxic therapy has been successful in achieving the cure of 10–30% of AML patients. Recently, attention has been focused on an alternative treatment for AML which seeks to change the malignant cell programme. A cardinal question is whether the leukaemic cells are capable of maturation, which might eliminate the malignant cell clone by 'death through differentiation', or whether the defect is not susceptible to correction.

Studies on regulatory events in normal and leukaemic haematopoiesis are facilitated by the use of a number of myeloid cell lines which were established from leukaemic patients[1,2]. These cell lines have the capacity to undergo differentiation along either the granulocytic or the monocytic pathway, and a variety of distinct morphological, antigenic, histochemical and functional markers of maturation emerge as the leukaemia cells undergo differentiation. Several substances, such as physiological compounds, polar-planar drugs and cytotoxic agents, have been identified as inducers of *in vitro* leukaemic cell differentiation[3]. The study of these substances can provide more insight into how the differentiation process functions and, most importantly, into the potential use of certain differentiation-inducing compounds in the therapy of acute leukaemias.

This chapter focuses on the role of physiological compounds, in particular on the retinoids, vitamin D compounds and tumour necrosis factor alpha (TNFα). We will discuss *in vitro* as well as *in vivo* data.

RETINOIDS

Retinoids are derivatives of the fat-soluble vitamin A. This substance is metabolized to aldehyde which in turn is further oxidized irreversibly to retinoic acid. Initially, the biological significance of vitamin A became clear by its corresponding deficiency disease with the major consequences of night blindness and xerophthalmia[4,5]. A role of retinoids in haematopoiesis was proposed as early as in the twenties when anaemia was produced in animals intentionally depleted of vitamin A. Over the years, evidence has accumulated that retinoids, and in particular retinoic acid, are of key importance in normal cell growth and differentiation as well as in morphogenesis[4–8]. In addition, retinoids were shown to inhibit growth and to induce differentiation of malignant cells[9] and to suppress carcinogenesis in animal models[10]. The most dramatic effects were reported on the induction of teratocarcinoma cells towards normal parietal entoderm[11] and the differentiation of the promyelocytic HL-60 leukaemia cells towards granulocytic cells[12]. We will concentrate on the role of retinoids in normal and abnormal haematopoiesis.

In vitro studies

All-*trans* retinoic acid stimulates the clonal growth of normal human granulocyte–monocyte and early erythroid precursors in the presence of haematopoietic growth factors[13,14]. Retinoids appear to enhance haematopoietic proliferation by increasing the responsiveness of the stem cells, though the precise mechanism of this enhancing effect is as yet unclear. Also, retinoids were shown to augment clonal growth of myeloid cells and to induce differentiation in myeloid cells from some myelodysplastic syndrome (MDS) patients[15,16].

In contrast to this stimulatory effect, retinoic acid inhibits proliferation and induces differentiation of cells from several human acute myeloid leukaemia cell lines[17]. The myeloblastic KG-1 line is very sensitive to all-*trans* retinoic acid with 50% inhibition of clonal growth in soft agar observed at 2×10^{-9} mol/L. The 50% inhibition of clonal growth of human promyelocytic leukaemia cells (HL-60) occurs at 2.5×10^{-8} mol/L. In contrast, clonal growth of human K562 erythroblasts and of the murine M1 myeloblasts is not affected by retinoic acid. Studies of differentiation have shown that all-*trans* and 13-*cis* retinoic acid are equally effective in inducing HL-60 cells to differentiate to granulocytes within 7 days of culture and that maximal differentiation (90%) occurs at 10^{-6} mol/L retinoic acid[12]. Continuous exposure to retinoids is necessary for optimal differentiation of HL-60 cells. Retinoic acid is unable to induce differentiation of the KG-1 cells even though these cells are very sensitive to the clonal growth-inhibiting properties of retinoic acid, demonstrating that growth inhibition of leukaemic myeloid cells is not necessarily associated with induction of differentiation[17].

Retinoids inhibit the *in vitro* proliferation of blast cells from some acute myelogenous leukaemic patients at pharmacologically achievable levels[17]. Retinoic acid inhibited the clonal growth of leukaemia cells from 5 out of 7 patients with acute myeloid leukaemia. A concentration of all-*trans* retinoic acid between 5×10^{-8} and 3×10^{-7} mol/L inhibited 50% clonal growth; and 10^{-6} mol/L retinoic acid inhibited 64–98% of the leukaemic colonies in sensitive patients. In a larger group of AML patients, a marked inhibition of clonogenic growth was observed in 17 out of 35 samples with 10^{-7} to 10^{-6} mol/L 13-*cis*-retinoic acid[18]. However, exposure to the drug at the same concentrations resulted in enhanced growth in ten samples. All-*trans* retinoic acid (10^{-6} mol/L) triggered *in vitro* differentiation of blast cells from only 2 out of 21 acute myelogenous leukaemic patients[19]. Each of the responsive samples was obtained from patients with promyelocytic leukaemia (M3, FAB). In a more recent *in vitro* study of leukaemic cells, 34 of 35 M3 samples differentiated in response to all-*trans* retinoic acid[20]. These findings suggest that blast cells from patients with promyelocytic leukaemia may be easily triggered to differentiate to granulocytes similar to HL-60 promyelocytes.However, the weight of evidence indicates that retinoids are not capable of inhibiting clonal growth or of inducing substantial maturation *in vitro* of most acute myelogenous leukaemia cells. They appear even to enhance the growth of certain myeloid leukaemic cells in a subgroup of the patients.

By examining a number of retinoids that differ in their ring, side chain and polar structure, we found that retinoic acid derivatives with a carboxyl group were significantly (10 times) more active than retinoids with a derivatized carboxyl moiety in inhibiting clonal growth and inducing differentiation of myeloid leukaemia cells[21]. Increasing alkyl group substitution on the lipophilic head of the retinoid skeleton also enhanced activity. Replacing the terminal acid group of tetrahydrobenzo[b]thiophene (TTNPB) by a hydrogen decreased activity in HL-60 cells by at least 10-fold. These retinoids also stimulated the clonal growth of normal human granulocyte-macrophage colony-forming cells (GM-CFC). Retinoids potent in their inhibition of leukaemic colony formation were also potent in their stimulation of normal GM-CFC colonies. These studies showed that both normal and leukaemic myeloid progenitors have a common structural requirement for either stimulation or inhibition of proliferation, respectively. The amide derivatives (retinamides) had no activity towards HL-60 and KG-1 cells, nor towards normal human GM-CFC. Retinamides are of interest because they are less toxic than retinoic acid, but still retain their biological activities in animal models[10,22,23]. In these models, they inhibit chemically induced carcinogenesis in the mammary gland and urinary bladder[23,24], and they reverse epithelial keratinization of hamster trachea[25-27]. The lack of activity in human cells could be explained by the absence of the necessary metabolizing systems in normal and leukaemic human haematopoietic cells. Probably, as a class, retinamides must be converted to retinoic acid to be active, and perhaps human haematopoietic cells cannot metabolize retinamides to retinoic acid.

The mechanism by which retinoids induce differentiation and inhibit leukaemic cell growth is not clear, but the following observations suggest that growth inhibition is probably more than a non-specific toxic effect.

(1) Concentrations of retinoic acid that inhibit clonal growth of leukaemia cells enhance clonal growth of normal human myeloid stem cells.

(2) Inhibition of growth of leukaemia cells occurs at very low concentrations of retinoic acid.

(3) The growth of K562 and M1 myeloid leukaemia cells is not affected by high concentrations of retinoic acid (10^{-5} mol/L).

One potential common pathway of retinoid action is by binding to a cytoplasmic retinoic acid binding protein (cRABP)[28]. This protein has been postulated as an intracellular mediator of action of retinoic acid. A positive correlation exists between binding of some retinoids to cRABP and their biological potency in various tissues[26,29]. The terminal carboxyl group seems to be essential for the binding of the retinoids to cRABP[29]. In previous studies, we and others were unable to find detectable cRABP in KG-1, HL-60, and acute myeloid leukaemic cells harvested from patients[17,18], which strongly indicates that cRABP does not mediate the action of retinoids on human leukaemic cells. Nevertheless, the rank order of potency of retinoid action on haematopoietic cells parallels the rank order of potency of retinoid action on other tissues that do contain cRABP. The exact role of cRABP remains obscure.

The recent identification of three different receptors for retinoic acid (RAR-α, RAR-β, RAR-γ and their role as transcriptional activators suggests that retinoids have a mode of action similar to that of steroid–thyroid–vitamin D hormones[30-35]. The RAR-α gene, which is expressed in many tissues, maps[36] to chromosome 17q22. It encodes a 462-amino-acid protein with a DNA-binding domain (C region) and a ligand-binding domain (E region). The RAR-β gene which is expressed in epithelial cells has been localized[37] to chromosome 3p24. The expression of the third RAR receptor, RAR-γ, seems to be restricted to skin[34]. The existence of at least three different RAR receptors for the same ligand suggests that each RAR mediates different effects of retinoic acid.

We, as well as others, have examined the expression of RAR-α in haematopoietic cells by Northern blot analyses[38-41]. All haematopoietic cells studied expressed RAR-α mRNA including KG-1 myeloblasts, HL-60 promyelocytes, ML3 myelomonoblasts, THP-1 and U937 monoblasts, K562 erythroblasts and also the T-lymphocyte line S-LB1. RAR-α steady-state RNA levels were not affected by induction of terminal differentiation to either granulocytes or macrophages. The half-life of RAR-α mRNA was short (0.7 hours), and inhibition of protein synthesis resulted in increased expression of the transcripts. Also, exposure to the ligand (all-*trans* retinoic acid) did not affect levels of RAR-α mRNA. These results indicate that RAR-α is constitutively expressed in various haematopoietic cells of different lineages and stages of differentiation, and that this expression is not affected by terminal differentiation either. Thus, paradoxically, these studies revealed no clear correlation between the expression of RAR-α (at the RNA level) and the sensitivity of leukaemic cells to retinoic acid.

Evidence that the retinoic acid-induced differentiation is directly mediated through the RAR-α was recently provided. A retinoic acid-resistant HL-60 subclone was shown to display RAR-α receptors with a decreased affinity for retinoic acid and fewer receptors per cell compared with nuclear receptors from the sensitive parent HL-60 cells[42]. Retroviral vector-mediated transduction of a single copy of the RAR-α gene into this retinoic acid-resistant subclone restored the sensitivity of these cells to the ligand. In a further study, K562 cells which are resistant to retinoic acid displayed RAR-α of the same molecular weight when compared with RAR-α of the retinoic acid-sensitive HL-60 cell line[43]. However, the receptor number was much lower in K562 cells (80 per cell) compared with the 550 receptors expressed in HL-60 cells. Most interestingly, transduction of a copy of the RAR-α gene into K562 cells resulted in increased numbers of RAR-α receptors (2000 per cell), diminished cell growth and decreased c-*myc* expression. Furthermore, these transduced cells accumulated in Go/G1. The decreased proliferation was not accompanied by differentiation. These studies strongly support the notion that, in leukaemic cells, the effects of retinoic acid are directly mediated by RAR-α. Nevertheless, the exact role and the target genes of RAR-α still remain to be determined, and also the question of how retinoic acid acts on normal haematopoietic cells remains unanswered. In this context, it is noteworthy that, in acute promyelocytic leukaemia, the RAR-α is translocated from chromosome 17 to a locus **myl** (for myelocytic leukaemia) on chromosome 15[44]. The t(15:17) translocation creates a fusion gene between the C-terminus of RAR-α and the amino-terminus of the new locus **myl**. The missing N-terminus of RAR-α is thought to be important for transactivation and target gene specificity based on the homology to the steroid hormone receptor family[45].

Clinical Studies

Studies in myelodysplastic syndrome patients

Several clinical trials have evaluated the use of 13-*cis* retinoic acid in patients with myelodysplastic syndromes (MDS)[46] and demonstrated an improvement of peripheral blood or bone marrow blast counts in 5 out of 15 patients[47], in 3 out of 15 patients[48], in 6 out of 15 patients[49] and in 2 out of 6 patients[50]. One patient with MDS with excess of blasts achieved a complete clinical response and a disappearance of cytogenetic abnormalities after 10 months of 13-*cis* retinoic acid therapy[51]. A randomized trial with low doses of 13-*cis* retinoic acid (20 mg/day) in MDS patients without excess of blasts and without sideroblasts demonstrated a better survival compared with the placebo group[52].

We performed a double-blind randomized trial of 13-*cis* retinoic acid vs placebo to determine whether the drug has a therapeutic effect in patients with MDS[53]. Sixty-eight patients were evaluable. About 50% of the patients in each group had refractory anaemia with excess of blasts (RAEB). The treatment group received a daily dose of 100 mg/m^2 13-*cis* retinoic acid for a period of up to 6 months. Only one-third of the patients from each group received treatment for 6 months. Two-thirds of the patients in the treatment group discontinued the treatment, toxicity being the reason in 20%. Major side-effects were either mild or moderate skin toxicity (>90% of the patients). No significant difference in the mean values of the haematological parameters was noted between the two treatment groups ($p > 0.05$). Thirty-one percent in the 13-*cis* retinoic acid group and 27% in the placebo group experienced progression of their disease. None in either group had a partial or complete response. Most of the progressions (17 patients) and all of the minor responses occurred in those patients who began treatment with the diagnosis of either RAEB or RAEB in transformation (RAEB-T). Further, no significant difference existed in progression-free survival between 13-*cis* retinoic acid and placebo groups ($p=0.89$). Thus our study did not find that 13-*cis* retinoic acid exerts a beneficial effect in patients with MDS, and also showed that toxicity is a major problem for long-term therapy with 13-*cis* retinoic acid. A more recent non-randomized and non-placebo-controlled study in sixty-six patients with MDS suggests that addition of α-tocopherol to 13-*cis* retinoic acid decreases toxicity and allows long-term therapy with retinoic acid, and that this regimen may decrease the rate of progression or transformation to acute leukaemia[54].

Studies in AML patients

The *in vitro* results indicate that, in acute promyelocytic leukaemia (M3, FAB)[55], induction of differentiation by retinoic acid may be an attractive alternative to conventional chemotherapy. Until recently, only a few cases of acute promyelocytic leukaemia with responses to 13-*cis* retinoic acid had been reported[56–60]. Two larger studies have now provided evidence that all-*trans* retinoic acid may be an effective treatment for acute promyelocytic leukaemia[61,62].

In the first study, twenty-four patients with acute promyelocytic leukaemia were treated with 45–100 mg m^{-2}day^{-1} all-*trans* retinoic acid[61]. Eight patients had been either non-responsive or resistant to previous chemotherapy; the other 16 patients were treated *ab initio* with all-*trans* retinoic acid. Remarkably, 23 patients achieved complete remission without undergoing bone marrow aplasia. One patient failed to respond to retinoic acid alone but attained complete remission after addition of low-dose cytosine arabinoside. This patient's cells were also resistant to induction of differentiation *in vitro* by retinoic acid. No exacerbation of haemorrhages was noted. Eight patients relapsed after two to five months of complete remission; the remaining patients were still in complete remission at one to 11 months.

Similar results were obtained in a second study of twenty-two patients with acute promyelocytic leukaemia who were treated with all-*trans* retinoic acid (45 mg m^{-2}day^{-1} for 90 days)[62]. Fourteen patients reached complete remission. One patient treated with retinoic acid for a third relapse did not respond to the drug; this patient's leukaemic cells also did not respond to retinoic acid *in vitro*. No patient experienced an exacerbation of disseminated intravascular coagulation. Durations of complete remissions, however, were short irrespective of the maintenance therapy applied. Nine patients relapsed after a median of 7 months. Taken together, these studies show that treatment with retinoic acid results in complete remissions in the majority of acute promyelocytic leukaemia patients without the hazards of aplasia. However, the duration of complete remission is short, indicating that this treatment modality does not eradicate the leukaemic clone. Thus, the place of retinoic acid in the treatment of M3 leukaemias still remains to be established. Possibly, retinoic acid therapy followed by an aggressive conventional consolidation therapy may yield better results; or, retinoic acid may be beneficial in the consolidation phase after conventional induction therapy. Trials are under way to address these questions.

1α, 25-DIHYDROXYVITAMIN D$_3$

The vitamin D endocrine system is a major regulator of calcium metabolism. The main sources of vitamin D are food and exposure to ultraviolet light. Recent evidence has indicated that 1α, 25-dihydroxyvitamin D$_3$ (1α,25(OH)$_2$D$_3$), which is the most active metabolite of vitamin D, can be synthesized in organs other than the kidney, and thus may play a wider biological role than previously appreciated (for review, see reference 63). Ectopic extrarenal 1α,25(OH)$_2$D$_3$ production in humans can occur under certain conditions. For example, γ-interferon-activated pulmonary and human bone marrow macrophages are able to synthesize 1α, 25(OH)$_2$D$_3$ from the 25(OH)D$_3$ metabolite[64,65].

Like retinoids, 1α,25(OH)$_2$D$_3$ may influence the differentiation and proliferation of various tissues, for example cancer and epidermal cells[63]. It also has an affect on haematopoiesis and the immune system. For instance, it decreases synthesis of cytokines by T-lymphocytes and fibroblasts[66–69]. The effects of the hormone on the proliferation and differentiation of haematopoietic cells will be discussed in more detail in the following section.

In vitro studies

The 1α,25(OH)$_2$D$_3$ induces cells from both a murine myeloid leukaemia line known as M1[70] and a human promyelocytic leukaemia line (HL-60)[71–74] to differentiate to monocyte macrophage-like cells. The cells, when cultured in 1α,25(OH)$_2$D$_3$ (10^{-7} to 10^{-10} mol/L), become adherent to charged surfaces, develop long filamented pseudopodia, stain positively for non-specific acid esterase, reduce nitro-blue tetrazolium, and acquire the ability to phagocytose yeast.

We have examined the effect of 1α,25(OH)$_2$D$_3$ on both clonal proliferation and differentiation of cells from eight myeloid leukaemic lines (Table 6.1)[75]. Fifty per cent inhibition of colony formation of the responsive lines occurred in a concentration range of 2×10^{-8} to 8×10^{-10} mol/L 1α,25(OH)$_2$D$_3$. These concentrations are comparable to those required for induction of differentiation

Table 6.1 Effects of 1,25(OH)$_2$D$_3$ and TNFα on leukaemic clonal growth

Cell line	Stage of Maturation	50% inhibitory concentration	
		1,25(OH)$_2$D$_3$ (mol/L)	TNFα (U/ml)
HL-60	Promyelocyte	8×10^{-10}	6
U-937	Monoblast	4×10^{-9}	12
THP-1	Monoblast	3×10^{-8}	No inhibition
HEL	Myeloblast/erythroblast	2×10^{-8}	No inhibition
HL-60 blast	Early myeloblast	No inhibition	7
KG-1a	Early myeloblast	No inhibition	150
KG-1	Myeloblast	No inhibition	45
K-562	Myeloblast/erythroblast	No inhibition	No inhibition

in liquid culture[70,74,76,77]. Cell lines which were induced to differentiate by $1\alpha,25(OH)_2D_3$ were always inhibited in their clonal growth by the compound. Differentiation was measured by their ability to reduce nitro-blue tetrazolium. The responsive cells were relatively more mature (HL-60, U937, THP1, HEL, M1) than the unresponsive cells (KG1A, KG-1, HL-60 blast, K562). The vitamin D-responsive progenitor cells differentiated *in vitro* and lost their potential for clonal growth. The vitamin D-unresponsive leukaemic cells did not differentiate and remained in the proliferative pool, giving rise to colonies of similar cells. The $1\alpha,25(OH)_2D_3$ also inhibited the clonal growth of leukaemic blast cells from myeloid leukaemic patients[76]. Ten out of 14 leukaemic patients had neoplastic cells that were at least 50% inhibited in their colony formation in the presence of 5×10^{-7} mol/L $1\alpha,25(OH)_2D_3$ and 5 of the 14 leukaemic patients manifested 50% inhibition of leukaemic colony formation at 5×10^{-9} mol/L $1\alpha,25(OH)_2D_3$. In contrast, normal human myeloid progenitor cells (GM-CFC) were stimulated to proliferate by concentrations of $1\alpha,25(OH)_2D_3$ that almost completely inhibited clonal growth of myeloid leukaemic cells[75,78]. The mechanism by which $1\alpha,25(OH)_2D_3$ exerts its effect on myeloid cells is as yet unclear. Indirect evidence suggests that differentiation is mediated through intracellular receptors[71,74,75]. The dissociation constant for the ligand[79] is in the range of 1 to 50×10^{-11} mol/L. HL-60 cells display[74] about 4000 receptors for $1\alpha,25(OH)_2D_3$ per cell. However, expression of $1\alpha,25(OH)_2D_3$ receptors is not sufficient for induction of differentiation. For example, the KG-1 myeloblasts have a comparable number of $1\alpha,25(OH)_2D_3$ receptors as do HL-60 cells, but are resistant to the differentiation-inducing effects of the compound. Furthermore, why $1\alpha,25(OH)_2D_3$ preferentially inhibits the proliferation *in vitro* of leukaemic, but not normal, human myeloid stem cells is still not clear. Differences in number or affinity of $1\alpha,25(OH)_2D_3$ receptors, or the activation of different genes and metabolic pathways, may account for this differential effect.

The receptor for $1\alpha,25(OH)_2D_3$ from several species has been recently cloned and characterized[80-82]. It shares structural homologies in the putative DNA-binding domain (C region) with all the other steroid hormone receptors and with the v-erbA oncogene[80]. Thus, like the retinoic acid receptors, the $1\alpha,25(OH)_2D_3$ receptor belongs to the steroid/thyroid hormone receptor supergene family[45]. As with the action of other steroid hormones, the $1\alpha,25(OH)_2D_3$ might passively enter the cell and interact with an intracellular receptor protein. This steroid–receptor complex would then bind to specific DNA-binding domains either to repress or to activate gene transcription[35]. We recently examined the expression of $1\alpha,25(OH)_2D_3$ receptor RNA and its modulation in various haematopoietic cells[83]. Except for B-lymphocytes, constitutive expression of a 4.6 kb transcript was observed in normal cells, such as macrophages and stimulated T-lymphocytes. Also, several leukaemic cells expressed the $1\alpha,25(OH)_2D_3$ receptor RNA, including KG-1 myeloblasts, HL-60 promyelocytes, ML-3 myelomonoblasts, U937 and THP-1 monoblasts, K562 erythroblasts and HTLV-1 transfected T-cells. In HL-60 cells, levels of $1\alpha,25(OH)_2D_3$ receptor RNA were not affected by exposure to high concentrations of the ligand (10^{-7} mol/L). Furthermore, induction of HL-60 cell differentiation along the monocytic or granulocytic pathways did not change steady-state RNA levels for the receptor. The half-life of the 4.6 kb transcript was short (one hour), and its accumulation increased when protein synthesis was inhibited. Further studies should now help to elucidate the physiological role of $1\alpha,25(OH)_2D_3$ receptor in normal and leukaemic haematopoietic cells.

Induction of hypercalcaemia is a limiting factor for the *in vivo* application of $1\alpha,25(OH)_2D_3$ (see *In vivo studies* below). Therefore, we, as well as others, have directed our attention to the development and study of new vitamin D compounds which induce differentiation and inhibit proliferation of leukaemic cells but do not induce hypercalcaemia[84–86]. We identified seven new analogues of $1\alpha,25(OH)_2D_3$ which are equivalent to or more potent than $1\alpha,25(OH)_2D_3$ in their capacity either to induce differentiation or to inhibit proliferation of leukaemic cells and to induce clonal growth of normal GM-CFC[84]. In contrast, these compounds were 10–15-fold less potent in their ability to stimulate intestinal absorption of calcium or mobilization of calcium from bone in vitamin-D-deficient chicks. Among them, the analogue $1\alpha,25(OH)_2$-16ene-23yne-D_3 was the most potent modulator of growth and differentiation of leukaemic cells. With HL-60 cells, a 50% inhibition (ED_{50}) of clonal growth was reached at 4×10^{-9} mol/L, whereas $1\alpha,25(OH)_2D_3$ had an ED_{50} of 16×10^{-9} mol/L. Also $1\alpha,25(OH)_2$-16ene-23yne-D_3 was the most potent inducer of HL-60 cell differentiation with an ED_{50} of approximately 14×10^{-9} mol/L compared with 30×10^{-9} mol/L for $1\alpha,25(OH)_2D_3$. We further examined the regulation of c-*myc* RNA. Expression of c-*myc* is associated with cellular proliferation[87]. $1\alpha,25(OH)_2$-16ene-23yne-D_3 was about ten-fold more potent than $1\alpha,25(OH)_2D_3$ at decreasing levels of c-*myc* RNA in HL-60 cells. As importantly, the new compound was found to be 30 and 50 times less potent in causing intestinal calcium absorption and bone marrow mobilization respectively, compared with $1\alpha,25(OH)_2D_3$.

In vivo studies

Initial studies have shown that 1α-hydroxyvitamin D_3 (a compound metabolized *in vivo* to $1\alpha,25(OH)_2D_3$) prolonged the life of SL mice injected with the M1 transplantable murine leukaemia cells for a mean of 23 days in controls and 34 days in treated mice[88]. We have performed a trial of oral administration of $1\alpha,25(OH)_2D_3$ (2 μg/day) in 19 patients with myelodysplastic syndromes (MDS)[89]. This dose results in serum concentrations of about 2×10^{-10} mol/L $1\alpha,25(OH)_2D_3$ in normal individuals[90]. A concentration of 2×10^{-10} mol/L $1\alpha,25(OH)_2D_3$ induces maturation of less that 20% of HL-60 promyelocytes *in vitro*[74,75]. The median duration of therapy with $1\alpha,25(OH)_2D_3$ was 12 weeks (range 4 to >20). The concentration of granulocytes, monocytes and platelets in the blood was not significantly different between the beginning and the end of the study. The percentage of myeloblasts in the marrow rose from a beginning median value of 10% (range 3–20%) to a significantly elevated ($p<0.0136$) ending median value of 15% (range 4–70%). Of a total of 19 patients, 6 had progressed to acute myelogenous leukaemia by the end of the study. During the study, 9 patients became hypercalcaemic. Thus, this study indicated that oral administration of $1\alpha,25(OH)_2D_3$ at the dosage administered to preleukaemic patients is ineffective and that hypercalcaemia develops before achievement of therapeutic concentrations of $1\alpha,25(OH)_2D_3$ in the sera.

Our recent *in vitro* studies on new vitamin D analogues[84] prompted us to develop *in vivo* models of acute myelogenous leukaemia[91]. We found that WEHI 3BD+, a murine myeloid leukaemia line, can be induced by either $1\alpha,25(OH)_2D_3$ or $1\alpha,25(OH)_2$-16ene-23yne-D_3 to lose clonal proliferative capacity as the cells terminally differentiate. A 50% inhibition of clonal growth of these cells was achieved at 2×10^{-8} mol/L $1\alpha,25(OH)_2$-16ene-23yne-D_3 and 5×10^{-8} mol/L $1\alpha,25(OH)_2D_3$. Most importantly, *in vivo* the $1\alpha,25(OH)_2$-16ene-23yne-D_3 was 10–25 times less active than $1\alpha,25(OH)_2D_3$ in causing hypercalcaemia, allowing higher concentrations of the new compound to be administered to animals in our leukaemia mouse model.

We examined three models of leukaemia that were dependent on the number of leukaemic cells injected. Mice that received intraperitoneally (ip) 2.5×10^{-5} leukaemic cells developed a fulminant leukaemia, resulting in death of all mice by day 26. Mice treated with $1\alpha,25(OH)_2D_3$ ($0.1\,\mu g$ ip every other day) had nearly the same survival. Those treated with $1\alpha,25(OH)_2$-16ene-23yne-D_3 ($1.6\,\mu g$ every other day) had a significantly longer survival ($p=0.003$), with the last mouse dying of leukaemia on day 50. Mice that received 1×10^5 leukaemic cells had an intermediate survival time (moderate leukaemia model). Eighty-six per cent of control mice were dead at day 100, whereas mice treated with $1\alpha,25(OH)_2$-16ene-23yne-D_3 ($0.8\,\mu g$ every other day) survived significantly longer ($p=0.0006$); only 53% were dead of leukaemia by day 100. Mice that received 1.5×10^4 leukaemic cells slowly developed leukaemia. This model of slowly progressive leukaemia is somewhat reminiscent of preleukaemia. Thirteen per cent of control mice were disease free at day 180; experimental animals that received $1\alpha,25(OH)_2$-16ene-23yne-D_3 ($1.6\,\mu g$ every other day) had a significantly longer survival ($p=0.028$) with 43% free of disease at day 180. Taken together, our study suggests that $1\alpha,25(OH)_2$-16ene-23yne-D_3 is most effective when the tumour burden is low. Thus, further studies should concentrate on the combination of this analogue with chemotherapy.

TUMOUR NECROSIS FACTOR ALPHA

Tumour necrosis factor alpha (TNFα) was discovered when mice bearing transplanted tumours developed haemorrhagic necrosis of these tumours when endotoxin was injected after priming with Bacillus Calmette Guerin (BCG)[92]. Activated monocytes/macrophages were identified as the main source of TNFα (for reviews, see references 93–98). More recently, mast cells have been shown to produce TNFα[99]. Growth of a variety of mouse and human tumour cells is inhibited by TNFα, whereas several types of normal cells from the same species are unaffected by exposure to the protein.

In vitro studies

The gene for human TNFα has been cloned and recombinant proteins synthesized[100–102]. TNFα has been shown to be identical to cachectin by molecular

172

cloning studies[103]. Recombinant or natural TNFα is, under denaturing conditions, a protein of 17 kDa. The most active form of TNFα is an approximately 55 kDa protein corresponding to a trimer[104]. In HL-60 cells, expression of TNFα mRNA is markedly increased during differentiation of the cells along the monocytic pathway. By 1–4 hours after treatment with phorbolesters (e.g. TPA) or other inducers of monocyte–macrophage differentiation (interferon α or γ, lymphotoxin, TNFα itself), HL-60 cells express high levels of TNFα mRNA, and TNFα expression returns to baseline levels within 8 hours[105]. The effect of TPA on expression of TNFα was inhibited by blockers of protein kinase C. We have observed a similar increase of TNFα mRNA levels 24–48 h after treatment of HL-60 cells with $1\alpha,25(OH)_2D_3$, with a decrease to baseline levels after 72 h.

We, as well as others, have found that TNFα inhibits clonal proliferation of leukaemic cell lines[106–109]. The concentration required for a 50% inhibition of colony formation in soft agar (ED_{50}) of 6 out of 9 myeloid leukaemia cell lines varied between 6 and 150 iu/ml (Table 6.1)[106]. Colony formation by sensitive lines was inhibited almost 100% at 1000 U/ml. Cell lines which did not reach a 50% inhibition at 10 000 U/ml TNFα, nevertheless, were still partially inhibited at this concentration. The effects observed are due to TNFα since a preincubation with a neutralizing monoclonal antibody could prevent 97±2% of the inhibition of HL-60 cells. In further experiments, we exposed HL-60 cells to TNFα for different periods of time, washed the cells three times, plated them in soft agar and counted viable cells. The cloning efficiency was drastically reduced after a short exposure to TNFα. For example, after a 3-hour exposure (at 37°C) to 50 U/ml TNFα, greater than 75% of colonies from HL-60 cells were inhibited. Thus, part of the growth-inhibitory action of TNFα on leukaemic cells might be explained by terminal differentiation. Indeed, low doses of TNFα (20 U/ml for 6 days) induced a partial differentiation of the HL-60 line with 25% of cells developing the ability to reduce nitro-blue tetrazolium and 8% of cells staining positively with non-specific acid esterase, and enzyme that is found in monocytes and macrophages. The viability of the cells on day 6 of culture was ≥90%. The TNFα was unable to induce differentiation of KG-1 myeloblasts or HL-60 variant blast cells and yet these cells were sensitive to the growth inhibitory action of TNFα in soft agar[106]. This suggest that induction of differentiation may be important but not the sole mechanism of growth inhibition.

We also studied the effect of TNFα on clonal growth inhibition of fresh leukaemic cells from patients[106]. Leukaemia cells from 12 out of 15 patients with myeloid leukaemia were sensitive to TNFα in the clonogenic assay, with an ED_{50} in the range of 20–2500 U/ml. The cells of 4 out of 5 cases of acute myelogenous leukaemia, 5 out of 6 cases of chronic myelogenous leukaemia in chronic phase, and 3 out of 4 cases of chronic myelogenous leukaemia in myeloid blast crisis responded to TNFα with a clonal growth inhibition. No obvious correlation could be observed between the *in vitro* response to TNFα and either the induction of remission or the survival in the 13 patients for whom follow-up was available.

TNFα has been reported to suppress clonal growth of normal human myeloid and erythroid progenitor cells[106,110,111]. We found that the degree of suppression strongly depended on the source of colony stimulating factors (CSF)) used in the assay[106]. A strong suppression of myeloid colonies by TNFα occurred in the presence of recombinant granulocyte CSF but recombinant granulocyte-macrophage CSF partially protected the myeloid progenitors from the inhibitory effects of TNFα. We also observed a similar protection of myeloid colony formation by T-lymphocyte-derived granulocyte-macrophage CSF against the suppressive influences of interferons. A recent study using highly purified CD34+ human haematopoietic progenitor cells also showed that the type of CSF was very important[112]. TNFα strongly potentiated interleukin-3 and granulocyte-macrophage CSF induced growth of haematopoietic progenitor cells. In contrast, TNFα inhibited the growth-promoting effect of granulocyte CSF. This study suggests that TNF may enhance earlier stages of myelopoiesis, but possibly may exert a suppressive effect on more differentiated precursor cells. Another study revealed that TNFα down-regulated the expression of granulocyte-CSF receptors on both acute myeloid leukaemia cells and granulocytes[113]. Thus, down-regulation of granulocyte-CSF receptor expression may be one mechanism by which TNFα suppresses granulocyte-CSF-dependent haematopoiesis.

A cooperative effect on growth and differentiation of various cell types can be observed when TNFα is combined with various other agents[114,115]. For example, we, as well as others, found that TNFα, in combination with recombinant interferons, produced in $vitro$ an additive or synergistic inhibition of growth and induction of differentiation of myeloid leukaemic cell lines and leukaemic cells from patients[106,109,116–121]. Also, either all-$trans$ retinoic acid or 1,25(OH)$_2$D$_3$ in combination with TNFα synergistically inhibited clonal growth and induced differentiation of HL-60 cells[117,120,122,123]. In addition, transforming growth factor β_1 (TGFβ_1) alone induces differentiation of the monocytic U937 cells into macrophage-like cells[124,125]. When combined with TNFα, TGFβ_1 additively or synergistically induced differentiation.

The mechanisms by which these agents act synergistically with TNFα are not understood. Interferon-γ[115,126] as well as retinoic acid[122] up-regulate expression of TNFα receptors. Several lines of evidence indicate that the induction of TNFα receptors by interferons or other agents is not a major mechanism of synergism. Firstly, the presence and the number of TNFα receptors on the cell do not necessarily predict whether a cell will be sensitive to TNFα. A TNFα-resistant cell line has been reported to have approximately the same number of TNFα receptors as a cell line sensitive to the cytotoxic effects of TNFα[114]. We noted no correlation between the number of TNFα receptors expressed on myeloid leukaemic cells and the biological sensitivity of these cell lines to the growth inhibitory action of the ligand[127]. Several cell lines, such as K562 and THP-1, were resistant to TNFα but expressed comparable numbers of receptors when compared with sensitive lines, such as HL-60. Secondly, although interferon-γ was maximally effective at inducing TNFα-receptors in a human cervical carcinoma cell line, enhancement of TNFα-mediated cytotoxicity was also observed with interferon-α and β which did not change receptor expression[128]. Similarly, enhancement of effects of TNFα by TGFβ_1 was not accompanied by increased receptor expression[124,125]. These studies suggest that interferons and other agents may affect TNFα-activity by mechanisms not related to receptor induction, but rather to post-receptor events.

At the molecular level, TNFα profoundly inhibited the expression of c-myc in HL-60 cells[129–132]. Time–response experiments showed that a 4-hour exposure to TNFα (100 U/ml) reduced c-*myc* mRNA accumulation in HL-60 cells by 95%, and a 50% reduction occurred within <1 hour[129]. Nuclear *in vitro* run-on studies revealed that this decrease in c-*myc* mRNA levels is due to a reduced rate of transcription. TNFα, by inhibiting the transcription of c-*myc*, causes a decrease in c-*myc* protein levels which, in turn, might contribute to the reduced proliferation and survival of HL-60 cells and neoplastic cells in general. These *in vitro* results suggested that TNFα might be of potential interest in the treatment of leukaemia and perhaps other tumours.

In vivo studies

The antitumour effects of TNFα have mostly been studied *in vitro*. Recent *in vivo* studies using mice showed that murine rTNFα did not cause a marked regression of SAI sarcoma cells in immunocompetent mice[133]. Almost lethal quantities of TNFα were required to cause tumour regression in the host. However, TNFα was able to induce haemorrhagic reactions, resulting in the destruction of >75% of the centre of the tumour. Interestingly, the haemorrhagic reaction was greatly reduced in T-cell-deficient animals. These results indicate that TNFα-mediated effects depend on host immunocompetence and that *in vivo* TNFα probably does not directly destroy SAI tumour cells. Further experiments revealed that exposure of rats for 7–10 days to sublethal doses of TNFα caused cachexia and anaemia, indicating that long-term application of TNFα to induce tumour regression may be intolerable to the host[134].

In a phase I trial to test the effects on humans *in vivo* [135], twenty patients with disseminated cancer received rTNFα in doses ranging from 1–200 μg/m^2 by alternating intramuscular and intravenous bolus injections with a minimal intervening period of 72 hours. Each patient received a maximum of eight treatments given twice weekly over four weeks. TNFα concentrations were achievable which *in vitro* inhibited virtually 100% of HL-60 cells growth. Only two of 16 patients who completed 4 weeks of therapy showed some evidence for tumour regression. A drop in haemoglobin levels and in thrombocyte counts was noted. So far, no trials have been reported concerning the effect of TNFα in leukaemic patients.

Taken together, despite very promising *in vitro* data, the *in vivo* results indicate that TNFα may not be an effective antitumour agent, at least when used as a single agent.

Acknowledgements

This work was supported in part by grants from the Swiss National Science Foundation (31–32524.91), the Roche Research Foundation and the Bernese Cancer League to A.T., and in part by US Public Health Service grants No. DK41936–02, CA26038–11, CA43277–05, CA33936–08, R86LA022, IRT370, the Weisz Family Foundation, 4E Leukaemia Fund in memory of Marilyn Levine and the Realtors of Real Estate Industry Division to H.P.K.

We thank Heidi Haag for her secretarial help.

175

References

1. Lubbert, M. and Koeffler, H. P. (1988).Myeloid cell lines: tools for studying differentiation of normal and abnormal hematopoietic cells. *Blood Rev.*, **2**, 121–133
2. Collins, S. J. (1987). The HL-60 promyelocytic cell line. Proliferation, differentiation, and cellular oncogene expression. *Blood*, **70**, 1233–1244
3. Koeffler, H. P. (1983). Induction of differentiation of human acute myelogenous leukaemia cells; therapeutic implications. *Blood*, **62**, 709–721
4. Bollag, W. (1983). Vitamin and retinoids: from inhibition to pharmacotherapy in dermatology and oncology. *Lancet*, 860–865
5. Goodman, D. (1984). Vitamin A and retinoids in health and disease. *N. Engl. J. Med.*, **310**, 1023–1031
6. Durston, A., Timmermans, J., Hage, W., Hendricks, H., de Vries, N., Heideveld, M. and Nieukoop, P. (1989). Retinoic acid causes an anteroposterior transformation on the developing central nervous system. *Nature*, **340**, 140–144
7. Maden, M. (1982). Vitamin A and pattern formation in the regenerating limb. *Nature*, **295**, 672–675
8. Slack, J. M. W. (1987). We have a morphogen. *Nature*, **327**, 553–554.
9. Sporn, M. B. and Roberts, A. B. (1983). Role of retinoids in differentiation and carcinogenesis. *Cancer Res.*, **43**, 3034–3040
10. Moon, R. C., McCormick, D. L. and Mehta, R. G. (1983). Inhibition of carcinogenesis by retinoids. *Cancer Res.*, **43** (suppl.), 2469s–2475s
11. Strickland, S. and Mahdavi, M. (1978). The induction of differentiation in teratocarcinoma cells by retinoic acid. *Cell*, **15**, 393–403
12. Breitman, T. R., Selonick, S. E. and Collins, S. J. (1980). Induction of differentiation of the human promyelocytic leukaemia cell line (HL-60) by retinoic acid. *Proc. Natl. Acad. Sci. USA*, **77**, 2936–2940
13. Douer, D. and Koeffler, H. P. (1982). Retinoic acid enhances colony-stimulating factor induced clonal growth of normal human myeloid progenitor cells in vitro. *Exp. Cell Res.*, **138**, 193–198.
14. Douer, D. and Koeffler, H. P. (1982). Retinoic acid enhances growth of early erythroid progenitor cells *in vitro*. *J. Clin. Invest.*, **69**, 1039–1042
15. Greenberg, P. L., Swanson, G., Picozzi, V., Morgan, R. and Hecht, F. (1985). Myelodysplastic syndromes (MDS): responses of hematopoietic precursors to 13-cis-retinoic acid (CRA) and 1,25 dihydroxyvitamin D_3 (Vit D). *Exp. Hematol.*, **13**, 377
16. Fabian, I., Shvartzmayer, S. and Nagler, A. (1987). In vitro growth and differentiation of marrow cells from myelodysplastic patients in the presence of a retinoidal benzoic acid derivative. *Leukemia Res.*, **11**, 635–640
17. Douer, D. and Koeffler, H. P. (1982). Retinoic acid inhibition of the clonal growth of human myeloid leukaemia cells. *J. Clin. Invest.*, **69**, 277–282
18. Lawrence, J., Conner, K., Kelly, M. A., Hanslerr, M. R., Wallace, P. and Bagby, G. C. Jr. (1987). Cis-retinoic acid stimulates the clonal growth of some myeloid leukaemic cells in vitro. *Blood*, **69**, 302–307
19. Breitman, T., Collins, S. and Keene, B. (1981). Terminal differentiation of human promyelocytic leukaemia cells in primary cultures in response to retinoic acid. *Blood*, **57**, 1000–1004
20. Chomienne, C., Ballerini, P., Balitrand, N., Daniel, M. T., Febaux, P., Castaigne S. and Degos, L. (1990). All-trans-retinoic acid in acute promyelocytic leukemia. II. In vitro studies: structure–function relationship. *Blood*, **76**, 1710–1717
21. Tobler, A., Dawson, M.I. and Koeffler, H. P. (1986). Retinoids: structure function relationship in normal and leukemic hematopoiesis. *J. Clin Invest*, **78**, 303–309
22. Sani, B. P. and Meeks, R G. (1983). Subacute toxicity of all-trans and 13-cis-isomers of N-ethylretinamide, N-2 hydroxyethyl retinamide, and N-4-hydroxyphenyl retinamide. *Toxicol. Appl. Pharmacol.*, **70**, 228–235
23. Moon, R. C., Thompson, H. T., Becci, P. T., Grubbs, C. T., Gander, R. T., Newton, D. L., Smith, J. M., Phillips, S. L., Henderson, W. R., Mullen, R. T., Brown, C. C. and Sporn, M. B. (1978). N-(4-hydroxyphenyl) retinamide, a new retinoid for prevention of breast cancer in the rat. *Cancer Res.*, **39**, 1339–1346
24. Moon, R. C., McCormick, D. L., Becci, P. J., Shealy, Y. F., Frickel, F., Faust, J. and Sporn, M.B. (1982). Influence of 15 retinoic acid amides on urinary bladder carcinogenesis in the mouse. *Carcinogenesis (London)*, **3**, 1469–1472

25. Newton, D. L., Henderson, W. R. and Sporn, M. B. (1980). Structure–activity relationship of retinoids in hamster tracheal organ culture. *Cancer Res.*, **40**, 3413–3425
26. Lotan, R., Neumann, G. and Lotan, D. (1980). Relationship among retinoic structure, inhibition of growth and cellular retinoic acid-binding protein in cultured S91 melanoma cells. *Cancer Res.*, **40**, 1097–1102
27. Sporn, M. B., Dunlop, N. M., Newton, D. L. and Henderson, W. R. (1976). Relationship between structure and activity of retinoids. *Nature*, **263**, 110–113
28. Chytil, F. and Ong, D. E. (1979). Cellular retinol- and retinoic acid-binding proteins in vitamin A action. *Fed. Proc.*, **38**, 2510–2514
29. Sani, B., Dawson, M. I., Hobbs, P. D., Chan, R. L.-S. and Schiff, L. J. (1984). Relationship between binding affinities to cellular retinoic acid-binding protein and biological properties of a new series of retinoids. *Cancer Res.*, **44**, 190–195
30. Gigure, V., Ong, E., Segui, P. and Evans, R. (1987)). Identification of a receptor for the morphogen retinoic acid. *Nature*, **330**, 624–629
31. Petkovich, M., Brand, N., Krust, A. and Chambon, P. (1987). A human retinoic acid receptor which belongs to the family of nucleic receptors. *Nature*, **330**, 444–450
32. Benbroock, D., Lernhardt, E. and Pfahl, M. (1988). A new retinoic acid receptor identified from a hepatocellular carcinoma. *Nature*, **333**, 669–672
33. Brand, N., Petkovich, M., Krust, A., Chambon, P., de The, H., Marchio, A., Tiollais, P. and Dejean, A. (1988). Identification of a second human retinoic acid receptor. *Nature*, **332**, 850–853
34. Zelent, A., Kust, A., Petkovich, M., Kastner, P. and Chambon, P. (1989). Cloning of a murine a and b retinoic acid receptor and a novel receptor g predominantly expressed in the skin. *Nature*, **339**, 714–717
35. Beato, M. (1989). Gene regulation by steroid hormones. *Cell*, **56**, 335–344
36. Mattei, M. G., Petkovich, M., Mattei, J. F., Brand, N. and Chambon, P. (1988). Mapping of the human retinoic acid receptor to the q21 band of chromosome 17. *Hum. Genet.*, **80**, 186–188
37. Mattei, M. G., de The, H., Mattei, J. F., Marchio, A., Tiollais, P. and Dejean, A. (1988). Assignment of the human hap receptor RAR b to the p24 band of chromosome 3. *Hum. Genet.*, **80**, 189–190
38. Kizaki, M., Koeffler, H. P., Lin, C.W. and Miller, C. (1990). Expression of retinoic acid receptor mRNA in hematopoietic cells. *Leukemia Res.*, **14**, 645–655
39. Largman, C., Detmer, K., Corral, J. C., Hack, F. M. and Lawrence, H. J. (1989). Expression of retinoic acid receptor alpha mRNA in human leukemia cells. *Blood*, **74**, 99–100
40. Gallagher, R. E., Said, F., Pua, I., Papenhausen, P. R., Paiettea, E. and Wiernik, P. H. (1989). Expression of retinoic acid receptor alpha mRNA in human leukemia cells with variable responsiveness to retinoic acid. *Leukemia*, **3**, 789–795
41. Wang, C., Curtis, J. E., Minden, M. A. and McMulloch, E. A. (1989). Expression of retinoic acid receptor gene in myeloid leukemic cells. *Leukemia*, **3**, 264–269
42. Collins, S. J., Robertson, K. A. and Mueller, L. (1990). Retinoic acid-induced granulocytic differentiation of HL-60 myeloid leukemia cells is mediated directly through the retinoic acid receptor (RAR-alpha). *Mol. Cell. Biol.*, **10**, 2154–2163
43. Robertson, K. A., Mueller, L. and Collins, S. J. (1991). Retinoic acid receptors in myeloid leukemia: characterization of receptors in retinoic acid-resistant K562 cells. *Blood*, **77**, 340–347
44. De The, H., Chomienne, C., Lanotte, M., Degos, L. and Dejean, A. (1990). The t(15;17) translocation of acute promyelocytic leukemia fuses the retinoic acid receptor alpha gene to a novel transcribed locus. *Nature*, **347**, 558–561
45. Evans, R. M. (1988). The steroid and thyroid hormone receptor supergene family. *Science*, **240**, 889–895
46. Bennett, J. M., Catovsky, D., Daniel, M. T., Flandrin, G., Galton, D. A. G., Gralnick, H. R. and Sultan, C. (1982). The French–American–British (FAB) Co-operative group: proposal for the classification of the myelodysplastic syndromes. *Br. J. Haematol.*, **51**, 189–199
47. Gold, E. J., Mertelsmann, R. H., Itri, L. M., Gee, T., Arlin, Z., Kempin, S., Clarkson, B. and Moore, M. A. S. (1983). Phase I trial of 13-cis retinoic acid in myelodysplastic syndromes. *Cancer Treat Rep.*, **67**, 981–986
48. Greenberg, B., Durie, B., Garnett, T. and Meyskens, F. (1985). Phase I-II study of 13-cis retinoic acid in myelodysplastic syndrome. *Cancer Treat. Rep.*, **69**, 1369–1376
49. Picozzi, V., Swanson, G., Morgan, R., Hecht, F. and Greenberg, P. (1986). 13-cis Retinoic acid treatment of myelodysplastic syndromes. *J. Clin. Oncol.*, **4**, 589–595

50. Kerndrup, G., Bendix-Hansen, K., Pedersen, B., Ellegaard, J. and Hokland, P. (1986). Primary myelodysplastic syndrome: treatment of six patients with 13-cis retinoic acid. *Scand. J. Haematol.*, **45**, 126–132

51. Abrahm, J. L., Besa, E. C., Hyzinski, M., Finan, J. and Nowell, P. (1986). Disappearance of cytogenetic abnormalities and clinical remission with 13-cis-retinoic acid in a patient with myelodysplastic syndrome: inhibition of growth of the patient's malignant monocytoid·clone. *Blood*, **67**, 1323–1327

52. Clark, R. E., Jacobs, A. and Lusch, C. J. (1987). Effect of 13-cis RA on the survival of patients with myelodysplastic syndrome. *Lancet*, **11**, 763–765

53. Koeffler, H. P., Heitjan, D., Mertelsmann, R., Kolitz, J., Schulman, P., Itri, L., Gunter, P. and Besa, E. (1988). Randomized study of 13-cis retinoic acid in the myelodysplastic disorders. *Blood*, **71**, 703–708

54. Besa, E. C., Abrahm, J. L., Bartholomew, M. J., Hyzinski, M. and Nowell, P. C. (1990). Treatment with 13-cis-retinoic acid in transfusion-dependent patients with myelodysplastic syndrome and decreased toxicity with addition of alpha-tocopherol. *Am. J. Med.*, **89**, 739–747

55. Bennett, J. M., Catovsky, D., Daniel, M. T., Flandrin, G., Galton, D. A. G., Gralnick, H. R. and Sultan, C. (1985). Proposed revised criteria for the classification of acute myeloid leukemia. A report of the French–American–British Cooperative Group. *Ann. Intern. Med.*, **103**, 626–629

56. Fontana, J. A., Rogers, J. S. and Durham, J. P. (1986). The role of 13-cis retinoic acid in the remission induction of a patient with acute promyelocytic leukemia. *Cancer*, **57**, 209–217

57. Daenen, S., Vellenga, E., van Dobbenburgh, O. A. and Halie, M. R. (1986). Retinoic acid as antileukemic therapy in a patient with acute promyelocytic leukemia and aspergillus pneumonia. *Blood*, **67**, 559–561

58. Flynn, P. J., Miller, W. J., Weisdorf, D. J., Arthur, D. C., Brunning, R. and Branda, R. F. (1983). Retinoic acid treatment of acute promyelocytic leukemia: in vitro and in vivo observations. *Blood*, **62**, 1211–1217

59. Nilsson, B. (1984). Probable in vivo induction of differentiation by retinoic acid in acute promyelocytic leukaemia. *Br. J. Haematol.*, **57**, 365–371

60. Chomienne, C., Ballerini, P., Balitrand, N., Amar, M., Bernard, J. F., Boivin, P., Daniel, M. T., Berger, R., Castaigne, S. and Degos, L. (1989). Retinoic acid therapy for promyelocytic leukemia. *Lancet, 2*, 746–747

61. Huang Meng-er, Ye Yu-chen, Chen-Shu-rong, Chai Jin-ren, Lu Jia-Xiang, Zhoa Lin, Gu Long-jun and Wang Zhen-yi (1988). Use of all-trans-retinoic acid in the treatment of acute promyelocytic leukemia. *Blood*, **72**, 567–572

62. Castaigne, S., Chomienne, C., Daniel, M. T., Ballerini, P., Berger R., Fenaux, P. and Degos, L. (1990). All-trans-retinoic acid as a differentiation therapy for acute promyelocytic leukemia. I. Clinical results. *Blood*, **76**, 1704–1709

63. Reichel, H., Koeffler, H. P. and Norman, A. W. (1990). The role of the vitamin D endocrine system in health and disease. *N. Engl. J. Med.*, **15**, 980–991

64. Reichel, H., Koeffler, H. P., Barbers, R. and Norman, A. W. (1987). Regulation of 1,25-dihydroxyvitamin D3 production by cultured alveolar macrophages from normal human donors and from patients with pulmonary sarcoidosis. *J. Clin. Endocrinol. Metab.*, **65**, 1201–1209

65. Reichel, H., Koeffler, H. P. and Norman, A. W. (1987). Synthesis in vitro of 1,25-dihydroxyvitamin D_3 and 24,25-dihydroxyvitamin D_3 by interferon-gamma-stimulated normal human bone marrow and alveolar macrophages. *J. Biol. Chem.*, **262**, 10931–10937

66. Tsoukas, C. D., Provvedini, D. M. and Manolagas, S. C. (1984). 1,25-Dihydroxyvitamin D_3: a novel immunoregulatory hormone. *Science*, **224**, 1438–1440

67. Reichel, H., Koeffler, H. P., Tobler, A. and Norman A. W. (1987). 1alpha,25-dihydroxyvitamin D_3 inhibits gamma-interferon synthesis by normal human peripheral blood lymphocytes. *Proc. Natl. Acad. Sci. USA*, **84**, 3385–3389

68. Tobler, A., Miller, C. W., Norman, A. W. and Koeffler, H. P. (1988). 1,25-Dihydroxyvitamin D_3 modulates expression of a lymphokine (granulocyte-macrophage colony-stimulating factor) posttranscriptionally. *J. Clin. Invest.*, **81**, 1819–1823

69. Tobler, A., Marti, H. P., Gimmi, C., Cachelin, A. B., Saurer, S. and Fey, M. F. (1991). Dexamethasone and 1,25-dihydroxyvitamin D_3, but not cyclosporine A inhibit production of granulocyte-macrophage colony-stimulating factor in human fibroblasts. *Blood*, **77**, 1912–1918

70. Abe, E., Miyaura, C., Sakagami, H., Takeda, M., Konno, K., Yamazaki, T., Yoshiki, S. and Suda T. (1981). *Proc. Natl. Acad. Sci. USA*, **78**, 4990–4994

71. Tanaka, H., Abe, E., Miyaura, C., Kuribayashi, T., Konno, K., Nishii, Y. and Suda, T. (1982). 1alpha, 25-dihydroxycholecalciferol and a human myeloid cell line (HL-60). The presence of a cytosol receptor and induction of differentiation. *Biochem. J.*, **204**, 713–719

72. Bar-Shavit, S., Teitelbaum, S. L., Reitsma, P., Hall, A., Pegg, L. E., Trial, J. and Kahn, A. J. (1983). Induction of monocytic differentiation and bone resorption by 1,25-dihydroxyvitamin D3. *Proc. Natl. Acad. Sci. USA*, **80**, 5907–5911

73. McCarthy, D. M., San Miguel, J. F., Ferake, H. C., Green, P. M., Zola, H., Catovsky, D. and Goldman, J. M. (1983). 1,25-dihydroxyvitamin D3 inhibits proliferation of human promyelocytic leukemia (HL-60) cells and induces monocyte–macrophage differentiation in HL-60 and normal human bone marrow. *Leukemia Res.*, **7**, 51–55

74. Mangelsdorf, D. J., Koeffler, H. P., Donaldson, C. A., Pike, J. W. and Haussler, M. R. (1984). 1,25-dihydroxyvitamin D3 induced differentiation in a human promyelocytic leukemia cell line (HL-60): receptor-mediated maturation to macrophage-like cells. *J. Cell. Biol.*, **98**, 391–398

75. Munker, R., Norman, A. and Koeffler, H. P. (1986). Vitamin D compounds. Effect on clonal proliferation and differentiation of human myeloid cells. *J. Clin. Invest.*, **78**, 1–8

76. Rigby, W. F. C., Shen, L., Ball, E. D., Juyre, P. M. and Fanger, M. W. (1984). Differentiation of a human monocytic cell line by 1,25-dihydroxyvitamin D3 (calcitriol): a morphologic, phenotypic, and functional analysis. *Blood,* **64**, 1110–1115

77. Matsui, T., Nakao, Y., Kobayashi, N., Kishihara, M., Ishizuka, S., Watanabe, S. and Fujita, T. (1984). Phenotypic differentiation-linked growth inhibition in human leukemia cells by active vitamin D3 analogues. *Int. J. Cancer*, **33**, 193–202

78. Koeffler, H. P., Amatruda, T., Ikekawa, N., Kobayashi, Y. and DeLuca, H. F. (1984). Induction of macrophage differentiation of human normal and leukemic myeloid stem cells by 1,25-dihydroxyvitamin D3 and its fluorinated analogues. *Cancer Res.* **44**, 5624–5628

79. Haussler, M. R. (1986). Vitamin D receptor: nature and function. *Ann. Rev. Nutr.*, **6**, 527–562

80. McDonell, D. P., Mangelsdorf, D. J., Pike, J. W., Haussler, M. R. and O'Malley, B. W. (1987). Molecular cloning of complementary DNA coding for the avian receptor for vitamin D. *Science*, **235**, 1214–1217

81. Burmester, J. K., Wiese, R. J., Maeda, N. and DeLuca, H. F. (1988). Structure and regulation of the rat 1,25-dihydroxyvitamin D3 receptor. *Proc. Natl. Acad. Sci. USA*, **85**, 9499–9502

82. Baker, A. R., McDonnell, D. P., Hughes, M., Crisp, T. M., Mangelsdorf, D. J., Haussler, M. R., Pike, J. W., Shine, J. and O'Malley, B. W. (1988). Cloning and expression of full-length cDNA coding human vitamin D receptor. *Proc. Natl. Acad. Sci. USA*, **85**, 3294–3298

83. Kizaki, M., Norman, A. W., Bishop, J., Lin, C.-W., Karmakar, A. and Koeffler, H. P. (1991). 1,25-dihydroxyvitamin D3 receptor RNA: expression in hematopoietic cells. *Blood*, **77**, 1238–1247

84. Zhou, J. Y., Norman, A. W., Lubbert, M., Collins, E. D., Uskokovic, M. R. and Koeffler, H. P. (1989). Novel vitamin D analogs that modulate leukemic cell growth and differentiation with little effect on either intestinal calcium absorption or bone calcium mobilization. *Blood*, **74**, 82–93

85. Abe, J., Morikawa, M., Miyamoto, K., Kaiho, S., Fukushima, M., Miyaura, C., Abe, E., Suda, T. and Nishii, Y. (1987). Synthetic analogues of vitamin D3 with an oxygen atom in the side chain skeleton. *FEBS Lett.*, **226**, 58–62

86. Ostrem, V.K., Tanaka, Y., Prahl, J., DeLuca, H. F. and Ikekawa, N. (1987). 24- and 26-homo-1,25-dihydroxyvitamin D3: preferential activity in inducing differentiation of human leukemia cells HL-60 in vitro. *Proc. Natl. Acad. Sci. USA*, **84**, 2610–2614

87. Studzinski, G. P., Brelvi, Z. S., Feldman, S. C. and Watt, R. A. (1986). Participation of c-myc protein in DNA synthesis of human cells. *Science*, **234**, 467–469

88. Honma, Y., Hozumi, M., Abe, E., Konno, K., Fukushima, M., Hata, S., Nishii, Y., DeLuca, H. F. and Suda, T. (1983). 1alpha,25–dihydroxyvitamin D3 and 1alpha-hydroxyvitamin D3 prolong survival time of mice inoculated with myeloid leukemia cells. *Proc. Natl. Acad. Sci. USA*, **80**, 201–204

89. Koeffler, H. P., Hirij. K. and Itri. L. (1985). 1,25-dihydroxyvitamin D3: in vivo and in vitro effects on preleukemic and leukemic cells. *Cancer Treat. Rep.*, **69**, 1399–1406

90. Adams, N., Gray, R. and Lemann J. (1982). Effects of calcitriol administration on calcium metabolism in healthy men. *Kindey Int.*, **21**, 90–97

91. Zhou, J. Y., Norman, A. W., Chen, D. L., Sun, G. W., Uskokovic, M. and Koeffler, H. P. (1990). 1,25-dihydroxy-16-ene-23-yne-vitamin D3 prolongs survival time of leukemic mice. *Proc. Natl. Acad. Sci. USA*, **87**, 3929–3932

92. Carswell, E. A., Old, L. J., Kassel, R. L., Green, S., Fiore, N. and Williamson, B. (1975). An endotoxin-induced serum factor that causes necrosis of tumors. *Proc. Natl. Acad. Sci. USA*, **72**, 3666–3670
93. Ruff, M. R. and Gifford, G. E. (1981). Tumor necrosis factor. In Pick (ed.) *Lymphokines*, Vol. 2, pp. 231–272 (New York : Academic Press)
94. Old, L. L. (1985). Tumor necrosis factor. *Science*, **230**, 630–632
95. Beutler, B. and Cerami, A. (1987). Cachectin: more than a tumor necrosis factor. *N. Engl. J. Med.*, **316**, 379–385
96. Beutler, B. and Cerami, A. (1989). The biology of cachectin/TNF – a primary mediator of the host response. *Annu. Rev. Immunol.*, **7**, 625–655
97. Old, L. L. (1987). Tumor necrosis factor. Another chapter in the long history of endotoxin. *Nature*, **330**, 602–603
98. Nathan, C. F. (1987). Secretory products of macrophages. *J. Clin. Invest*, **79**, 319–326
99. Gordon, J. R. and Galli, S. J. (1990). Mast cells as a source of both preformed and immunologically active TNF alpha/cachectin. *Nature*, **346**, 274–276
100. Pennica, D., Nedwin, G. E., Hayflick, J. S., Seeburg, P. H., Derynk, R., Palladino, M. A., Khor, W. J., Aggarwal, B. B. and Goedel, D. V. (1984). Human tumor necrosis factor: precursor structure, expression and homology to lymphotoxin. *Nature*, **312**, 724–729
101. Wang, A. M., Creasy, A. A., Ladner, M. B., Lin, L. S., Strickler, J., Van Arsdell, J. N., Yamamoto, R. and Mark, D. F. (1985). Molecular cloning of the complementary DNA for human tumor necrosis factor. *Science*, **228**, 149–154
102. Shirai, T., Yamaguchi, H., Ito, H., Todd, C. W. and Wallace, R. B. (1985). Cloning and expression in Escherichia coli of the gene for human tumor necrosis factor. *Nature*, **313**, 803–806
103. Beutler, B., Greenwald, D., Hulmes, J., Chang, M., Pan, Y.-C. E., Mathison, J., Ulevitch, R. and Cerami, A. (1985). Identity of tumor necrosis factor and the macrophage secreted factor cachectin. *Nature*, **316**, 552–554
104. Smith, R. A. and Baglioni, C. (1987). The active form of tumor necrosis factor is a trimer. *J. Biol. Chem.*, **262**, 6951–6954
105. Hensel, G., Mannel, D. N., Pfizenmaier, K. and Kroenke M. (1987). Autocrine stimulation of TNF alpha mRNA expression in HL-60 cells. *Lymphokine Res.*, **6**, 119–124
106. Munker, R. and Koeffler, H. P. (1987). In vitro action of tumor necrosis factor on myeloid leukemia cells. *Blood*, **69**, 1102–1108
107. Peetre, C., Gullberg, U., Nilsson, E. and Olsson, I. (1986). Effects of recombinant tumor necrosis factor on proliferation and differentiation of leukemic and normal hemopoietic cells in vitro. Relationship to cell surface receptor. *J. Clin. Invest.*, **78**, 1694–1700
108. Murase, T., Hotta, T., Saito, H. and Ohno, R. (1987). Effect of recombinant human tumor necrosis factor on the colony growth of human leukemia progenitor cells and normal hematopoietic progenitor cells. *Blood*, **69**, 467–472
109. Beran, M., McCredie, K. B., Keating, M. J. and Gutterman, J. U. (1988). Antileukemic effect of recombinant tumor necrosis factor in vitro and its modulation by alpha and gamma interferons. *Blood*, **72**, 728–738
110. Broxmeyer, H. E., Williams, D. E., Lu, L., Cooper, S., Anderson, S. L., Beyer, G. S., Hoffman, R. and Rubin, B. (1986). The suppressive influence of human tumor necrosis factors on bone marrow hematopoietic progenitor cells from normal donors and patients with leukemia: synergism of tumor necrosis factor and interferon-gamma. *J. Immunol.*, **136**, 4487–4495
111. Murphy, M., Perussia, B. and Trinchieri, G. (1988). Effects of recombinant tumor necrosis factor, lymphotoxin, and immune interferon on proliferation and differentiation of enriched hematopoietic precursor cells. *Exp. Hematol.*, **16**, 131–138
112. Caux, C., Saeland, S., Favre, C., Duvert, V., Mannoni, P. and Banchereau, J. (1990). Tumor necrosis factor-alpha strongly potentiates interleukin-3 and granulocyte-macrophage colony-stimulating factor-induced proliferation of human CD34+ hematopoietic progenitor cells. *Blood*, **75**, 2292–2298
113. Elbaz, O., Budel, L. M., Hoogergrugge, H., Touw, I. P., Delwel, R., Mahmoud, L. A. and Loewenberg, B. (1991). Tumor necrosis factor downregulates granulocyte-colony-stimulating factor receptor expression on human myeloid leukemia cells and granulocytes. *J. Clin. Invest.*, **87**, 838–841
114. Sugarman, B. J., Aggarwal, B. B., Hass, P. E., Figari, I. S., Palladino, M. A. and Shepard, H. M. (1985). Recombinant human tumor necrosis factor-alpha: effects on proliferation of normal and transformed cells in vitro. *Science*, **230**, 943–945

115. Aggarwal, B. B., Eessalu, T. E. and Hass, P. E. (1985). Characterization of receptors for human necrosis factor and their regulation by gamma-interferon. *Nature*, **318**, 665–667

116. Williamson, B. D., Carswell, E. A., Rubin, B. Y., Pendergast, J. S. and Old, L. J. (1983). Human tumor necrosis factor produced by human B cell lines: synergistic cytotoxic interaction with human interferon. *Proc. Natl. Acad. Sci. USA*, **80**, 5397–5401

117. Trinchieri, G., Rosen, M. and Perussia, B. (1987). Retinoic acid cooperates with tumor necrosis factor and immune interferon in inducing differentiation and growth inhibition of the human promyelocytic leukemic cell line HL-60. *Blood*, **69**, 1218–1224

118. Geissler, K., Tricot, G., Leemhuis, T., Walker, E. and Broxmeyer, H. E. (1989). Differentiation-inducing effect of recombinant human tumor necrosis factor alpha and gamma-interferon in vitro on blast cells from patients with acute myeloid leukemia and myeloid blast crisis of chronic myeloid leukemia. *Cancer Res.*, **49**, 3057–3062

119. Trinchieri, G., Kobayashi, M., Rosen. M., Louden, R., Murphy, M. and Perussia, B. (1986). Tumor necrosis factor and lymphotoxin induce differentiation of human myeloid cell lines in synergy with immune interferon. *J. Exp. Med.*, **164**, 1206–1225

120. Weinberg, B. and Larrick. J. W. (1987). Receptor mediated monocytoid differentiation of human promyelocytic cells by tumor necrosis factor: synergistic actions with interferon-gamma and 1,25-dihydroxyvitamin D3. *Blood*, **70**, 994–1002

121. Rao, K. M. K., Miskukonis, M. A., Cohen, H. J. and Weinberg, B. (1988). Cooperative effect of tumor necrosis factor and gamma-interferon on chemotactic peptide receptor expression and stimulus induced actin polymerization in HL-60 cells. *Blood*, **71**, 1062–1067

122. Tobler, A., Munker R., Heitjan, D. and Koeffler, H. P. (1987). In vitro interaction of recombinant human tumor necrosis factor and all-trans-retinoic acid with normal and leukemic hematopoiesis. *Blood*, **70**, 1940–1946

123. Trinchieri, G., Rosen, M. and Perussia, B. (1987). Induction of differentiation of human myeloid cell lines by tumor necrosis factor in cooperation with 1alpha-dihydroxyvitamin D3. *Cancer Res.* **47**, 2236–2242

124. Kamijo, R., Takeda, K., Nagumo, M. and Konno, K. (1990). Effects of combinations of transforming growth factor-beta1 and tumor necrosis factor on induction of differentiation of human myelogenous leukemic cell lines. *J. Immunol.*, **144**, 1311–1316

125. De Benedetti, F., Falk, L. A., Ellingsworth, L. R., Ruscetti, F. W. and Faltynek, C. R. (1990). Synergy between transforming growth factor beta and tumour necrosis factor-alpha in the induction of monocytic differentiation of human leukemic cell lines. *Blood*, **75**, 626–632

126. Tsujimoto, M., Yip, Y. K. and Vilcek, J. (1986). Interferon-gamma enhances expression of cellular receptors for tumor necrosis factor. *J. Immunol.*, **136**, 2441–2444

127. Munker, R., DiPersio, J. and Koeffler, H. P. (1987). Tumor necrosis factor: receptors on hematopoietic cells. *Blood*, **70**, 1730–1734

128. Aggarwal, B. B. and Eessalu, T.E. (1987). Induction of receptors for tumor necrosis factor-alpha by interferons is not a major mechanism for their synergistic cytotoxic response. *J. Biol. Chem.*, **262**, 1000–1007

129. Tobler, A., Johnston, D. and Koeffler, H. P. (1987). Recombinant human tumor necrosis factor alpha regulates c-myc expression in HL-60 cells at the level of transcription. *Blood*, **70**, 200–205

130. Kroenke, M., Schlueter, C. and Pfizenmaier, K. (1987). Tumor necrosis factor inhibits MYC expression in HL-60 cells at the level of transcription. *Proc. Natl. Acad. Sci. USA*, **84**, 469–473

131. Bergamaschi, G., Carlo-Stella, C., Cazzola, M., De Fazio, P., Pedrazzoli, P., Peverali, F. A. and Della-Valle, G. (1990). Tumor necrosis factor alpha downregulates c-myc RNA expression and induces monocytic differentiation in myeloblastic leukemia. *Leukemia*, **4**, 426–430

132. Schachner, J., Blick, M., Freireich, E., Gutterman, J. and Beran, M. (1988). Suppression of c-*myc* and c-*myb* expression in myeloid cell lines treated with recombinant tumor necrosis factor-alpha. *Leukemia*, **11**, 749–753

133. Havell, E. A., Fiers, W. and North, R. (1988). The antitumor function of tumor necrosis factor (TNF). *J. Exp. Med.*, **167**, 1067–1085

134. Tracey, K. J., Wei, H., Manogue, K. R., Fong, Y., Hesse, D. G., Nguyen, H. T., Kuo, G. C., Beutler, B., Cotran, R. S., Cerami, A. and Lowry, S. F. (1988). Cachectin/tumor necrosis factor induces cachexia, anemia, and inflammation. *J. Exp. Med.* **167**, 1211–1227

135. Blick, M., Sherwin, S. A., Rosenblum, M. and Gutterman, J. (1987). Phase I study of recombinant tumor necrosis factor in cancer patients. *Cancer Res.*, **47**, 2986–2989

7
Angiosuppression

T.-P. D. FAN and S. BREM

INTRODUCTION

Angiogenesis is the growth of new blood vessels. The term was coined in 1935 by Hertig[1] to describe neovascularization in the developing placenta. However, it is now recognized that angiogenesis is not only an important physiological process, but also plays a major role in angiogenic diseases[2] such as diabetic retinopathy[3], atherosclerosis[4], rheumatoid arthritis[5], and cancer[6].

It is becoming clear that angiogenesis is not simply controlled by the presence of a single factor, but rather by the balance of several angiogenic inducers and inhibitors[2,7-15] from tumours and/or normal cells (see Tables 7.1 and 7.2). Furthermore, the composition of the extracellular matrix and the activity of endothelial enzymes also play a critical part. In physiological angiogenesis, such as that of embryonic development, the down-regulation of endothelial cell proliferation is concomitant with neovascularization, lest the embryo become a haemangioma[16]. For these reasons, the term 'angiosuppression' was introduced to describe the physiological or pharmacological down-regulation of angiogenesis[17].

This chapter aims to review the development of the concept that tumour growth and metastasis are angiogenesis-dependent and to highlight recent advances in the search of angiogenesis inhibitors. The principle of angiosuppression will be evaluated with particular reference to its therapeutic potential in cancer treatment.

EARLY STUDIES ON TUMOUR ANGIOGENESIS

For over 100 years solid tumours have been known to be associated with an increased vascular supply, but detailed studies of tumour angiogenesis only began about 50 years ago. In 1939, Ide et al.[18] surmised that "it is probable that tumours may be elaborating a vessel growth stimulating substance". Algire et al.[19] then showed that tumour implants begin to grow in size only after the initial vascularization occurs, implying that the capacity of tumours to stimulate perpetual growth of new capillaries from the host may be the fundamental difference between the malignant cell and the normal cell from which it arose. In

1966, Folkman et al.[20] reported that, when tumours are grown in isolated perfused organs where blood vessels do not proliferate, they reach a maximum size of only 1–2 mm^3. However, on transplantation to mice these tumours induce vascularization and expand rapidly to 1–2 cm^3. This finding suggested that, when a tumour is held in the 'prevascular' state, tumour growth may be suppressed. By 1970, Tannock's experiments[21,22] demonstrated that within a solid tumour the [^{3}H]thymidine labelling index of tumour cells is inversely proportional to the distance from the nearest open capillary. He proposed that the doubling time of the tumour is a function of the labelling index of the vascular endothelial cells.

FOLKMAN'S HYPOTHESIS

Based on the data cited above, Folkman[23] proposed the hypothesis that "tumour growth is angiogenesis dependent". *In its simplest terms, this hypothesis can be stated as follows: once tumour take has occurred, every increase in tumour cell population must be preceded by an increase in new capillaries converging on the tumour*[2].

In an important series of experiments, Gimbrone et al.[24] showed that tumours suspended in the aqueous fluid of the anterior chamber of the eye remained viable, avascular, and limited in size (<1 mm^3). However, if they were implanted on the iris vessels, they induced neovascularization and grew rapidly, reaching 16 000 times their original volume within two weeks. Thus, tumour dormancy can be achieved when neovascularization is prevented[25]. Taking these observations a step further, Folkman pioneered in 1972 the concept that an anti-angiogenesis strategy might be a new therapeutic approach for the treatment of solid tumours[26].

EVIDENCE THAT TUMOUR GROWTH AND METASTASIS ARE ANGIOGENESIS DEPENDENT

Over the last 20 years, many lines of evidence have accumulated supporting Folkman's hypothesis[6,27].

(1) In the chick chorioallantoic membrane (CAM), the [^{3}H]thymidine labelling index of the vascular endothelial cells reaches a peak on day 5 and decreases with age, with an abrupt reduction on day 11[28]. Tumours implanted on the chick chorioallantoic membrane are often restricted in growth during the avascular phase (≤72 hours), but rapid growth begins within 24 hours after vascularization. In older embryos, tumours grow at slower rates in parallel with the reduced rates of endothelial cell growth[29].

(2) When implanted in the avascular cornea, tumour growth is slow and becomes exponential only after vascularization[30]. Human retinoblastomas metastatic to the vitreous or the anterior chamber are similarly avascular, viable, and growth-restricted[6].

(3) Denekamp and Hobson showed that there is a major difference in proliferation rates of vascular endothelial cells lining the blood vessels in tumours and in normal tissues[31,32]. After a single injection of [³H]thymidine, the endothelial cells in various murine tumours reveal 1–33% labelling. Similar high values are observed for human tumour endothelium labelled *in vitro* or *in vivo*. In contrast, only 0.01–0.1% of endothelial cells in most normal tissues are labelled.

(4) Tumour cells injected subcutaneously into mice grow and become vascularized at about $0.4\,mm^3$; afterwards there is a rapid increase in tumour-associated neovasculature that reaches a plateau of about 1.5% of the tumour volume, a four-fold increase of the vascular density of normal subcutaneous tissue[33]. The tumour infiltrates surrounding connective tissue and expands into the newly formed vessels in that tissue.

(5) Using transgenic mouse models, Folkman *et al.* have provided insights into the switch to the angiogenic state in tumours. Hyperplastic pancreatic islet cells become angiogenic *in vitro* at the same time that they are neovascularized *in vivo*. The angiogenic lesions expand swiftly into large vascularized tumours that eventually kill the mice[34]. In another model, the transition of a non-angiogenic fibroma to a highly angiogenic fibrosarcoma occurs when an endothelial mitogen is first released[35]. Thus, the induction of angiogenesis precedes gross tumour formation and correlates with the transition from hyperplasia to neoplasia.

(6) Vascular casts of metastases to the rabbit liver show that these tumours are avascular up to 1 mm in diameter. Larger tumours are invariably vascularized[36]. Several recent reports have also generated evidence for the regulatory role of angiogenesis in cancer metastasis[37–41]. For example, the intensity of neovascularization in melanomas can predict the probability of metastasis[40,41]. In a quantitative study on microvessel density in biopsy specimens from women with invasive breast cancer, the intensity of angiogenesis correlates with expansion of the tumour mass and metastatic disease[42]. Thus, quantitation of angiogenesis may prove valuable in identifying patients with breast carcinomas and other malignancies at high risk and to initiate aggressive therapy, including angiosuppression.

(7) Recent experiments have begun to yield *direct* evidence for the role of angiogenesis in tumour growth[43–46]. For example, Gross *et al.*[43–45] isolated a human colon carcinoma that lacks high-affinity receptors for basic fibroblast growth factor (bFGF) and for which bFGF is not mitogenic *in vitro*. However, when this tumour is grown in nude mice, intraperitoneal administration of bFGF leads to intense neovascularization of the tumour as well as a two-fold increase in tumour size. In contrast, tumour growth is significantly retarded in animals given neutralizing monoclonal antibodies to bFGF. Autoradiography of tumour sections revealed that receptors for bFGF are on the vascular endothelium[45].

Subsequent to the demonstration that glioma cells have high level of expression of multiple immunoreactive forms of bFGF and high affinity receptors for bFGF, Gross *et al.* showed that both human (SNB-19) and rat C6 glioma cells contained message for both bFGF and the high affinity bFGF receptors, FGFR1 (*flg*) and FGFR2. In addition, SNB-19 cells also contained message for bFGF-related oncogenic proteins, FGF-1, FGF-5 and FGF-7. These findings suggest that expression of members of the FGF family, besides acidic and bFGF, may be significant in brain neoplasms[45]. The expression of angiogenic growth factor genes in human gliomas *in situ* may contribute to their growth and progression[46,47].

ANGIOGENIC FACTORS

Using a transparent chamber in the hamster cheek pouch, Greenblatt and Shubik[48] observed that tumour fragments separated from the connective tissue stroma by a Millipore filter could still induce capillary proliferation in the host, providing the first clear evidence that tumour angiogenesis is mediated by a diffusible factor(s) derived from the growing tumour. Folkman *et al.*[49] subsequently isolated from human and animal tumours a polypeptide that caused neovascularization, and suggested that tumour cells release a tumour angiogenesis factor (TAF) to elicit new capillary formation and maintain the growth of tumours.

Due to the difficulties in the purification and chemical identification of TAF, progress in this area was slow up to about 1984[50]. A major advance in the purification of endothelial cell mitogens came as a result of the discovery by Shing *et al.* that an angiogenic factor derived from rat chondrosarcoma has strong heparin affinity[51]. Subsequently, several angiogenic factors were purified to homogeneity using heparin-affinity chromatography, their amino acid sequences were determined and their genes were cloned. It is now clear that there are a multitude of angiogenic factors (Table 7.1). These factors appear to fall into two groups, when evaluated according to their putative targets[2]: (i) Some (e.g. bFGF, VEGF) act directly on vascular endothelial cells to stimulate migration, proliferation and/or tube formation. (ii) Others (e.g. TNF-α, TGF-β) act indirectly by mobilizing host cells such as macrophages to release endothelial cell growth factors.

The large number of angiogenic factors implies biochemical redundancy in angiogenesis[121]. Angiogenic factors are also found in multiple tissues including hypothalamus[122], pineal gland[123], salivary glands[61,62], synovial fluid[5], wound fluid[124], myocardial infarcts[125], vitreous humour from diabetic retinopathy[3,107] and tumours[2,49,51,58,79,118]. Tumour cells produce their own angiogenic factors but also attract a variety of inflammatory cells (e.g. mast cells, macrophages and occasionally lymphocytes) that generate further angiogenic modulators[68].

ANGIOGENESIS IS A MULTI-STEP PROCESS

Angiogenesis is a complex process involving the intricate interplay between cells, soluble factors and extracellular matrix components. Elegant studies on angiogenesis *in vitro* show that endothelial cells can express all the information

Table 7.1 Angiogenic factors

Factor	Angiogenic activity in vivo	EC migration	EC proliferation	Tube formation	References
Polypeptides					
Basic fibroblast growth factor (bFGF)	CAM, hamster cheek pouch, rat sponge implants	+	+	+	51–55
Acidic fibroblast growth factor (aFGF)	CAM, rat sponge implants	+	+	0	56, 57
Angiogenin	CAM, rabbit cornea	0	0/+	ND	58–60
Epidermal growth factor (EGF)	Hamster cheek pouch	+	+	ND	61, 62
Transforming growth factor-α (TGF-α)	Hamster cheek pouch	+	+	ND	61, 62
Transforming growth factor-β (TGF-β)	Subcutaneous injection in mice	–	–	+	63–67
Tumour necrosis factor-α (TNF-α)	CAM, rat cornea	+	–	+	68–70
Human angiogenesis factor (h-AF)	CAM	ND	0	ND	71
Angiotropin	CAM, rabbit cornea, rabbit skin	+	–	+	72, 73
Platelet-derived endothelial cell growth factor (PD-ECGF)	CAM, PD-ECGF-transfected tumour cells induce highly vascular tumours	+	+	ND	74
Vascular endothelial growth factor/vascular permeability factor (VEGF/VPF)	CAM, rat and rabbit cornea	ND	+	ND	75–79
Interleukin 1α (IL-1α)	Rabbit cornea, rat brain, rat sponge implants	0	+/–	ND	80–87
Interleukin 4 (IL-4)	ND	ND	+	ND	88
Erythropoietin	ND	+	+	ND	89
Granulocyte-colony stimulating factor (G-CSF) and granulocyte-macrophage colony stimulating factor (GM-CSF)	ND	+	+	ND	90
Angiotensin II	Rabbit cornea, CAM, rat sponge implants	+	+	ND	91–93
Substance P	Rabbit cornea, rat sponge implants	ND	+	ND	85, 94
Calcitonin gene related peptide (CGRP)	Rat sponge implants	ND	+	ND	85, 95
Bradykinin	Rat sponge implants	ND	ND	ND	85, 87

Table 7.1 *continued*

Factor	Angionic activity in vivo	EC migration	EC proliferation	Tube formation	References
Lipids					
Prostaglandin E_1/E_2	Rabbit cornea	ND	ND	+	96–98
Leukotriene C_4	ND	+	–	+	99
Platelet-activating factor	Rat sponge implants	+	+	ND	100–102
1-butyryl-glycerol (monobutyrin)	CAM	+	–	ND	103
Erucamide	CAM, rat cornea	ND	0	ND	104
Other compounds					
Endothelial stimulating angiogenesis factor (ESAF)	CAM, cornea, sponge implants	+	+	ND	5, 105–108
Heparin	CAM	+	ND	ND	109, 110
Hyaluronic acid fragment (4-25 disaccharide)	CAM, rat sponge implants	+	+	ND	111, 112 Fan *et al.* (unpublished)
Fibrinogen	Rat sponge implants	ND	ND	ND	82
Fibrin	Guinea pig plastic chambers	ND	ND	+	113, 114
Laminin	Rat sponge implants	ND	ND	+	82, 115
Adenosine	CAM	+	+	ND	116, 117
Nicotinamide	Rabbit cornea	0	ND	ND	118
Histamine	CAM	ND	ND	ND	119
Spermine and spermidine	CAM	ND	ND	ND	120

Key: + = stimulation; – = inhibition; 0 = no effect; ND = not determined; EC = endothelial cell.

necessary to construct a capillary tube and assemble a vascular network[126]. Because endothelial cells play a crucial role in neovascularization, their biology has been extensively reviewed[127–133].

Eight fundamental, sequential steps in the angiogenesis process are:

(1) The initial vascular response of *dilation and hyperpermeability*; endothelial cells retract with a decrease in endothelial junctions; the cells appear 'reactive'.

(2) Basement membrane dissolution caused by *activation of proteases*, including plasminogen activator and type IV collagenase.

(3) *Migration of endothelial cells* from the vascular wall, through perivascular connective tissue and parenchyma, towards the angiogenic stimulus.

(4) *Proliferation of endothelial cells* behind the leading front of migrating endothelial cells.

(5) *Formation of capillary tubules and loops* derived from anastomoses of proximate sprouts.

(6) The newly formed capillary tubules then differentiate further and *synthesize a basement membrane*. Until these newly formed blood vessels fully develop a basement membrane with supporting cells, they are leaky, as in granulation tissue.

(7) *Migration of perivascular cells*, e.g. pericytes and fibroblasts, to the sites of the capillary loops.

(8) *Further tissue remodelling*, regression, and rearrangement of newly formed capillaries; contraction of capillaries by fibroblasts and myofibroblasts.

ANGIOSUPPRESSION AS A POTENTIAL ANTICANCER STRATEGY

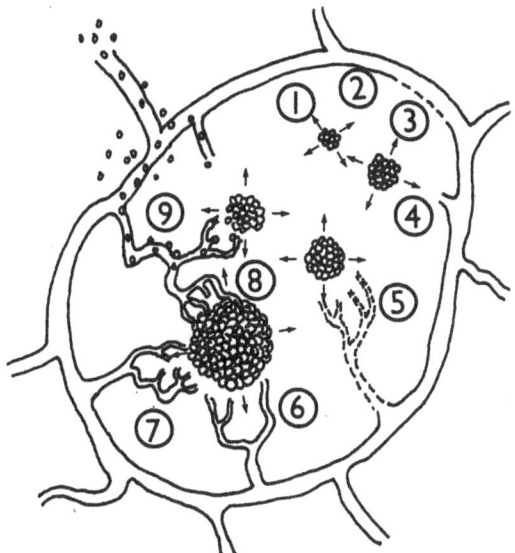

Figure 7.1   Possible targets for pharmacological intervention of tumour angiogenesis

Target	Examples of inhibitors
1 Production of angiogenic factors	Glucocorticoids, gold salts
2 Binding of angiogenic factors to receptors	Suramin, bFGF antibody, PF4, distamycin A analogues
3 Basement membrane degradation	Minocycline, PF4, medroxyprogesterone, cartilage-derived inhibitor, TIMP, vitreous-derived inhibitor
4 Endothelial cell migration	Angiostatic steroids, AGM-1470, thrombospondin, CDPGYIGSR-NH₂. Gly-Arg-Gly-Asp-Ser
5 Endothelial cell proliferation	Angiostatic steroids, D-penicillamine, gold salts, interferon-γ, tumour necrosis factor-α, DS-4152
6 Capillary tube formation	Interferon-γ, cyclic YIGSR peptide Gly-Arg-Gly-Asp-Ser
7 Basement membrane synthesis	Angiostatic steroids, GPA 1734, proline analogues
8 Vessel penetration to tumour	Not identified yet
9 Metastasis	Angiostatic steroids, AGM-1470, TIMP

Figure 7.1 further illustrates the discrete steps in angiogenesis that could be altered pharmacologically:

(1) Blocking expression, synthesis and/or release of angiogenic factor(s).
(2) Neutralization of the activity of released angiogenic factors.
(3) Inhibition of proteases that cause dissolution of basement membrane.
(4) Prevention of endothelial cell migration.
(5) Prevention of endothelial cell proliferation.
(6) Interference with tube formation.
(7) Inhibition of basement membrane biosynthesis.
(8) Prevention of vessels from penetrating a tumour.
(9) Metastasis

For an angiosuppressive agent to be most useful clinically, it should effectively and specifically inhibit one or more steps in new blood vessel formation with low toxicity. The well-characterized angiogenesis inhibitors are listed in Table 7.2, highlighting known mechanisms of action. Certain molecules act as potent suppressors of tumour growth, invasion, and metastasis, while no data exist for others.

Table 7.2 Angiogenic inhibitors

Factor	Nature	Main Action(s)	Anti-Tumour Effect	References
Steroids				
Glucocorticoids	Anti-inflammatory and immunosuppressive agents	Inhibit production and action of IL-1β Inhibit collagenous protein synthesis	Yes	134–147
Angiostatic steroids	Steroids with distinct structure on D ring	Cause dissolution of BM Inhibit EC proliferation Inhibit EC migration	Yes	134–147
Progestogens				
Medroxyprogesterone acetate	Synthetic	Inhibits collagenase and plasminogen activator	Yes	148, 149
Angiostatic antibiotics				
Herbimycin A	Benzenoid ansamycin	Induces malignant cells to express differentiated phenotype	ND	150–152
Minocycline	Semisynthetic tetracycline	Inhibits collagenase Inhibits EC proliferation	Yes	153
AGM-1470	Fumagillin analogue	Inhibits EC migration proliferation and collagenase	Yes	154–156

Table 7.2 *continued*

Factor	Nature	Main Action(s)	Anti-Tumour Effect	References
Angiostatic polysaccharides				
SP-PG	Sulphated polysaccharide/ peptidoglycan	Inhibits EC proliferation	Yes	141
DS-4152	Sulphated polysaccharide/ peptidoglycan	Inhibits EC proliferation	Yes	142
SCM-chitin III	Sulphated polysaccharide	Inhibits type IV collagenase and EC migration	Yes	157
Krestin	Protein-bound plant polysaccharide	Inhibits EC collagen synthesis	Yes	158, 159
Vitamin derivatives				
Retinoids	Natural or synthetic	Induce cell differentiation	ND	160, 161
Vitamin D_3 analogues	Active metabolites of vitamin D_3	Induce cell differentiation	ND	162, 163
Interferons				
Interferon-α 2a	Recombinant protein, 18.5 kD	Inhibits EC migration May also inhibit growth factor production by spindle cells	Yes	164–166
Interferon-β	21 kD glycoprotein	May inhibit production of angiogenic factors from tumour cells	Yes	167
Interferon-γ	50 kD glycoprotein	Down-regulates aFGF receptors; inhibits EC growth and capillary formation	ND	166–172
Cytokines				
Tumour necrosis factor-α	17 kD polypeptide	Cytotoxic and cytostatic against tumour cells Activation of neutrophils; Bifunctional modulaton of EC functions Inhibits EC proliferation (and stimulates angio-genesis; dose dependent)	Yes	68, 70, 172–176
Transforming growth factor-β	25 kD homodimer	Bifunctional modulator of EC migration and proliferation	ND	2, 63–67, 86, 177

Table 7.2 *continued*

Factor	Nature	Main Action(s)	Anti-Tumour Effect	References
Platelet-related products				
Platelet Factor 4	28 kD tetrameric protein	Binds heparin Inhibits EC growth and migration Inhibits collagenase	Yes	178–180
Thrombospondin	450 kD adhesive glycoprotein	Inhibits capillary EC migration	ND	181–184
Platelet-activating factor (PAF) antagonists	Synthetic	PAF receptor antagonism	ND	100
Modulators of extracellular matrix turnover				
BM synthesis inhibitors	Synthetic	Inhibit collagen synthesis	Yes	160, 185–190
CDPGYIGSR-NH$_2$	Synthetic laminin peptide	Inhibits EC migration	ND	191–195
Arg-Gly-Asp containing peptide	Synthetic peptide	Inhibits EC migration and capillary formation	ND	196
Cartilage-derived inhibitor (CDI)	28 kD polypeptide	Inhibits collagenase Inhibits EC migration and proliferation	ND	197–201
TIMP	8.5 kD glycoprotein	Inhibits metallo-proteinases, EC migration and proliferation	ND	120, 202–206
TIMP-2	21 kD glycoprotein	Inhibits collagenase IV, EC migration and proliferation	ND	120, 204, 206
Vitreal inhibitor	5.7 kD glycoprotein	Inhibits matrix metalloproteinases, EC proliferation	ND	207–210
Hyaluronic acid	High molecular weight glycosaminoglycan	Inhibits EC proliferation	ND	111, 112, 114
Polycationic and polyanionic compounds				
Protamine	4.3 kD arginine-rich cationic protein	Binds heparin Blocks heparin-induced EC migration Inhibits EC proliferation	Yes	178
Suramin	1.4 kD polyanionic compound	Binds to various growth factors, cell membrane and intra-cellular enzymes	Yes	143, 211–221 Takano *et al.* (unpublished)
Distamycin A analogues	Sulphonic derivatives of distamycin	Inhibit binding of bFGF and PDGF-b to their receptors	Yes	222, 223

Table 7.2 *continued*

Factor	Nature	Main Action(s)	Anti-Tumour Effect	References
Others				
Gold salts	Synthetic anti-rheumatic agents	Inhibit EC mitosis Inhibit production of angiogenic factors by macrophages Inhibit angiogenesis in sponge implants	ND	224, 225 Fan *et al.* (unpublished)
D-penicillamine	Synthetic anti-rheumatic agent	Chelates copper Inhibits EC proliferation Inhibits collagenase, collagen biosynthesis, and plasminogen activator	Yes	17, 44, 226, 227
RNAse inhibitor	51 kD protein	Inhibits angiogenin-induced angiogenesis	ND	228

BM = basement membrane; EC = endothelial cell; ND = not determined

ANGIOSTATIC STEROIDS AND HEPARIN

Corticosteroids, at high doses administered locally or systemically, can cause partial regression of blood vessels. At the doses required, however, systemic immunosuppression, electrolyte imbalance, and other serious problems occur. In the presence of heparin, low doses of cortisone block angiogenesis in the chorioallantoic membrane, cause tumour regression, and prevent metastasis[134]. A unique feature of angiostatic steroids is that they are effective only in the presence of heparin or a non-anticoagulant fragment of heparin[110,135]. Other groups reported that heparin does not enhance the action of angiostatic steroids[136–138]. The difference can be due to the heterogeneity of heparin preparations (e.g. composition, molecular size, position of substituents and sequence)[139]. Recently, effective heparin substitutes have been identified, e.g. a synthetic inhibitor of arylsulphatase[140], a polysaccharide-peptidoglycan from *Arthrobacter*[141,142], suramin[143] and β-cyclodextrin tetradecasulphate (β-CD-14S)[139]. When administered with a steroid, β-CD-14S is 100 to 1000 times more effective than heparin in inhibiting angiogenesis in the chick chorioallantoic membrane assay[139].

The immunosuppressive and metastasis-promoting effects of glucocorticoids prompted a search for angiosuppressive steroids devoid of hormonal activity, i.e. true angiostatic steroids[135]. Structure–activity studies show that the angio-suppressive activity is associated with the pregnane structure and by the structure of the D ring. To date, tetrahydrocortisol is the most potent naturally occurring angiostatic steroid[135]. Effective synthetic angiostatic steroids such as U-24067 and U-42129 are being developed as potential anticancer drugs[143].

The mechanism of action of angiostatic steroids is not fully understood, although at least four possibilities exist: (i) Induction of capillary basement membrane dissolution and endothelial cell rounding[144,144a]. (ii) Inhibition of collagenous protein synthesis[145]. (iii) Inhibition of microvascular endothelial cell migration[146]. (iv) Inhibition of the formation and effects of cytokines and/or angiogenic factors. Glucocorticoids are known to reduce inflammatory response by multiple mechanisms. In addition to blocking eicosanoid synthesis via the production of phospholipase A_2-inactivating proteins such as lipocortin, they also inhibit the transcription of the interleukin-1β (IL-1β) gene and decrease the stability of IL-1β mRNA, and suppress the expression of basic fibroblast growth factor by cultured cells[147,147a].

MEDROXYPROGESTERONE

Medroxyprogesterone acetate is an anticancer drug used in the treatment of mammary carcinoma. When locally applied in sustained polymer to rabbit V2 carcinoma or mouse B-16 melanoma implanted in the rabbit cornea, it blocked neovascularization and growth of the tumours[139]. The inhibitory responses were accompanied by significant reduction in collagenolytic activity released into culture medium by explants of the two tumours. Recently medroxyprogesterone was shown to inhibit extracellular and cell-associated activity of plasminogen activator of bovine endothelial cells, but not their growth[149]. Furthermore, it diminished the high level of endothelial plasminogen activator induced by bFGF or phorbol myristate acetate (PMA).

ANGIOSUPPRESSIVE ANTIBIOTICS

Herbimycin A

Herbimycin A is the first example of an angiostatic antibiotic. Isolated from cultures of *Streptomyces* species, when applied to the chick chorioallantoic membrane, herbimycin A has powerful angiosuppressive activity at 0.1–10 μg per egg, 200-fold more active than medroxyprogesterone acetate. The mechanism of action is unknown. It can convert avian sarcoma virus-transfected cells to a normal phenotype concomitant with inhibition of p60v-*src* kinase activity. Herbimycin A might induce angiosuppressive activity by selectively reducing the activity of certain oncogene products related to tyrosine kinase[151,152].

Minocycline

Recent studies on the control mechanism of angiogenesis have stressed the importance of enzyme-mediated remodelling of the extracellular matrix in capillary growth and proliferation. Minocycline is a semi-synthetic tetracycline with anti-collagenase activity. It also significantly prolongs the doubling time of bovine retinal endothelial cells but not C6 glioma, F98 glioma, or 9L gliosarcoma tumour lines[153]. *In vivo*, minocycline inhibits tumour angiogenesis in the rabbit cornea[153]. Since anti-collagenase agents could be used to inhibit pathological collagenolysis, sparing physiological proteolysis, they should be considered as potentially important anti-neoplastic agents[153].

Fumagillin and AGM-1470

Ingber *et al.* recently observed that, in contrast to other fungal contaminants that produce total detachment and death of capillary endothelial cells, one fungus consistently produced a local gradient of endothelial cell rounding. Cells that were only a few cell diameters away spread normally. Further work led to the isolation and identification of the fungus as *Aspergillus fumigatus fresenius*. The active fraction purified from large-scale fungal cultures was identified as a naturally secreted antibiotic fumagillin, commonly used to treat amoebiasis in man. At $0.5\,ng\,ml^{-1}$, fumagillin results in a half-maximal inhibition of endothelial cell proliferation in the presence of saturating levels of basic FGF. At a concentration above $2\,\mu g$ per chorioallantoic membrane, fumagillin inhibits angiogenesis. It also suppresses tumour-induced neo-vascularization in the mouse dorsal air sac. However, fumagillin produces severe weight loss, thus limiting its usefulness as an inhibitor of tumour growth. This led to the synthesis and discovery of a subset of fumagillin analogues that retain the potent anti-angiogenic activity of fumagillin without the side-effects.

AGM-1470 is the most potent fumagillin analogue[154]. Given systemically in mice, there is a sustained inhibition of growth of solid tumours including Lewis lung carcinoma, B16 melanoma and Engelbreth–Holm Swarm sarcoma. More recent studies[155] show that tumours M27 and H59 (derived from Lewis lung carcinoma) in the lungs of the AGM-1470-treated mice are smaller and essentially avascular compared to tumours in the lungs of saline-treated mice. In the mouse sponge implantation assay, systemically administered AGM-1470 inhibits neovascularization induced by bFGF. Taken together, these data show that AGM-1470 suppresses tumour growth and metastasis and that this effect is primarily by inhibition of angiogenesis.

In vitro, AGM-1470 produces half-maximal cytostatic inhibition of endo-thelial cell proliferation at $\sim 10\,pg\,ml^{-1}$, about 50 times more potent than the fumagillin parent. Much higher concentrations ($>1\,\mu g\,ml^{-1}$) are required to cause cytotoxicity. Furthermore, $100\,pg\,ml^{-1}$ AGM-1470 is sufficient to inhibit migration of bovine capillary endothelial cells, while half-maximal inhibition of migration of M27 carcinoma cells requires much higher doses, approx-imately $30\,ng\,ml^{-1}$. In the rat, AGM-1470 selectively inhibits the capillary-like tube formation of endothelial cells with a minimal effect on non-endothelial cell growth[156]. Thus the sensitivity of endothelial cells to AGM-1470 adds further evidence that the tumour microvasculature is the prime target of its action.

ANGIOSTATIC POLYSACCHARIDES

DS-4152

DS-4152 is a sulphated polysaccharide-peptidoglycan complex, isolated from the culture supernatant of an *Arthrobacter* species[142]. It inhibits angiogenesis and tumour growth in the chick chorioallantoic membrane and enhances the angiosuppressive activity of steroids by 2–100-fold. In contrast to heparin and its fragments that are angiostatic only when applied in combination with a steroid, DS-4152 inhibits angiogenesis in the absence of a steroid. Furthermore, the anticoagulant activity of DS-4152 is markedly lower than that of heparin, although its angiosuppressive activity is more potent. Repeated subcutaneous treatment with heparin causes haemorrhagic death of mice, but DS-4152 suppresses tumour growth without reducing body weight.

Sulphated chitin derivatives

Unlike heparin, which is a structurally heterogeneous sulphated polysaccharide composed of repeated units of glucosamine and uronic acid, chitin is a homogeneous polysaccharide composed of *N*-acetylglucosamine residues. SCM-chitin III is a group of chemically modified chitin derivatives containing 6-*O*-sulphate and 6-*O*-carboxymethyl groups. SCM-chitin III significantly inhibits the lung tumour colonization of B16-BL6 melanoma in experimental and spontaneous lung metastasis models[157]. SCM-chitin III inhibits tumour-associated angiogenesis in mice. The chitin derivatives inhibit the activity of type IV collagenase and heparanase more potently than heparin. Thus, it is possible that SCM-chitin III may act as an inhibitor of type IV collagenase. SCM-chitin III also prevents the invasion of endothelial cells through Matrigel and the migration to fibronectin-substrate *in vitro*, suggesting that the inhibition of tumour angiogenesis by chitin may be due to the inhibition of endothelial cell migration modulated by the extracellular matrix.

Krestin

Krestin is a protein-bound polysaccharide isolated and purified from mycelia of the CM-101 strain of *Coriolus versicolor*. Administered intraperitoneally, Krestin markedly inhibits tumour-induced neovascularization. Krestin has no direct effect on endothelial cell proliferation or migration, but it significantly reduces the synthesis of collagen by microvascular endothelial cells *in vitro*[158,159].

VITAMIN DERIVATIVES

Retinoids

The angiosuppressive property of herbimycin suggested that agents that induce malignant cells to differentiate might also affect activation/differentiation

196

coupling of endothelial cells in neovascularization. To test this hypothesis, Oikawa *et al.*[161] examined the angiosuppressive potential of retinoids, a group of compounds known to modify the differentiation of human promyelocytic leukaemia cells, mouse embryonic carcinoma cells and human neuroblastoma cells (see Chapter 6). Several retinoid derivatives exhibited potent angio-suppressive activity in the chorioallantoic membrane assay[161]. Based on the dose required to achieve half-maximal inhibition, the rank order of inhibitory activity is Ch55 (synthetic chalcone carboxylic acid) > retinoic acid > herbimycin A > retinyl acetate. The order of potency correlates with the ability of these compounds to induce cell differentiation *in vitro*.

Vitamin D_3 analogues

Like retinoids, vitamin D_3 analogues induce differentiation[162] (see Chapter 6). In the picomolar range, the active metabolite of vitamin D_3, $1\alpha,25$-dihydroxyvitamin D_3 ($1,25(OH)_2D_3$), and a synthetic vitamin D_3 analogue, 22-oxa-$1\alpha,25$-dihydroxyvitamin D_3, inhibit angiogenesis of the chick embryo chorioallantoic membrane.

Both angiostatic vitamin D_3 analogues and retinoids exhibit similar biological activities: (i) inhibition of the induction of epidermal ornithine decarboxylase by the tumour promoter, PMA, (ii) their effects are mediated by intracellular receptors, and (iii) result in an increased number of $1,25(OH)_2D_3$ receptors. Thus, it appears that the two angiostatic vitamins could act by common mechanisms. Analogues of vitamin A and D_3 may be promising angiogenesis antagonists. Indeed, $1,25(OH)_2D_3$ inhibits the growth of human tumour xenografts in mice[163].

INTERFERONS

Successful treatment of an angiogenic disease[229] is exemplified by the dramatic results of interferon α for the treatment of haemangioendotheliomas[164], and the remarkable clinical efficacy of interferon α-2a in the treatment of pulmonary capillary haemangiomatosis – a previously fatal disease marked by excessive proliferation of blood vessels[165].

Although interferon γ inhibits capillary tube formation *in vitro*, interferon α actually produces the opposite effect[166]. Interferon α could suppress the production of autocrine growth factor(s) from the spindle cells observed in pulmonary neovascular lesions (cf. spindle cells in Kaposi's sarcoma[230,231]). Tumour cells treated with homologous interferon are significantly less competent to initiate angiogenesis than untreated cells[167]. Furthermore, interferon β impairs the ability of L1210 leukaemia cells (resistant to the anti-proliferative effects of interferons) to induce angiogenesis. Thus interferons might inhibit production or release of angiogenic factors from tumour cells.

In contrast, the action of interferon γ appears to be directed against endothelial cells[166,168-170]. It inhibits aFGF-induced endothelial cell proliferation[169] by the down-regulation of the FGF receptors, evidenced by a concomitant reduction in binding of aFGF to the endothelial cell surface. Interferon γ also blocks IL-2-induced endothelial cell growth[170].

PLATELET-RELATED PRODUCTS

Platelet factor 4

Platelet factor 4 (PF4) is a platelet alpha-granule protein that is released from platelets during aggregation. Like protamine, PF4 has high affinity for heparin and is angiosuppressive[178]. Recombinant human PF4 (rHuPF4) and several analogues inhibit blood vessel proliferation in the chick chorioallantoic membrane[179], as well as the growth of murine melanoma and human colon carcinoma in nude mice[180]. The angiosuppressive activity of PF4 is associated with the carboxyl-terminal, heparin-binding domain. The inhibitory effects can be abrogated by the addition of heparin, suggesting that *in vivo* sulphated polysaccharides might modulate the angiosuppressive activity of PF4. *In vitro*, PF4 (5–50 μg ml^{-1}) inhibits growth factor-stimulated endothelial cell proliferation, an action that can be reversed by re-addition of growth factor. The migration of human endothelial cells is also inhibited by rHuPF4 within the same concentration range. Fibroblasts, keratinocytes and several human and murine tumour cell lines are insensitive to rHuPF4.

Thrombospondin

Thrombospondin is a high-molecular-weight, ubiquitous adhesive glycoprotein, stored in platelet alpha-granules, synthesized by cultured fibroblasts, macrophages, tumour cells, and endothelial cells[184]. The angiosuppressive property of a 140-kD fragment of thrombospondin was discovered in the conditioned media of hamster and hamster-hybrid cells[181]. The inhibitor seems to be produced by cells when they are expressing an active cancer suppressor gene. Subsequent studies[182] established that the secreted inhibitor was biochemically similar to and immunologically cross-reactive with thrombospondin. In addition, human thrombospondin inhibits endothelial cell migration *in vitro* and angiogenesis *in vivo*, as does the hamster protein, Gp140. Both proteins sensitize smooth muscle cells to stimulation by EGF. Thus thrombospondin is likely to be involved in the normal physiological down-regulation of angiogenesis[183,184]. The suppressor and the thrombospondin genes are located on different chromosomes. Thrombospondin may be one of a number of target molecules through which a tumour suppressor gene could act to restrain tumour growth. The loss of this inhibitory activity occurs concomitantly with expression of both angiogenesis and tumourigenesis[184].

Platelet-activating factor antagonists

Platelet-activating factor (PAF) is a fatty acid derivative that increases vascular permeability, induces platelet aggregation and promotes leucocyte chemotaxis. PAF stimulates (i) endothelial cell proliferation, (ii) endothelial cell migration and (iii) collagenase production by fibroblasts[101]. Daily administration of 10^{-10} moles PAF, but not lyso-PAF, into subcutaneous sponge implants in rats enhances their neovascularization. Conversely, three structurally unrelated PAF antagonists produce a dose-related (1–100 μg per day) inhibition of angiogenesis[100]. Preliminary histological studies show that vascularity and cellularity of the implanted sponges are modulated by these compounds. Taken together, these observations suggest a role for PAF antagonists in the modulation of angiogenesis.

MODULATORS OF EXTRACELLULAR MATRIX TURNOVER

Recent studies have emphasized the importance of basement membranes in vascular development[160,185]. Basement membranes are mainly composed of collagen IV, fibronectin, heparan sulphate proteoglycan and laminin. These molecules regulate the attachment, migration, proliferation and organization of isolated endothelial cells. Identification of extracellular matrix metabolism as a control point in neovascularization may provide a novel approach for the development of angiosuppressive regimens[160,185–196].

Basement membrane biosynthesis inhibitors

Basement membrane is an essential component of all blood vessels and its biosynthesis is one of the final steps of angiogenesis. Thus, selective inhibition of basement membrane biosynthesis would be expected to prevent angiogenesis. For example, proline analogues and an inhibitor of prolyl hydroxylase (α,α-dipyridyl) that interferes with triple helix formation and collagen deposition cause the regression of growing capillaries in the chorioallantoic membrane. Furthermore, an inhibitor of collagen cross-linking (β-aminopropionitrile) is also angiosuppressive. Co-administration of proline analogues, angiostatic steroids and heparin lead to complete inhibition of angiogenesis and larger and more extensive avascular zones in the chick chorioallantoic membrane than do steroid-heparin combinations[160]. Independently, Maragoudakis et al.[188] discovered the angiosuppressive effect of two collagen biosynthesis inhibitors: (i) GPA 1734 blocks the hydroxylation of proline and lysine in the formation of collagen IV, and inhibits angiogenesis in the chick chorioallantoic membrane; (ii) D609 inhibits basement membrane biosynthesis by an unknown mechanism and also prevents angiogenesis. Both inhibitors also have anti-tumour effects in rats bearing Walker 256 carcinosarcoma[189].

Laminin analogues

The known functions of laminin include cell adhesion, migration, differentiation and growth. Graf et al. demonstrated that an active site for these functions consists of nine sequential amino acids: Cys-Asp-Pro-Gly-Tyr-Ile-Gly-Ser-Arg-(CDPGYIGSR)[191]. This polypeptide inhibits the bioactivity of laminin by competing for cell surface receptors. The pentapeptide, YIGSR, prevents both the formation of lung tumour colonies by blocking the binding of tumour cells to basement membranes[192] and the differentiation of endothelial cells into capillary-like structures[193–195]. A synthetic laminin peptide, CDPGYIGSR-NH$_2$, inhibits both angiogenesis and solid tumour growth[195]. The synthetic peptide also suppresses embryonic angiogenesis in the chorioallantoic membrane and the growth of the solid tumour form of Sarcoma 180, but not the ascitic form, consistent with its role as an angiosuppressive agent. Furthermore, the peptide inhibits pulmonary metastasis both when administered with pretreated 3LL cells and when the treatment starts after intravenous injection with 3LL cells. *In vitro*, CDPGYIGSR-NH$_2$ suppresses the migration of vascular endothelial cells induced by tumour-conditioned medium but neither the proliferation of endo-thelial cells nor that of tumour cells. Thus, the solid tumour growth inhibition by CDPGYIGSR-NH$_2$ is due to inhibition of endothelial cell migration rather than a direct effect on cell growth.

Arg-Gly-Asp-containing synthetic peptide

The endothelial response to the extracellular matrix is, in part, mediated by integrins, a family of cell membrane receptors that bind to extracellular matrix molecules. Many receptors belonging to the integrin family recognize poly-peptide domains containing the Arg-Gly-Asp (RGD) amino acid sequence. The RGD sequence is present in fibronectin, laminin, collagen and thrombospondin. Gly-Arg-Gly-Asp-Ser (GRGDS), a synthetic peptide containing the RGD sequence, inhibits endothelial cell migration and angiogenesis *in vitro*[196].

Tissue inhibitor of metalloproteinases; cartilage and vitreous inhabitors

During angiogenesis, proteases are crucial for the escape of the endothelial cells from the parent venule, and for allowing tumour cells to migrate into and out of microvasculature in the process of metastasis. Thus, protease inhibitors could have great potential in limiting the aberrant neovascularization in tumours.

In 1975, Brem and Folkman observed that an implant of neonatal scapular cartilage blocked angiogenesis in the rabbit corneal pocket assay[197]. Local infusion of a partially purified cartilage extract on to corneas led to almost complete inhibition of neovascularization induced by an implant of V2 car-cinoma[198]. *In vitro*, the inhibitor suppresses endothelial cell growth, but has no effect on tumour cell growth[199,200]. Subsequently, a 28 kD inhibitor of mammalian collagenase has been isolated from bovine cartilage, that not only inhibits the proliferation and migration of capillary endothelial cells *in vitro* but also arrests angiogenesis in the chorioallantoic membrane assay[201]. The cartilage-derived inhibitor (CDI) has homology to a collagenase inhibitor isolated, sequenced and cloned from several sources – tissue inhibitor of metalloproteinases (TIMP)[202–204]. The exact relation between CDI and TIMP is under active study. TIMP and TIMP-2 are considered to be tumour- and metastasis-suppressor gene products [202–204] capable of blocking polyamine-induced angiogenesis and tumour invasion[120,206].

Another source of angiogenic inhibitors is the vitreous humour[25, 207–210]. The two glycoproteins (3.5 kD and 5.7 kD) isolated from the vitreous inhibit collagenase, microvessel endothelial cell proliferation and angiogenesis on the chick yolk sac membrane[209, 210].

GOLD SALTS

Gold salts have been used in the treatment of rheumatoid arthritis for many years; however, their mechanism of action has not been established. Angiosuppression may account for their beneficial effects. Gold sodium thiomalate and auranofin inhibit dose-dependently the proliferation of endothelial cells[224], and sponge-induced angiogenesis in rats (Fan and Andrade, unpublished data). Gold sodium thiomalate and auranofin potently reduce or completely inhibit the production of macrophage-derived angiogenic activity[225]. Thus, gold salts are among the first compounds that act directly on the macrophage to cause a decrease in the production of angiogenic factors. Whether gold salts can inhibit tumour growth or prevent metastasis remains an open question.

D-PENICILLAMINE

D-Penicillamine inhibits proliferation of endothelial cells *in vitro* and angiogenesis *in vivo*[226]. The inhibitory action of D-penicillamine[17] is thought to

Table 7.3 Copper-binding angiogenesis factors

Factor	Reference
Angiogenin	59
Angiotropin	73
Gly-His-Lys	97
Fibroblast growth factor (acidic and basic)	232
Tumour necrosis factor-α	233
Heparin	234
Ceruloplasmin	235
Mammary tumour-derived growth factor	236
Endothelial stimulating factor	237
Transforming growth factor-β	Folkman *et al.* (unpublished)
Vascular permeability factor	Connolly DT *et al.* (unpublished)
Platelet-activating factor	Sorensen *et al.* (unpublished)

be related to (i) removal of copper, a trace metal bound to numerous angiogenic molecules (Table 7.3); (ii) inhibition of collagen biosynthesis; and (iii) inhibition of proteolytic enzymes, e.g. collagenase[227] and plasminogen activator[44].

Copper depletion and penicillamine treatment (CDPT) effectively inhibit tumour growth by a selective reduction of endothelial cell turnover of approximately 50%[17]. Because a small change in a mitotic regulatory circuit, with time, leads to a major change in the overall growth of a cell population[238], a subtotal reduction in endothelial cell mitotic rate may be sufficient to suppress neovascularization. The intracerebral nodules of CDPT-treated V2 carcinomas[17] show a remarkable histological resemblance to dormant V2 carcinomas maintained artificially in the avascular state by anatomic separation from an available blood supply. Despite proximity to preformed vessels, the carcinoma is consigned pharmacologically to the angiosuppressed state, demonstrating the feasibility of therapeutic suppression within a vascularized organ such as the brain.

PRACTICAL CONSIDERATIONS

Initiation of angiosuppression therapy

Angiosuppression, because it arrests tumour growth at the tiny prevascular stage, will reduce tumour burden and therefore be effective in combination with other forms of adjuvant therapy[239,240] (chemotherapy, immunotherapy, radiation therapy and hyperthermia) that work best when the tumour cell population is small[241,242]. A larger tumour mass is more resistant to cancer chemotherapy, in part, because of 'pharmacological sanctuaries' of cell populations compartmentalized in areas of increasing tumour–blood distance and slower proliferative rates[242,243].

Even in an established tumour, most of the endothelium is non-cycling and statin-positive[244]. The vascular tree exists as a quiescent monolayer of endothelial cell with a non-terminal, differentiated phenotype that can be 'switched' into the mitotic cycle by the local release of angiogenic mitogens[245]. Although malignant human brain tumours are well vascularized, only a small fraction of vascular endothelial cells are actually replicating at a given moment[246]. By contrast, continuous labelling of small, 3.5–5.0 mm experimental tumours shows that between 25 and 100% of the endothelial cells replicate during a one-week period[31]. In the copper-depletion experiments, it was necessary to pretreat the animals; acute therapy was ineffective[17]. This could be due to the time required to remove an angiogenic stimulus, such as copper salts in the tissues; alternatively, angiosuppression may be more effective against smaller, younger, proliferative tumours about to acquire new vessels, in contrast to non-proliferative, preformed, well-differentiated microvessels within the scaffold of an established tumour.

Side-effects and toxicity

Given the structural, chemical, and biological diversity of angiogenic inhibitors, each agent would be expected to have individual side-effects. For example, inhibitors of collagen biosynthesis[160,188,189] could predispose to osteoporosis. Likewise, inhibition of tumour growth by rHuPF4 occurs only at high concentrations (2–5 µmol/L) that might limit therapeutic application due to side-effects or toxicity[178–180]. However, as a class of compounds, the toxicity of angiosuppression should be less daunting than conventional chemotherapy. The turnover of normal endothelium is estimated to be 10–3000 times longer than parenchymal cells, and does not vary between slow turnover tissues (e.g. lung and brain) and those where the parenchyma is rapidly turning over, e.g. jejunum[32]. Therefore, angiosuppression might not have the gastrointestinal toxicity of conventional anti-mitotic chemotherapy.

Because of the importance of angiogenesis to both wound healing and tumour growth, there is concern that wound healing might be impaired. It has been observed, however, that scalp[17] and flank[44] wounds heal well in animals receiving copper depletion and D-penicillamine treatment, possibly because of the involvement of separate non-mitogenic angiogenic factors[124]. A relatively minor problem, nevertheless, might be alopecia, because angiogenesis is important in the cyclical growth of the hair follicle[247]. Furthermore, we observed shedding of hair in a few angiosuppressed rabbits.

Angiogenesis is essential for normal ovulatory function[248]; therefore, chronic angiosuppression might render female patients oligomenorrhoeic and infertile. Placental endothelium has a high [^{3}H] thymidine labelling index[31,249]. Thus, angiosuppression will be of limited use in pregnant patients.

The effects on the vascular infrastructure of an established tumour once angiosuppression begins are not well understood. There have been only rare reports of regression of established tumours by angiosuppression. Acute vascular injury, or even infarction, might be undesirable for a large established tumour, and could lead to necrosis and swelling, with unwanted clinical consequences.

The recently discovered angiogenic protein, VPF (VEGF)[75–79], also acts as a permeability factor, but the effects of angiosuppressive agents on vascular permeability are unknown. For brain tumours, the tumour-associated vasogenic oedema is a major cause of morbidity; any treatment that blocked the hyperpermeability of brain tumour vessels would be welcome. On the other hand, angiosuppression may increase cerebral oedema[17]. Tumour vessels are bidirectional conduits that not only permit the influx of metabolites and serum proteins, but also return interstitial proteins to the systemic circulation[250]. Angiogenesis often appears in areas previously oedematous. The increased permeability and vasogenic oedema has been suggested to represent a *forme fruste* of angiogenesis in the brain[17]. Oedema resulting from angiosuppression has not been reported in organs except the brain; extracerebral tissues contain lymphatics that can clear the interstitial proteins.

Therapeutic plurality of angiosuppressives

Given the 'redundancy in angiogenic regulation', i.e. the multiplicity of angiogenic stimulators and inhibitors, Zetter suggested that tissues that require an angiogenic response elaborate multiple mechanisms to provoke such a response[121]. It follows logically that an angiosuppressive agent, to be truly effective, may need to inhibit more than one angiogenic molecule, pathway, or circuit. Such a 'therapeutic plurality' could account for the efficacy of D-penicillamine as an angiosuppressive agent, because it works at several postulated points in the angiogenesis cascade[17].

Combination therapy

The current management of hypertension illustrates the distinct advantage of combination therapy to potentiate efficacy and minimize toxicity. Angiogenesis is a multistep process: an angiosuppressive molecule may readily synergize with another. For example, angiostatic steroids can be augmented by using an anti-collagen agent[160], an inhibitor of arylsulphatase[140], or suramin[143]. Because dissolution of the basement membrane and endothelial cell migration are primary steps in neovascularization, the combination of agents that block plasminogen activator and collagenase IV (e.g. medroxyprogesterone, minocycline, or TIMP) with another that inhibits endothelial cell movement (e.g. SCM-chitin III, PF4, AGM-1470) may prove more useful than single agents alone. Furthermore, CDPGYIGSR, which has been shown to inhibit the morphological differentiation of endothelial cells into capillary-like structures, may synergize with compounds that inhibit basement membrance collagen biosynthesis (e.g. GPA 1743 and D609). The combination of a sulphated polysaccharide-peptidoglycan complex and the anti-oestrogen tamoxifen results in angiosuppression and tumour inhibition in tamoxifen-resistant as well as tamoxifen-sensitive tumours in nude mice[251].

Denekamp has recently reviewed several systemic and local vasculature-related strategies for causing vascular collapse in tumours[252]. Patients may benefit from angiosuppressives together with agents that cause selective, localized coagulation within a solid tumour[253], or therapy that increases interstitial pressure[240]. For example, flavone acetic acid induces a coagulopathy in tumour-bearing mice[254], and tumour vascular shutdown[255]. Furthermore, the combination of flavone acetic acid and TNF-α results in greater growth delay in murine tumours than would be predicted on the basis of the activity of either agent alone[256]. Thus the combination of angiosuppressives with flavone acetic acid might be an effective anti-cancer regimen.

Finally, future exploitations in the combination of angiosuppression with chemotherapy, immunotherapy, radiation therapy, photodynamic therapy, hyperthermia[239] or tumour blood flow modification[240] are expected to generate new modalities effective in specific types of cancer.

Pharmacokinetics and drug delivery

Most drugs act by first-order kinetics, but the pharmacokinetics for angio-suppressive drugs remain to be determined. For example, dexamethasone as an angiosuppressive drug has a bell-shaped dose–response curve[144a]. Variables, including the route of administration, tissue absorption and distribution, drug metabolism, biliary and kidney clearance, and equilibrium constants for protein binding in the plasma and for non-specific binding in tissue[257], all need to be considered.

Because angiogenesis is a local process, polymer implants in patients may prove valuable in releasing angiosuppressive agents in high concentration directly at the tumour site, analogous to the polymeric implants in rabbits that have been used successfully in the cornea to inhibit angiogenesis[140,144a,153]. Slow-release, biodegradable polymers containing standard chemotherapy (BCNU) are now being used in patients with malignant gliomas[258]. Further development of these polymers for the release of angiosuppressive drugs for various forms of tumours is being actively pursued[259,260]. Langer[261] reported that, by altering the hydrophobicity of the polymer backbone, release times from 1 week to 6 years can be accomplished. Methods of enhancing release on-demand of drugs may be facilitated using magnets or ultrasound.

Systemic angiosuppression[17,44,154,262,263] has proved successful in inhibiting tumour growth; it has the advantage of reaching nearly all areas of the tumour and the host organ through the microcirculation, whereas an implant could thwart disease locally, but allow residual cells to escape and form new colonies at the edge of the therapeutic zone. Because the final effect of an angiogenic polypeptide, e.g. FGF or TNF-α, depends on the route of administration[264], an angiosuppressive agent could have different actions dependent on whether it is given intravascularly (systemically) or extravascularly (locally). The variability of the endothelial response to angiogenic polypeptides is also determined by cell density, the isoform of the growth factor, the concentration of the mitogen, the three-dimensional growth pattern, the size and site of the parent vessel, the composition of the extracellular matrix, and the availability and interactions with other growth factors and inhibitors[265].

Length of treatment

Angiosuppression, because it is not cytotoxic to tumour cells, does not destroy tiny, dormant colonies, and therefore remains a long-term treatment[229]. Therefore, combination therapy with low doses of multiple angiosuppressives might limit toxicity related to chronic therapy. However, if the levels of the drug become subtherapeutic, and if remaining tumour is not eradicated by other means, then a clinical recurrence would ensue. The ideal schedule might be first to surgically excise the primary tumour, decreasing the tumour burden, and removing a large depot of angiogenic substances that could overwhelm an inhibitor. Many angiogenesis inhibitors have little or no effect on non-growing vessels, e.g. the vessels that exist in the CAM older than 11–12 days[266]. These established vessels could be removed surgically with the tumour or targeted using therapies taking advantage of the selective vulnerability of the endothelium, e.g. radiation therapy, hyperthermia, or monoclonal antibodies.

Screening of angiogenic inhibitors

Current methodology for the identification of angiogenic inhibitors includes *in vitro* tests that examine the effect of a potential inhibitor on endothelial cell migration, proliferation, tube formation and/or protease production. Substances showing inhibitory actions are further scrutinized for their angiosuppressive activities using *in vivo* assays such as the corneal micropocket technique, the chick embryo chorioallantoic membrane, or sponge implant models[11].

Animal tumour models have been used in the screening of anticancer agents for several decades. Differences may exist between the endothelial response in different vascular beds or different species. For example, tumour necrosis factor and flavone acetic acid are more effective in murine[255,256] than in human cancer[267]. Consequently, the relevance of some tumour models has been questioned[252]. Theoretically, a small inoculum of syngeneic, slow-growing, differentiated tumour cells should be used in the establishment of tumour models, because tumours that are antigenic can be cured by killing 2–3 logs of cells, whereas syngeneic tumours, like human tumours, require the killing of 8–10 logs. There is also a need for a quantitative method to screen potential inhibitors reproducibly and rapidly *in situ* in vascularized tissue. Because endothelial cell proliferation is a key step in angiogenesis, Brien *et al.* developed a rapid immunocytochemical method to measure angiogenesis in the brain using a monoclonal antibody to bromodeoxyuridine[268].

For future clinical trials, it would be of immense benefit to have a serum marker or protein to measure angiogenic activity in the circulation. Indeed, Watanabe *et al.* recently developed a sensitive immunoassay to detect human fibroblast growth factor[269]. Using this assay, 16 of 31 patients with renal cell carcinoma showed elevated serum bFGF[270]. Furthermore, the elevated serum levels of basic FGF but not acidic FGF correlate with tumour stage and histological grade[270]. This discovery will certainly stimulate further development of diagnostic and prognostic angiogenic markers for cancer screening and angiosuppression.

Lessons from suramin trials

One putative angiosuppressive agent, suramin, is already in clinical trials for cancer therapy. Suramin is a 1.4 kD, polyanionic compound[211,212] that is the prototype of anticancer drugs that work by binding growth factors[213,214,271], including angiogenic molecules, VEGF[215], PDGF[213], EGF[272], and FGF[216]. The autocrine transformation by chimeric signal peptide-basic FGF is reversed by suramin[234]. Suramin reverts the malignant phenotype induced by the Simian sarcoma virus[217], an acutely transforming retrovirus with a capacity to induce experimental sarcomas and gliomas. Suramin can replace heparin in angio-suppression experiments[218], suppress tumour growth rates[213,218] and increase the lifespan of mice inoculated with B16 melanoma[218]. Basic FGF-induced neovascularization *in vivo* and the bFGF-induced growth of human prostatic cells *in vitro* is specifically inhibited by suramin[219].

In addition to the preclinical evidence of growth factor antagonism and angiosuppressive activity, suramin also binds to a wide variety of intracellular and cell membrane enzymes[220] as well as to histones, globulins, fibrinogen and albumin. Furthermore, it is an anti-parasitic, immunosuppressive, demyelinating, and adrenocorticolytic agent; thus, its actions are hardly confined to angio-suppression. Not surprisingly, its toxicity is formidable – serious infections, peripheral neuropathy, coagulopathy, a fatigue–malaise syndrome, or skin rash. Tested in 35 patients with metastatic prostatic cancer refractory to hormonal manipulation, its objective response was modest, with only three patients showing complete disappearance of soft tissue tumours, and a few others showing partial, temporary, or variable, site-related responses[220]. In a second trial[221], suramin was found to be inactive when administered to 12 patients with metastatic renal cell carcinoma by continuous parental infusion to a peak plasma level greater than $200 \mu g$ ml^{-1}. No objective radiographic responses were observed, although greater than 40% necrosis of multiple tumour sites and haemorrhages were noted in one patient, and suspected to be related to angiogenesis inhibition[221]. Unfortunately, there was no measure of angiogenesis activity either clinically or in the tissues examined at autopsy, but the need for optimization of the drug administration is emphasized.

The use of suramin, from these Phase 1 studies, is complicated by a narrow therapeutic window: no response occurred with peak plasma concentrations $<200 \mu g/ml$, yet toxicities become prohibitive in concentrations $>300 \mu g/ml$[213,273]. Contrary to the short-term treatment initially used, suramin associated with major (>50% decrease in tumour mass) antitumour activity with prolonged administration of suramin at optimal serum levels where careful prospective monitoring corrects for individual variability [273] and the pharmacodynamics of suramin[272,273]. Of equal concern is that subtherapeutic concentrations of suramin ($<200 \mu g/ml$) may potentially stimulate tumour growth[273]. Finally, suramin may have either a stimulating or an inhibitory effect on epithelial tumours predicated on the pattern of growth factor expression. For tumours that express both TGF-α and EGF-receptor (EGF-R), suramin may be growth inhibitory. Because suramin induces an increase in soluble TGF-α, an angiogenic molecule, as well as enhances EGF-R autophosphorylation and tyrosine phosphorylation of lower molecular weight proteins, it may be expected to stimulate the growth of certain other malignancies[274]. In the future, tissue typing for growth factor and receptor expression in individual tumours, as well as a clear understanding of the specific autocrine system affected by the drug, may guide the selection and optimal use of growth factor antagonists.

FUTURE DIRECTIONS

Receptor modulation of angiogenic growth factors

The success of β-blockers and antihistamines in the treatment of cardiac and allergic disorders undoubtedly makes receptor blockade of growth factors on endothelial cells an attractive strategy. This approach would include direct-acting (e.g. bFGF, IL-4) and indirect-acting angiogenic factors (e.g. TNF-α and TGF-β).

The functional domains of bFGF for stimulation of endothelial cell proliferation have been identified and synthetic analogues have been synthesized. In an elegant study, the mitogenic activity of human bFGF has been dissociated from its plasminogen activator-inducing function by the deletion of amino acid residues 27–32[275]. Other bioactive bFGF mutants could be synthesized using recombinant DNA technology.

An IL-1 inhibitor from human monocyte-conditioned medium has been purified; it binds to the IL-1 receptor but has no IL-1-like activity, even at very high concentrations, and is therefore a pure receptor antagonist[276]. Candidates for future receptor antagonists are PD-ECGF[74], VEGF/VPF[75–77], and angiotropin[72]. Unlike bFGF and many other growth factors/cytokines that are pleiotropic, these three molecules are endothelial cell-specific and therefore more selective.

Another important area of research is to define the role of neuropeptides in angiogenesis and tumour growth[85,94,95,277,278]. For example, both substance P and calcitonin gene-related peptide (CGRP) are mitogenic for endothelial cells[94,95] and substance P is angiogenic in the rabbit cornea[94]. In a rat sponge model, substance P, CGRP, vasoactive intestinal polypeptide, bradykinin and angiotensin II are angiogenic[85,87]. Furthermore, the activities of substance P, bradykinin and angiotensin II can be blocked by antagonists at receptor subtypes (Table 7.4). These data suggest that, in malignant diseases associated

Table 7.4 Inhibition of angiogenic activities of neuropeptides in sponge implants by specific receptor antagonists

Neuropeptide	Antagonist	Receptor subtype	References
Substance P	L-668,169	NK_1	Fan *et al.* (unpublished)
Bradykinin	des-Arg^9,[Leu^8]-BK	B_1	87
Angiotensin II	losartan (DuP 753)	AT_1	92a

with high levels of these neuropeptides, activation of distinct receptor subtypes in the vasculature could lead to aberrant neovascularization. In such situations, specific receptor antagonists such as losartan could provide an effective treatment.

Human small-cell lung cancer produces bombesin/gastrin-releasing peptide that acts as an autocrine growth factor[279]. [D-Arg^1,D-Phe^5,D-Trp^{7,9},Leu^{11}]-

substance P, a potent bombesin antagonist, inhibits the growth of human small-cell lung cancer cells *in vitro*[280]. Bombesin/gastrin-releasing peptide may also stimulate exocrine pancreatic cancer cells[281] while a bombesin/gastrin releasing peptide antagonist strongly inhibits the growth of experimental pancreatic tumours[282]. Future work should determine whether bombesin/gastrin-releasing peptide functions as an angiogenic factor.

A related strategy is to target tumour cells expressing bFGF receptors. Pilot studies with bFGF-SAP (a conjugate of bFGF and saporin-6, a ribosome-inactivating protein) show that the conjugate selectively inhibits protein synthesis leading to the death of bFGF receptor-bearing tumour cells *in vitro*. A single intravenous injection of $0.125 \, mg \, kg^{-1}$ bFGF-SAP is sufficient to produce a tumour growth delay of 25 days[283]. Because bFGF receptors are widely distributed and not confined to endothelial cells, this approach might produce toxicity. However, the problem may be overcome by improved dosing schedules using low doses of bFGF receptor-specific mitotoxins.

Recently Gross *et al.*[45] demonstrated that two monoclonal antibodies generated against human recombinant bFGF block bFGF-induced proliferation of cultured human glioma cells. Furthermore, one of these antibodies inhibits angiogenesis *in vivo* and retards rat C6 glioma growth in nude mice. Similarly, Hori *et al.* reported a bFGF monoclonal antibody that inhibits angiogenesis and tumour growth[284]. Thus, growth factor-directed approaches may generate novel therapeutic agents to antagonize angiogenic factors at the receptor level.

Another exciting development is that antisense oligonucleotides can be designed to hybridize to specific mRNA sequences, a novel approach that inhibits the gene expression of cellular and viral proteins. For example, antisense oligonucleotides are capable of specifically inhibiting the expression of the cell adhesion molecule ICAM-1 in a cell culture system[285]. Antisense oligodeoxynucleotides also suppress the bFGF expression and growth of transformed astrocytes[286]. Thus it is highly probable that antisense oligonucleotide technology will generate powerful angiosuppressives by directly interfering with the genetic programme for angiogenesis.

Targeting of tumour vasculature

Denekamp[287] proposed that selective targeting of tumour vasculature provides a fresh approach in cancer treatment based on the differences between tumour and normal vasculature outlined in Table 7.5. Human tumours often grow as cords with zones of peripheral necrosis, indicating that the vascular bed is insufficient. One endothelial cell segment subtends about 3000 tumour cells in such cords; thus the occlusion and/or damage of capillaries would lead to an 'avalanche' of tumour cell death[287]. Consistent with this proposal are the dramatic effects of vascular occlusion on experimental tumours[288] and the clinical success of photodynamic therapy[289] and hyperthermia[239,249,290]. Anti-endothelial approaches to therapy via the tumour vasculature may differ conceptually and technically from anti-angiogenesis[291,292]. Vascular-mediated injury should be effective for large tumours, while angiosuppression might be most effective against small tumours[293].

Table 7.5 Differences between tumour and normal blood vessels (modified from Denekamp[249])

Normal vasculature	Tumour vasculature
three-dimensionally adequate	three-dimensionally inadequate leading to nutritional deprivation, hypoxic cells, acidic cells and areas of necrosis
innervated	not innervated
collateral potential	no collateral potential
well-constructed walls	poor wall structure; few capillaries, but more sinuses
can increase blood flow in response to demand	abnormal response to vasoactive stimuli
vessels have endothelial cells that proliferate slowly	vessels have endothelial cells that proliferate rapidly
can withstand 90% depletion of endothelium (arterioles)	

Because the degree of endothelial cell proliferation in the tumour vascular bed is up to 100 times that found in the normal quiescent vasculature, Denekamp originally proposed that a general anti-endothelial cell monoclonal antibody coupled to a phase-specific cytotoxic drug could be used to target the proliferating endothelial cells of the tumour vasculature[31]. Systemically administered anti-endothelial antibodies, however, cause organ-specific damage[294,295]. It may be more appropriate to generate monoclonal antibodies that recognise only proliferating endothelial cells and not endothelium *per se*. Accordingly, Clarke and West[296] identified several proteins specifically expressed by human endothelial cells stimulated by mitogens or tumour-conditioned media. Furthermore, they produced two monoclonal antibodies that stain the tumour vessels but do not cross-react with vessels of normal tissues. Wang *et al.*[297] also developed a monoclonal antibody that binds preferentially to tumour vasculature. Thus it is possible to produce monoclonal antibodies to endothelial-specific, cell surface proliferation-related antigens expressed only in the presence of tumour-derived mitogenic stimuli. The antibodies could be conjugated with glucose oxidase[298], immunotoxins[299] or angiosuppressive agents, or used in enzyme-activated therapy[300]. Such strategies are expected to achieve preferential destruction of the endothelial cells responding to the tumour-induced stimulus.

The vasculature contains organ-specific differences among microvascular endothelial cells, e.g. surface antigens on endothelial cells, response to growth factors and expression of cell adhesion molecules[301] that can affect angiosuppression[17]. These differences might relate to the process of preferential organ metastasis[302–305]. However, in contrast to tumour cell heterogeneity[306], the phenotypic diversity of microvascular endothelial cells[307] should be therapeutically surmountable because the endothelial cells are a genetically stable, normal diploid subpopulation, in contrast to the transformed, tumorigenic cells that have arisen by one or a series of genetic changes that confer growth advantage, and acquisition of drug resistance to genetically unstable tumour cell subpopulations[243].

Signal transduction of growth factors

The large number of angiogenic factors, the biochemical redundancy, and multiple mechanisms might make angiosuppressive therapy formidable. However, growth factors such as FGF, EGF and TGF-α act using receptors with a common intrinsic tyrosine kinase mediator[308]. In cancer, signalling pathways that mediate the normal functions of growth factors are often subverted. Tyrosine analogues such as tyrphostins have been shown to block phosphorylation of tyrosine residues and cell proliferation at non-toxic concentrations[309]. Future work to design drugs that selectively inhibit tyrosine kinases may lead to the discovery of safe angiosuppressives.

Protein kinase C is an enzyme that plays a vital role in signal transduction[310]. For example, protein kinase C activators inhibit the growth-promoting effect of angiogenic mitogens on capillary endothelial cells[311]. There is a good correlation between the ability of phorbol esters to activate protein kinase C and their tumour-promoting potential. Thus, active tumour-promoting phorbol esters (e.g. PMA) stimulate the production by endothelial cells of proteases involved in basement membrance degradation and invasion of the underlying collagen matrix to form an extensive network of capillary-like tubules[312]. Phorbol esters stimulate angiogenesis *in vivo*, suggesting a role for activation of protein kinase C in the induction of angiogenesis[313]. Thus, interference with signal transduction of angiogenic factors may represent an effective means for clinical management of malignant neoplasms.

Suppressor genes and their products

As normal cells develop into tumours that require angiogenesis, they undergo a series of genetic changes that are mainly responsible for the emergence of the malignant phenotype[34,35,243,314–316]. Among these changes is the functional inactivation of both alleles of genes known as cancer- or tumour-suppressor genes[184]. Active suppressor genes in normal cells are thought to play a role in controlling growth, differentiation and modulation of angiogenesis activity. For example, the metalloproteinase inhibitor, TIMP, is now considered to be a tumour-suppressor gene product[205]. Because growth-factor gene expression is a manifestation of oncogenic change, Ross[317] questioned, "Is it possible that expression of genes encoding these growth factors might be useful as early markers of the transition from a hyperplastic state to a pre-neoplastic or frankly neoplastic state?" Angiogenesis is a marker of neoplastic transformation of experimental[314] and human[315,316] hyperplastic tissues. Genetically engineered cells express the angiogenic phenotype *in vitro* simultaneous with conversion to the malignant phenotype[34,35].

Retinoic acid, an angiogenic inhibitor[161], may function to up-regulate the angiogenesis suppressor gene, and therefore maintain the suppressed non-angiogenic phenotype[318]. Further work, using angiosuppressive agents, will help identify the genes responsible for the angiogenic phenotype. Because of its contiguity with the bloodstream, the endothelium provides an ideal target for retroviral vector transduction for the purpose of gene therapy[319–321]. Such technology could be used to produce genetically engineered endothelial cells for the delivery of suppressor genes and their products to inhibit tumour angiogenesis and metastasis.

CONCLUSION

Research in tumour angiogenesis has progressed rapidly in recent years, marked by four phases: (1) the study of the pathophysiology of tumour–host interactions to reveal the link between tumour blood flow and its internal milieu[322]; (2) the paradigm of neoplastic and neovascular interdependence, regulated by a chemical substance, a 'tumour angiogenesis factor'[23,26,27]; (3) the explosion in the New Biology that has led to the purification, cloning, and widespread availability of several classes of angiogenic polypeptide growth factors, receptor antagonists, monoclonal antibodies, oncogenes, and suppressive oncogenes [2,10–15,184,245,323–325]; and (4) the successful clinical treatment of an angiogenic disease using interferon-α[164,165,229] and the call for clinical trials on cancer patients using inhibitors of angiogenesis, with the promise of less toxicity than standard chemotherapy[12,15,17,153–157,243,249–252,266,291,301].

Angiosuppression is no longer a theoretical possibility but a practical reality. However, the precarious initial experience with suramin illustrates the problems ahead in bringing angiosuppression from the laboratory to the clinic. It should be remembered that the first trials for the current mainstay of adjuvant chemotherapy were equally frustrating, as noted by Burchenal, "Historically, first trials are perilous and can set back an entire field, especially if the first drugs are too weak, given in too small a dose, and for far too short a period"[241].

Although the continual recruitment of new blood vessels is necessary for the expansive growth of solid malignant tumours, angiogenesis is not, by itself, sufficient to convert a benign tumour to a malignant one. Multiple cellular pathways, e.g. activation of proteases, are involved in the development of the malignant phenotype. Certain benign tumours, e.g. haemangiomas, adrenal adenomas, meningiomas, and acoustic schwannomas, are highly angiogenic. It is conceivable that angiosuppression, if the toxicity is mild, might also be useful for certain benign neoplasms. Furthermore, experience gained from oncology and tumour biology could be readily applied to other angiogenic diseases[2]: atherosclerosis[4], diabetic retinopathy[326], arthritis[327], and psoriasis[328,329].

The field of angiogenesis research and endothelial biology has enjoyed spectacular growth during the past decade. Since the plenary lecture on "Angiogenesis" by Judah Folkman at the Eleventh International Congress of Pharmacology in Amsterdam (July 1990), at least three international meetings* on this and related topics have been convened, reflecting the worldwide interest and high expectations created. It is no longer a question 'if' angiosuppression

---

*   *Vasculature as a Target for Anti-cancer Therapy*, the 16th L.H. Gray Conference, Manchester, United Kingdom, 17–21 September 1990;
International Symposium on Angiogenesis, St. Gallen, Switzerland, 13–15 March 1991;
Angiogenesis in Health and Diseases, NATO Advanced Study Institute, Porto Hydra, Greece, 16–27 June 1991.

will work, but rather a therapeutic challenge to define the indications, the dosage, the scheduling, the drug delivery systems, the synergisms and antagonisms of drug combinations, and the clinical indices of efficacy[330]. Meticulous design of clinical trials will help validate this new approach to cancer treatment. Further insights into the mechanisms of action emerging from microvascular research and biotechnology will facilitate the development of safe and effective angiosuppressive agents. Much more work remains; the final chapter, however, of angiogenesis research should be the most rewarding as it is translated to the clinical level.

Acknowledgements

We thank Dr Cliff Murray and Professor Juliana Denekamp of the Cancer Research Campaign Gray Laboratory for critically reviewing this manuscript, Dr De-En Hu for valuable suggestions and Eleanora DiMango for editorial assistance. The research performed in the authors' laboratories was funded by the British Heart Foundation, the Wellcome Trust (to T.-P. D. Fan) the Medical Research Council of Canada, the Cancer Research Society, and the Northwestern Memorial Foundation (to S. Brem).

REFERENCES

1. Hertig, A. T. (1935). Angiogenesis in the early human chorion and the primary placenta of the Macaque monkey. *Contrib. Embryol.*, **25**, 37–81
2. Folkman, J. and Klagsbrun, M. (1987). Angiogenic factors. *Science*, **235**, 442–447
3. West. D. C. and Kumar, S. (1988). Endothelial cell proliferation and diabetic retinopathy. *Lancet*, **1**, 715–716
4. Alpern-Elran, H., Morog, N., Robert, F., Hoover, G., Kalant, N. and Brem, S. (1989). Angiogenic activity of the atherosclerotic carotid artery plaque. *J. Neurosurg.*, **70**, 942–945
5. Brown, R., Weiss, J. B., Tomlinson, I. W., Phillips, P. and Kumar, S. (1980). Angiogenic factor from synovial fluid resembling that from tumours. *Lancet*, **1**, 682–685
6. Folkman, J. (1990). What is the evidence that tumors are angiogenesis dependent? *J. Natl. Cancer Inst.*, **82**, 4–6
7. Auerbach, R. (1980). Angiogenesis-inducing factors: a review. In Pick, E. (ed.) *Lymphokines*. Vol. 4, pp. 69–88. (New York: Academic Press)
8. Gullino, P. M. (1981). Angiogenic factors. In Basseiga, R. (ed.) *Tissue Growth Factors.* Handbook of Experimental Pharmacology, Vol. 57, pp. 427–449. (Berlin, Heidelberg: Springer-Verlag)
9. Hudlicka, O. and Tyler, K. R. (1986). *Angiogenesis. The Growth of the Vascular System,* Academic Press, London
10. Doctrow, S. R. and Kulakowski, E. C. (1989). Angiogenesis modulators – new drugs for controlling blood vessel growth? *Drug News Perspect.*, **2**, 74–81
11. Klagsbrun, M. and Folkman, J. (1990). Angiogenesis. In Sporn, M. B. and Roberts, A. B. (eds.) *Peptide Growth Factors and Their Receptors II, Handbook of Experimental Pharmacology.* Vol. 95/II pp. 549–586. (Berlin, Heidelberg: Springer-Verlag)
12. Maione, T. E. and Sharpe, R. J. (1990). Development of angiogenesis inhibitors for clinical applications. *Trends Pharmacol. Sci.*, **11**, 457–461
13. Klagsbrun, M. and D'Amore, P. A. (1991). Regulators of angiogenesis. *Annu. Rev. Physiol.*, **53**, 217–239
14. Bicknell, R. and Harris, A. L. (1991). Novel growth regulatory factors and tumour angiogenesis. *Eur. J. Cancer*, **27**, 781–785

15. Moses, M. A. and Langer, R. (1991). Inhibitors of angiogenesis. *Biotechnology*, **9**, 630–634

16. Noden, D. M. (1989). Embryonic origins and assembly of blood vessels. *Am. Rev. Resp. Dis.*, **140**, 1097–1103

17. Brem, S., Zagzag, D., Tsanaclis, A. M. C., Gately S., Elkouby, M.-P. and Brein, S. E. (1990). Inhibition of angiogenesis and tumour growth in the brain. Suppression of endothelial cell turnover by penicillamine and the depletion of copper, an angiogenic cofactor. *Am. J. Pathol.*, **137**, 1121–1142

18. Ide, A. G., Harvey, R. A. and Warren, S. L. (1939). Role played by trauma in the dissemination of tumour fragments by the circulation; Tumour studied: Brown-Pearce rabbit epithelioma. *Arch. Pathol.*, **28**, 851–860

19. Algire, G. H., Chalkley, Legallais, F. Y. and Park, H. D. (1945). Vascular reactions of normal and malignant tumors *in vivo*. I. Vascular reactions of mice to wounds and to normal and neoplastic transplants. *J. Natl. Cancer Inst.*, **6**, 73–85.

20. Folkman, J., Cole, P. and Zimmerman, S. (1966). Tumor behavior in isolated perfused organs: *in vitro* growth and metastasis of biopsy material in rabbit thyroid and canine intestinal segment. *Ann. Surg.*, **164**, 491–502

21. Tannock, I. F. (1968). The relation between cell proliferation and the vascular system in a transplanted mouse mammary tumour. *Br. J. Cancer*, **22**, 258–273

22. Tannock, I. F. (1970). Population kinetics of carcinoma cells, capillary endothelial cells, and fibroblasts in a transplanted mouse mammary tumor. *Cancer Res.*, **30**, 2470–2476

23. Folkman, J. (1971). Tumor angiogenesis: therapeutic implications. *N. Engl. J. Med.*, **285**, 1182–1186

24. Gimbrone, M. A. Jr., Leapman, S. B., Cotran, R. S. and Folkman, J. (1972). Tumor dormancy *in vivo* by prevention of neovascularization. *J. Exp. Med.*, **136**, 261–276

25. Brem, S., Brem, H., Folkman, J., Finkelstein, D. and Patz, A. (1976). Prolonged tumor dormancy by prevention of neovascularization in the vitreous. *Cancer Res.*, **36**, 2807–2812

26. Folkman, J. (1972). Anti-angiogenesis: new concept for the therapy of solid tumors. *Ann. Surg.*, **175**, 409–416

27. Folkman, J. and Cotran, R. S. (1976). Relation of vascular proliferation to tumor growth. *Int. Rev. Exp. Pathol.*, **16**, 207–248.

28. Ausprunk, D. H., Knighton, D. and Folkman, J. (1974). Differentiation of vascular endothelium in the chick chorioallantois: a structural and autoradiographic study. *Devel. Biol.*, **38**, 237–248

29. Knighton, D., Ausprunk, D., Tapper, D. and Folkman, J. (1977). Avascular and vascular phases of tumour growth in the chick embryo. *Br. J. Cancer*, **35**, 347–356

30. Gimbrone, M. A. Jr., Cotran, R. S. and Folkman, J. (1974). Tumor growth neovascularization: an experimental model using rabbit cornea. *J. Natl. Cancer Inst.*, **52**, 413–427

31. Denekamp, J. and Hobson, B. (1982). Endothelial cell proliferation in experimental tumours. *Br. J. Cancer*, **46**, 711–720

32. Hobson, B. and Denekamp, J. (1984). Endothelial proliferation in tumours and normal tissues: continuous labelling studies. *Br. J. Cancer*, **49**, 405–413

33. Thompson, W. D., Shiach, K. J., Fraser, R. A., McIntosh, L. C. and Simpson, J. G. (1987). Tumours acquire their vasculature by vessel incorporation, not vessel ingrowth. *J. Pathol.*, **151**, 323–332

34. Folkman, J., Watson, K., Ingber, D. and Hanahan, D. (1989). Induction of angiogenesis during the transition from hyperplasia to neoplasia. *Nature*, **339**, 58–61

35. Kandel, J., Bossy-Wetzel, E., Radvanyi, F., Klagsbrun, M., Folkman, J. and Hanahan, D. (1991). Neovascularization is associated with a switch to the export of bFGF in the multistep development of fibrosarcoma. *Cell*, **66**, 1095–1104

36. Lien, W. and Ackerman, N. (1970). The blood supply of experimental liver metastases. II. A microcirculatory study of normal and tumor vessels of the liver with the use of perfused silicone rubber. *Surgery*, **68**, 334–340

37. Folkman, J. (1987). What is the role of angiogenesis in metastasis from cutaneous melanoma? *Eur. J. Cancer Clin. Oncol.*, **23**, 361–363

38. Blood, C. H. and Zetter, B. R. (1990). Tumor interactions with the vasculature: angiogenesis and tumor metastasis. *Biochim. Biophys. Acta*, **1032**, 89–118

39. Mahadevan, V. and Hart, I. R. (1990). Metastasis and angiogenesis. *Rev. Oncol.*, **3**, 97–103

40. Srivastava, A., Laidler, P., Hughes, L. E., Woodstock, J. and Shedden, E. J. (1986). Neovascularisation in human cutaneous melanoma: a quantitative morphological and Doppler ultrasound study. *Eur. J. Cancer Clin. Oncol.*, **22**, 1205–1209

41. Srivastava, A., Laidler, P., Davis, R. P., Horgan, K. and Hughes, L. E. (1988). The prognostic significance of tumor vascularity in intermediate-thickness (0.76–4.0 mm thick) skin melanoma: a quantitative histologic study. *Am. J. Pathol.*, **133**, 419–423

42. Weidner, N., Semple, J. P., Welch, W. and Folkman, J. (1991). Tumor angiogenesis and metastasis-correlation in invasive breast carcinoma. *N. Engl. J. Med.*, **324**, 1–8

43. Gross, J. L., Herblin, W. F., Dusak, B. A., Czerniak, P., Diamond, M. and Dexter, D. L. (1990). Modulation of solid tumor growth *in vivo* by bFGF. *Proc. Am. Assoc. Cancer Res.*, **31**, 79 (Abstr. 469)

44. Gross, J. L., Hertel, D., Herblin, W. F., Neville, M. and Brem, S. S. (1991). Inhibition of basic fibroblast growth factor-induced angiogenesis and glioma tumor growth *in vivo*. *Proc. Am. Assoc. Cancer Res.*, **32**, 57 (Abstr. 338)

45. Gross, J. L., Herblin, W. F., Ediscoog. K., Horlick, R. and Brem, S. S. (1992). Tumor growth regulation by modulation of basic fibroblast growth factor. In Steiner, R., Weisz, P.B. and Langer, R. (eds.) *Angiogenesis. Key Principles – Science – Technology – Medicine*. pp. 421–427. (Basel: Birkhäuser Verlag AG)

46. Maxwell, M., Naber, S. P., Wolfe, H. J., Hedley-Whyte, E. S., Galanopoulos, T., Neville-Golden, J. and Antoniades, H. N. (1991). Expression of angiogenic growth factor genes in primary human astrocytomas may contribute to their growth and progression. *Cancer Res.*, **51**, 1345–1351

47. Zagzag, D., Miller, D. C., Sato, Y., Rifkin, D. B. and Burstein, D. E. (1990). Immuno-histochemical localization of basic fibroblast in astrocytomas. *Cancer Res.*, **50**, 7393–7398

48. Greenblatt, M. and Shubik, P. (1968). Tumor angiogenesis: transfilter diffusion studies in the hamster by transparent chamber technique. *J. Natl. Cancer Inst.*, **41**, 111–124

49. Folkman, J., Merler, E., Abernathy, C. and Williams, G. (1971). Isolation of a tumor factor responsible for angiogenesis. *J. Exp. Med.*, **133**, 275–288

50. Marx, J. L. (1987). Angiogenesis research comes of age. *Science*, **237**, 23–24

51. Shing, Y., Folkman, J., Sullivan, R., Butterfield, C., Murray, J. and Klagsbrun, M. (1984). Heparin affinity: purification of a tumor-derived capillary endothelial cell growth factor. *Science*, **223**, 1296–1298

52. Gospodarowicz, D., Cheng, J., Lui, G.-M., Baird, A. and Bohlen, P. (1984). Isolation of brain fibroblast growth factor by heparin-Sepharose affinity chromatography: identity with pituitary fibroblast growth factor. *Proc. Natl. Acad. Sci. USA*, **81**, 6963–6967

53. Davidson, J. M., Klagsbrun, M., Hill, K. E., Buckley, A., Sullivan, R., Brewer, P. A. and Woodward, S. C. (1985). Accelerated wound repair, cell proliferation, and collagen accumulation are produced by a cartilage-derived growth factor. *J. Cell Biol.*, **100**, 1219–1225

54. Sprugel, K. H., McPherson, J. M., Clowes, A. W. and Ross, R. (1987). Effects of growth factors *in vivo*. I. Cell ingrowth into porous subcutaneous chambers. *Am. J. Pathol.*, **129**, 601–613

55. Montesano, R., Vassalli, J.-D., Baird, A., Guillemin, R. and Orci. L. (1986). Basic fibroblast growth factor induces angiogenesis *in vitro*. *Proc. Natl. Acad. Sci. USA*, **83**, 7297–7301

56. Thomas, K. A., Rios-Candelore, M. R., Gimenez-Gallego, G., DiSalvo, J., Bennet, C., Rodkey, J. and Fitzpatrick, S. (1985). Pure brain-derived acidic fibroblast growth factor is a potent angiogenic vascular endothelial cell mitogen with sequence homology to interleukin 1. *Proc. Natl. Acad. Sci. USA*, **82**, 6409–6413

57. Thompson, J. A., Anderson, K. D., DiPietro, J. M., Zweibel, J. A., Zametta, M., Anderson, W. F. and Maciag, T. (1988). Site-directed neovessel formation *in vivo*. *Science*, **241**, 1349–1352

58. Fett, W. J., Strydom, D. J., Lobb, R. R., Alderman, E. M., Bethune, J. L., Riordan, J. F. and Vallee, B. L. (1985). Isolation and characterization of angiogenin, an angiogenic protein from human carcinoma cells. *Biochemistry*, **24**, 5480–5486.

59. Badet, J., Soncin, F., Guitton, J.-D., Lamare, O., Cartwright, T. and Barritault, D. (1989). Specific binding of angiogenin to calf pulmonary artery endothelial cells. *Proc. Natl. Acad. Sci. USA*, **86**, 8427–8431

60. Chamoux, M., Dehouck, M. P., Fruchart, J. C., Spik, G., Montreuil, J. and Cecchelli, R. (1991). Characterization of angiogenin receptors on bovine brain capillary endothelial cells. *Biochem. Biophys. Res. Commun.*, **176**, 833–839

61. Schreiber, A. B., Winkler, M. E. and Derynck, R. (1986). Transforming growth factor-α: a more potent angiogenic mediator than epidermal growth factor. *Science*, **232**, 1250–1253

62. Grotendorst, G. R., Soma, Y., Takehara, K. and Charette, M. (1989). EGF and TGF-alpha are potent chemoattractants for endothelial cells and EGF-like peptides are present at sites of tissue regeneration. *J. Cell Physiol.*, **139**, 617–623

215

63. Roberts, A. B., Sporn, M. B., Assoian, R. K., Smith, J. M., Roche, N. S., Wakefield, L. M., Heine, U. I., Liotta, L. A., Falanga, V., Kehrl, J. H. and Fauci, A. S. (1986). Transforming growth factor type beta: rapid induction of fibrosis, and angiogenesis *in vivo* and stimulation of collagen formation *in vitro*. *Proc. Natl. Acad. Sci. USA*. **83**, 4167–4171

64. Mustoe, T. A., Pierce, G. F., Thomason, A., Gramates, P., Sporn, M. B. and Deuel, T. F. (1987). Accelerated healing of incisional wounds in rats induced by transforming growth factor-β. *Science*, **237**, 1333–1336

65. Frater-Schroder, M., Muller, G., Birchmeier, W. and Bohlen, P. (1986). Transforming growth factor-beta inhibits endothelial cell proliferation. *Biochem. Biophys. Res. Commun.*, **137**, 295–302

66. Muller, G., Behrens, J., Nussbaumer, U., Bohlen, P. and Birchmeier, W. (1987). Inhibitory action of transforming growth factor beta on endothelial cells. *Proc. Natl. Acad. Sci. USA*, **84**, 5600–5604

67. Heimark, R. L., Twardzik, D. R. and Schwartz, S. M. (1986). Inhibition of endothelial cell regeneration by type-beta transforming growth factor from platelets. *Science*, **233**, 1078–1080

68. Leibovich, S. J., Polverini, P. J., Shepard, H. M., Wiseman, D. M., Shively, V. and Niseir, N. (1987). Macrophage-induced angiogenesis is mediated by tumour necrosis factor-α. *Nature*, **329**, 630–632

69. Frater-Schroder, M., Risau, W., Hallman, R., Gautshi, R. and Bohen, P. (1987). Tumor necrosis type-α, a potent inhibitor of endothelial cell growth *in vitro*, is angiogenic *in vivo*. *Proc. Natl. Acad. Sci. USA*, **84**, 5277–5281

70. Sato, N., Sawasaki, Y., Haranaka, K., Satomi, N., Nariuchi, H. and Goto, T. (1985). Growth inhibitory and cytotoxic action of rabbit tumour necrosis factor against bovine capillary endothelial cells *in vitro*. *Proc. Jpn. Acad.*, **61**, Ser. B. 471–474

71. Schulze-Osthoff, K., Fruhbeis, B., Overwien, B., Hilbig, B. and Sorg, C. (1987). Purification and characterization of a novel human angiogenic factor (h-AF). *Biochem. Biophys. Res. Commun.*, **146**, 945–952

72. Hockel, M., Sasse, J. and Wissler, J. H. (1987). Purified monocyte-derived angiogenic substance (angiotropin) stimulates migration, phenotypic changes, and 'tube formation' but not proliferation of capillary endothelial cells *in vitro*. *J. Cell. Physiol.*, **133**, 1–13

73. Hockel, M., Jung, W., Vaupel, P., Rabes, H., Khaledpour, C. and Whissler, J. H. (1988). Purified monocyte derived angiogenic substance (angiotropin) induces controlled angiogenesis associated with regulated tissue proliferation in rabbit skin. *J. Clin. Invest.*, **82**, 1075–1090

74. Ishikawa, F., Miyazono, K., Hellman, U., Drexler, H., Wernstedt, C., Hagiwara, K., Usuki, K., Takaku, F., Risau, W. and Heldin, C.-H. (1989). Identification of angiogenic activity and the cloning and expression of platelet-derived endothelial cell growth factor. *Nature*, **338**, 557–562

75. Gospodarowicz, D., Abraham, J. A. and Schilling, J. (1989). Isolation and characterization of a vascular endothelial cell mitogen produced by pituitary-derived folliculo stellate cells. *Proc. Natl. Acad. Sci. USA*, **86**, 7311–7315

76. Ferrara, N. and Henzel, W. J. (1989). Pituitary follicular cells secrete a novel heparin-binding growth factor specific for vascular endothelial cells. *Biochem. Biophys. Res. Commun.*, **161**, 851–858

77. Connolly, D. T., Heuvelman, D. M., Nelson, R., Olander, J. V., Eppley, B. L., Delfino, J. J., Siegel, N. R., Leimgruber, R. M. and Feder, J. (1989). Tumor vascular permeability factor stimulates endothelial cell growth and angiogenesis. *J. Clin. Invest.*, **84**, 1478–1489

78. Jakeman, L. B., Winer, J., Bennett, G. L., Altar, A. and Ferrara, N. (1992). Binding sites for vascular endothelial growth factor are localized on endothelial cells in adult rat tissues. *J. Clin. Invest.*, **89**, 244–253

78a. Dvorak, H. F., Sioussat, T. M., Brown, L. F., Berse, B., Nagy, J. A., Manseau, E. J., Van De Water, L. and Serger, D. R. (1991). Distribution of vascular permeability factor (vascular endothelial growth factor) in tumors: concentration in tumor blood vessels. *J. Exp. Med.*, **174**, 1275–1278

79. Levy, A. P., Tamargo, R., Brem, H. and Nathans, D. (1989). An endothelial cell growth factor from the mouse neuroblastoma cell line NB41. *Growth Factors*, **2**, 9–19

80. Prendergast, R. A., Lutty, G. A. and Dinarello, C. A. (1987). Interleukin-1 induces corneal neovascularisation. *Fed. Proc.*, **46**, 1200

81. Giulian, D., Woodward, J., Young, D. G., Krebs, J. F. and Lachman, L. B. (1988). Interleukin-1 injected into mammalian brain stimulates astrogliosis and neovascularization. *J. Neurosci.*, **8**, 2485–2490

82. Mahadevan, V., Hart., I. R. and Lewis, G. P. (1989). Factors influencing blood supply in wound granuloma quantitated by a new *in vivo* technique. *Cancer Res.*, **49**, 415–419

83. Ben Ezra, D., Hemo, I., and Maftzir, G. (1990). *In vivo* angiogenic activity of interleukins. *Arch. Ophthalmol.*, **108**, 573–576

84. Cozzolino, F., Torcia, M., Aldinucci, D., Ziche, M., Almerigogna, F., Bani, D. and Stern, D. M. (1990). Interleukin-1 is an autocrine regulator of human endothelial cell growth. *Proc. Natl. Acad. Sci. USA*, **87**, 6487–6491

84a. Detmar, M., Tenorio, S., Hettmannsperger, U., Ruszczak, Z. and Orfanos, C. E. (1992). Cytokine regulation of proliferation and ICAM-1 expression of human dermal microvascular endothelial cells in vitro. *Invest. Dermatol.*, **98**, 147–153

85. Fan, T.-P. D. and Hu, D.-E.(1991). Modulation of angiogenesis by inflammatory polypeptides. *Int. J. Radiat. Biol.*, **60**, 71

86. Fan, T.-P. D., Frost, E. E. and Wren, A. D. (1992). A multichannel wounding device for the study of vascular repair *in vitro*. In Steiner, R., Weisz, P. B. and Langer, R. (eds.) *Angiogenesis. Key Principles – Science – Technology – Medicine*. pp. 315–320. (Basel: Birkhauser Verlag AG)

87. Hu, D.-E. and Fan, T.-P. D. (1991). Synergistic interaction between bradykinin and interleukin–1 in angiogenesis. *Br. J. Pharmacol.*, **104**, 83P

88. Toi, M., Harris, A. L. and Bicknell, R. (1991). Interleukin-4 is a potent mitogen for capillary endothelium. *Biochem. Biophys. Res. Commun.*, **174**, 1287–1293

89. Anagnostou, A., Lee, E. S., Kessimian, N., Levinson, R. and Steiner, M. (1990). Erythropoietin has a mitogenic and positive chemotactic effect on endothelial cells. *Proc. Natl. Acad. Sci. USA*, **87**, 5978–5982

90. Bussolino, F., Wang, J. M., Defilippi, P., Turrini, F., Sanavio, F., Edgell, C.-J. S., Aglietta, M., Aresse, P. and Mantovani, A. (1989). Granulocyte- and granulocyte-macrophage colony stimulating factors induce human endothelial cells to migrate and proliferate. *Nature*, **337**, 471–473

91. Fernandez, L. A., Twickler, J. and Mead, A. (1985). Neovascularization produced by angiotensin II. *J. Lab. Clin. Med.*, **105**, 141–145

92. Le Noble, F. A. C., Hekking, J. W. M., Van Straaten, H. W. M., Slaaf, D. W. and Struyker Boudier, H. A. J. (1991). Angiotensin II stimulates angiogenesis in the chorioallantoic membrane of the chicken embryo. *Eur. J. Pharmacol.*, **195**, 305–306

92a. Fan, T.-P.D. and Hu, D. E. (1992). Losartan (DuP 753) blocks the angiogenic effect of angiotensin II in rats. *FASEB J.*, **6** A937, (Abstr. 4)

93. Ariza, A., Fernandez, L. A., Inagami, T., Kim, J. H. and Manuelidis, E. E. (1988). Renin in glioblastoma multiforme and its role in neovascularization. *Am. J. Clin. Pathol.*, **90**, 437–441

94. Ziche, M., Morbidelli, L., Pacini, M., Geppetti, P., Alessandri, G. and Maggi, C. A. (1990). Substance P stimulates neovascularization *in vivo* and proliferation of cultured endothelial cells. *Microvasc. Res.*, **40**, 264–278

95. Haegerstrand, A., Dalsgaard, C.-J., Jonzon, B., Larsson, O. and Nilsson, J. (1990). Calcitonin gene-related peptide stimulates proliferation of human endothelial cells. *Proc. Natl. Acad. Sci. USA*, **88**, 3299–3303

96. Ben Ezra, D. (1978). Neovasculogenic ability of prostaglandins, growth factors and synthetic chemoattractants. *Am. J. Ophthalmol.*, **86**, 455–461

97. Ziche, M., Jones, J. and Gullino, P. M. (1982). Role of prostaglandin E_1 and copper in angiogenesis. *J. Natl. Cancer Inst.*, **69**, 475–481

98. Form, D. M. and Auerbach, R. (1983). PGE_2 and angiogenesis. *Proc. Soc. Exp. Biol. Med.*, **172**, 214–218

99. Kanayasu, T., Nakao-Hayashi, J., Asuwa, N., Morita, I., Ishii, T., Ito, H. and Murota, S.-I. (1989). Leukotriene C_4 stimulates angiogenesis in bovine carotid artery endothelial cells *in vitro. Biochem. Biophys. Res. Commun.*, **159**, 572–578

100. Smither, R. L. and Fan, T.-P. D. (1990). PAF antagonists inhibit angiogenesis in a rat sponge model. *Br. J. Pharmacol.*, **99**, 87P

101. Smither, R. L. and Fan, T.-P. D. (1992). Effects of platelet-activating factor on endothelial cells and fibroblasts *in vitro*. In Steiner, R., Weisz, P. B. and Langer, R. (eds.) *Angiogenesis. Key Principles – Science – Technology – Medicine*. pp. 230–234. (Basel: Birkhauser Verlag A G)

102. Bussolino, F., Camussi, G., Aglietta, M., Braquet, P., Bosia, A., Pescarmona, G., Sanavio, F., D'Urso, N. and Marchisio, P. C. (1987). Human endothelial cells are target for platelet-activating factor. I. Platelet-activating factor induces changes in cytoskeleton structures. *J. Immunol.*, **131**. 2397–2403

103. Dobson, D. E., Kambe, A., Block, E., Dion, T., Lu, H., Castellot, J. J. Jr. and Spiegelman, B. M. (1990). 1-Butyryl-glycerol: a novel angiogenesis factor secreted by differentiating adipocytes. *Cell*, **61**, 223–230

104. Wakamatsu, K., Masaki, T., Itoh, F., Kondo, K. and Sudo, K. (1990). Isolation of fatty acid amide as an angiogenic principle from bovine mesentery. *Biochem. Biophys. Res. Commun.*, **168**, 423–429

105. Weiss, J. B., Brown, R. A., Kumar, S. and Phillips, P. (1979). An angiogenic factor isolated from tumours: a potent low molecular weight compound. *Br. J. Cancer*, **40**, 493–496

106. Hill, C. R., Kissun, R. D., Weiss, J. B. and Garnder, A. (1983). Angiogenic factor in vitreous from diabetic retinopathy. *Experientia*, **39**, 583–585

107. Taylor, C. M. and Weiss, J. B. (1989). Raised endothelial cell stimulating angiogenesis factor in diabetic retinopathy. *Lancet*, **2**, 1329

108. Odedra, R. and Weiss, J. B. (1991). Low molecular weight angiogenesis factors. *Pharmacol. Ther.*, **49**, 111–124

109. Azizkhan, R. G., Azizkhan, J. C., Zetter, B. R. and Folkman, J. (1980). Mast cell heparin stimulates migration of capillary endothelial cells *in vitro*. *J. Exp. Med.*, **152**, 931–944

110. Folkman, J. (1985). Regulation of angiogenesis: a new function of heparin. *Biochem. Pharmacol.*, **34**, 905–909

111. West, D. C., Hampson, I. N., Arnold, F. and Kumar, S. (1985). Angiogenesis induced by degradation products of hyaluronic acid. *Science*, **228**, 1324–1326

112. West, D. C. and Kumar, S. (1989). The effect of hyaluronate and its oligosaccharides on endothelial cell proliferation and monolayer integrity. *Exp. Cell Res.*, **183**, 179–196

113. Montesano, R., Mouron, P. and Orci, L. (1985). Vascular outgrowths from tissue explants embedded in fibrin or collagen gels: a simple *in vitro* model of angiogenesis. *Cell Biol. Int. Rep.*, **9**, 869–875

114. Dvorak, H. F., Harvey, V. S., Estrella, P., Brown, L. F., McDonagh, J, and Dvorak, A. M. (1987). Fibrin gels induce angiogenesis. Implications for tumor stroma generation and wound healing. *Lab. Invest.*, **57**, 673–686

115. Grant, D. S., Tashiro, K.-I., Segui-Real, B., Yamada, Y., Martin, G. R. and Kleinman, H. K. (1989). Two different laminin domains mediate the differentiation of human endothelial cells into capillary-like structures *in vitro*. *Cell*, **58**, 933–943

116. Dusseau, J. W., Hutchins, P. M. and Malbasa, D. (1986). Stimulation of angiogenesis by adenosine on the chick chorioallantoic membrane. *Circ. Res.*, **59**, 163–170

117. Meininger, C. J., Schelling, M. E. and Granger, H. J. (1988). Adenosine and hypoxia stimulate proliferation and migration of endothelial cells. *Am. J. Physiol.*, **255**, H554–H562

118. Kull, F. C., Brent, D. A., Parikh, I. and Cuatrecasas, P. (1987). Chemical identification of tumor-derived angiogenic factor. *Science*, **236**, 843–845

119. Thompson, W. D. and Brown, F. I. (1987). Quantitation of histamine-induced angiogenesis in the chick chorioallantoic membrane: mode of action of histamine is indirect. *Int. J. Microirc. Clin. Exp.*, **6**, 343–357

120. Takigawa, M., Nishida, Y., Suzuki, F., Kishi, J., Yamashita, K. and Hayakawa, T. (1990). Induction of angiogenesis in chick yolk-sac membrane by polyamines and its inhibition by tissue inhibitors of metalloproteinases (TIMP and TIMP-2). *Biochem. Biophys. Res. Commun.*, **171**, 1264–1271

121. Zetter, B. R. (1988). Angiogenesis: State of the art. *Chest*, **93** (suppl. 3), 159S–166S

122. Maciag, T., Cerundolo, J., Ilsley, S., Kelly, P. R. and Forand, R. (1979). An endothelial cell growth factor from bovine hypothalamus; identification and partial characterization. *Proc. Natl. Acad. Sci. USA*, **76**, 5674–5678

123. Taylor, C. M., McLaughlin, B., Weiss, J. B. and Smith, I. (1988). Bovine and human pineal glands contain substantial quantities of endothelial cell stimulating angiogenesis factor. *J. Neural Trans.*, **71**, 79–83

124. Banda, M. J., Knighton, D. R., Hunt, T. K. and Werb, Z. (1982). Isolation of a nonmitogenic angiogenesis factor from wound fluid. *Proc. Natl. Acad. Sci. USA*, **79**, 7773–7777

125. Kumar, S., West, D., Shahabuddin, S., Arnold, F., Haboubi, N., Reid, H. and Carr, T. (1983). Angiogenesis factor from human myocardial infarcts. *Lancet*, **2**, 364–368

126. Folkman, J. and Haudenschild, C. C. (1980). Angiogenesis *in vitro*. *Nature*, **288**, 551–556

127. Ausprunk, D. H. and Folkman, J. (1977). Migration and proliferation of endothelial cells in preformed blood vessels during tumor angiogenesis. *Microvasc. Res.*, **14**, 53–65

128. Sholley, M. M., Gimbrone, M. A. Jr. and Cotran, R. S. (1977). Cellular migration and replication in endothelial regeneration. A study using irradiated endothelial cultures. *Lab. Invest.*, **36**, 18–25

129. Gross, J. L., Moscatelli, D. and Rifkin, D. B. (1983). Increased capillary endothelial cell protease activity in response to angiogenic stimuli *in vitro*. *Proc. Natl. Acad. Sci. USA*, **80**, 2623–2627

130. Folkman, J. (1984). What is the role of endothelial cells in angiogenesis? *Lab. Invest.*, **51**, 601–604

131. Folkman, J. (1986). How is blood vessel growth regulated in normal and neoplastic tissue? – G. H. A. Clowes Memorial Award Lecture. *Cancer Res.*, **46**, 467–473

132. Furcht, L. T. (1986). Critical factors controlling angiogenesis: cell products, cell matrix and growth factors. *Lab. Invest.*, **55**, 505–509

133. Montesano, R., Pepper, S. and Orci, L. (1990). Angiogenesis *in vitro*: morphogenetic and invasive properties of endothelial cells. *NIPS*, **5**, 75–79

134. Folkman, J., Langer, R., Linhardt, R. J., Haudenschild, C. and Taylor, S. (1983). Angiogenesis inhibition and tumor regression caused by heparin or a heparin fragment in the presence of cortisone. *Science*, **221**, 719–725

135. Crum, R., Szabo, S. and Folkman, J (1985). A new class of steroids inhibits angiogenesis in the presence of heparin or a heparin fragment. *Science*, **230**, 1375–1378

136. Penhaligon, M. and Camplejohn, R. (1985) Combination of heparin plus cortisone treatment of two transplanted tumors in C3H/He mice. *J. Natl. Cancer Inst.*, **74**, 869–873

137. Ziche, M., Ruggiero, M., Pasquali, F. and Chiarugi, V. P. (1985). Effects of cortisone with and without heparin on angiogenesis induced by prostaglandin E_1 and by S180 cells, and on the growth of murine transplantable tumors. *Int. J. Cancer*, **35**, 549–552

138. Teale, D. M., Underwood, J. C. E., Potter, C. W. and Rees, R. C. (1987). Therapy of spontaneously metastatic HSV-2 induced hamster tumours with cortisone acetate administered with or without heparin. *Eur. J. Clin. Oncol.*, **23**, 93–100

139. Folkman, J., Weisz, P. B., Joullie, M. M., Li, W. W. and Ewing, W. R. (1989). Control of angiogenesis with synthetic heparin substitutes. *Science*, **243**, 1490–1493

140. Chen, N. T., Corey, E. J. and Folkman, J. (1988). Potentiation of angiostatic steroids by a synthetic inhibitor of arylsulphatase. *Lab Invest.*, **59**, 453–455

141. Inoue, K., Korenaga, H., Tanaka, N. G., Sakamoto, N. and Kadoya, S. (1988). The sulfated polysaccharide-peptidoglycan complex potently inhibits embryonic angiogenesis and tumor growth in the presence of cortisone acetate. *Carbohyd. Res.*, **181**, 135–142

142. Tanaka, N. G., Sakamoto, A., Inoue, K., Korenaga, H., Kadoya, S., Ogawa, H. and Osada, Y. (1989). Antitumor effects of an antiangiogenic polysaccharide from an *Arthrobacter* species with or without a steroid. *Cancer Res.*, **49**, 6727–6730

143. Wilks, J. W., Scott, P. S., Vrba, L. K. and Cocuzza, J. M. (1991). Inhibition of angiogenesis with combination treatments of angiostatic steroids and suramin. *Int. J. Radiat. Biol.*, **60**, 73–77

144. Ingber, D. E., Madri, J. A. and Folkman, J. (1986). A possible mechanism for inhibition of angiogenesis by angiostatic steroids: induction of capillary basement membrane dissolution. *Endocrinology*, **119**, 1768–1775

144a. Folkman, J. and Ingber, D. E. (1987). Angiostatic steroids: Method of discovery and mechanism of action. *Ann. Surg.*, **206**, 374–383

145. Maragoudakis, M. E., Sarmonika, M. and Panoutsacopoulou, M. (1989). Antiangiogenic action of heparin plus cortisone is associated with decreased collagenous protein synthesis in the chick chorioallantoic membrane. *J. Pharmacol. Exp. Ther.*, **251**, 679–682

146. Stokes, C. L., Weisz, P. B., Williams, S. K. and Lauffenburger, D. A. (1990). Inhibition of microvascular endothelial cell migration by β-cyclodextrin tetradecasulfate and hydrocortisone. *Microvasc. Res.*, **40**, 279–284

147. Lee, S. W., Tsou. A.-P., Chan, H., Thomas, J., Petrie, K., Eugui, E. M. and Allison, A. C. (1988). Glucocorticoids selectively inhibit the transcription of the interleukin 1β gene and decrease the stability of interleukin 1β mRNA. *Proc. Natl. Acad. Sci. USA*, **85**, 1204–1208

147a. Gay, C. G. and Winkles, J. A. (1991). Interleukin 1 regulates heparin-binding growth factor 2 gene expression in vascular smooth muscle cells. *Proc. Natl. Acad. Sci. USA*, **88**, 296–300

148. Gross, J., Azizkhan, R. G., Biswas, C., Bruns, R. R., Hsieh, D. S. T. and Folkman, J. (1981). Inhibition of tumor growth, vascularization, and collagenolysis in the rabbit cornea by medroxyprogesterone. *Proc. Natl. Acad. Sci. USA*, **78**, 1176–1180

149. Ashino-Fuse, H., Takano, Y., Oikawa, T., Shimamura, M. and Iwaguchi, T. (1989). Medroxyprogesterone acetate, an anti-cancer and anti-angiogenic steroid, inhibits the plasminogen activator in bovine endothelial cells. *Int. J. Cancer*, **44**, 859–864

150. Oikawa, T., Hirotani, K., Shimamura, M., Ashino-Fuse, H. and Iwaguchi, T. (1989). Powerful antiangiogenic activity of herbimyċin A (named angiostatic antibiotic). *J. Antibiotics*, **42**, 1202–1204

151. Uehara, Y., Murakami, Y., Mizuno, S. and Kawai, S. (1988). Inhibition of transforming activity of tyrosine kinase oncogenes by herbimycin A. *Virology*, **164**, 294–298

152. Uehara, Y., Murakami, Y., Suzukake-Tsuchiya, K., Moriya, Y., Sano, H., Shibata, K. and Omura, S. (1988). Effects of herbimycin derivatives on src oncogene function in relation to antitumor activity. *J. Antibiotics*, **41**, 831–834

153. Tamargo, R. J., Bok, R. A. and Brem, H. (1991). Angiogenesis inhibition by minocycline. *Cancer Res.*, **51**, 672–675

154. Ingber, D., Fujita, T., Kishimoto, S., Sudo, K., Kanamaru, T., Brem, H. and Folkman, J. (1990). Synthetic analogues of fumagillin that inhibit angiogenesis and suppress tumour growth. *Nature*, **348**, 555–557

155. Brem, H., Ingber, D., Muirhead, W., Panigrahy, D., Blood, C. H., Urioste, S., Bradley, D. and Folkman, J. (1992). Suppression of tumor metastasis by AGM 1470. In Maragoudakis, M. E. (ed.) *Angiogenesis in Health and Diseases*. (New York, Plenum Publishing)

156. Kusaka, M., Sudo, K., Fujita, T., Marui, S., Itoh, F., Ingber, D. and Folkman, J. (1991). Potent anti-angiogenic action of AGM-1470: comparison to the fumagillin parent. *Biochem. Biophys. Res. Commun.*, **174**, 1070–1076

157. Murata, J., Saiki, I., Makabe, T., Tsuta, Y., Tokura, S. and Azuma, I. (1991). Inhibition of tumour-induced angiogenesis by sulfated chitin derivatives. *Cancer Res.*, **51**, 22–26

158. Kumar, S. (1990). Modulation of tumour growth by a protein-bound plant polysaccharide. *J. Clin. Res. Clin. Oncol.*, **116**, 872

159. Kumar, S., Saitoh, K. and Kumar, P. (1992). Antiangiogenesis strategies in cancer therapy with special reference to Krestin. In Steiner, R., Weisz, P. B. and Langer, R. (eds.) *Angiogenesis. Key Principles – Science – Technology – Medicine*. pp. 463–470. (Basel: Birkhauser Verlag AG)

160. Ingber, D. and Folkman, J. (1988). Inhibition of angiogenesis through modulation of collagen metabolism. *Lab. Invest.*, **59**, 44–51

161. Oikawa, T., Hirotani, K., Nakamura, O., Shudo, K., Hiragun, A. and Iwaguchi, T. (1989). A highly potent antiangiogenic activity of retinoids. *Cancer Lett.*, **48**, 157–162

162. Oikawa, T., Hirotani, K., Ogasawara, H., Katayama, T., Nakamura, O., Iwaguchi, T. and Hiragun, A. (1990). Inhibition of angiogenesis by vitamin D$_3$ analogues. *Eur. J. Pharmacol.*, **178**, 247–250

163. Eisman, J. A., Barkla, D. H. and Tutton, P. J. M. (1988). Suppression of *in vivo* growth of human cancer solid tumour xenografts by 1,25-dihydroxyvitamin D$_3$. *Cancer Res.*, **47**, 21–25

164. Orchard, P. J., Smith, C. M. III, Woods, W. G., Day, D. L., Dehner, L. P. and Shapiro, R. (1989). Treatment of haemangioendotheliomas with alpha interferon. *Lancet*, **2**, 565–567

165. White, C. W., Sondheimer, H. M., Crouch, E. C., Wilson, H. and Fan, L. L. (1989). Treatment of pulmonary hemangiomatosis with recombinant interferon alfa-2a. *N. Engl. J. Med.*, **320**, 1197–1200

165a. Ezekowitz, R. A. B., Mulliken, J. B. and Folkman, J. (1992). Interferonalfa-2a therapy for life-threatening hemangiomas of infancy. *N. Engl. J. Med.*, **326**, 1456–1463

166. Maheshwari, R. K., Srikantan, V., Bhartiya, D., Kleinman, H. K. and Grant, D. S. (1991). Differential effects of interferon gamma and alpha on in vitro model of angiogenesis. *J. Cell. Physiol.*, **146**, 164–169

167. Sidky, Y. A. and Borden, E. C. (1987). Inhibition of angiogenesis by interferons: effects on tumor- and lymphocyte-induced vascular responses. *Cancer Res.*, **47**, 5155–5161

168. Tsuruoka, N., Sugiyama, M., Tawaragi, Y., Tsujimoto, M., Nishihara, T., Goto, T. and Sato, N. (1988). Inhibition of *in vitro* angiogenesis by lymphotoxin and interferon-gamma. *Biochem. Biophys. Res. Commun.*, **155**, 429–435

169. Friesel, R., Komoriya, A. and Maciag, T. (1987). Inhibition of endothelial cell proliferation by gamma-interferon. *J. Cell Biol.*, **104**, 689–696

170. Hicks, C., Breit, S. N. and Penny, R. (1989). Response of microvascular endothelial cells of biological response modifiers. *Immunol. Cell. Biol.*, **67**, 271–277

171. du P. Heyns, A., Eldor, A., Vlodavsky, I., Kaiser, N., Fridman, R. and Panet, A. (1985). The antiproliferative effect of interferon and the mitogenic activity of growth factors are independent cell cycle events: Studies with vascular smooth muscle cells and endothelial cells. *Exp. Cell. Res.*, **161**, 297–306

172. Saegusa, Y., Ziff, M., Welkovich, L., Cavender, D. (1990). Effect of inflammatory cytokines on human endothelial cell proliferation. *J. Cell Physiol.*, **142**, 488–495

173. Palladino, M. A. Jr., Patton, J. S., Figari, I. S. and Shalaby, R. (1987). Possible relationships between in vivo antitumour activity and toxicity of tumour necrosis factor-alpha. In Bock, G. and Marsh, J. (eds.) *Tumour Necrosis Factor and Related Cytotoxins*. Ciba Foundation Symposium, Vol. **131**, pp. 21–38. (New York, John Wiley & Sons)

174. Haranaka, K., Satomi, N., Sakurai, A. and Haranaka, R. (1987). Antitumour effects of tumour necrosis factor: cytotoxic or necrotizing activity and its mechanism. In Bock, G. and Marsh, J. (eds.) *Tumour Necrosis Factor and Related Cytotoxins*. Ciba Foundation Symposium, Vol. **131**, pp. 140–149. (New York, John Wiley & Sons)

175. Ito, A., Sato, T., Iga, T. and Mori, Y. (1990). Tumor necrosis factor bifunctionally regulates matrix metalloproteinases and tissue inhibitor of metalloproteinases (TIMP) production by human fibroblasts. *FEBS Lett.*, **269**, 93–95

176. Fajardo, L. F., Kwan, H. H., Kowalski, J., Priunas, S. D. and Allison, A. C. (1992). Dual role of tumor necrosis factor-α in angiogenesis. *Am. J. Pathol.*, **140**, 539–544

177. Yang, E. Y. and Moses, H. L. (1990). Transforming growth factor β1-induced changes in cell migration, proliferation, and angiogenesis in the chicken chorioallantoic membrane, *J. Cell Biol.*, **111**, 731–741

178. Taylor, S. and Folkman, J. (1982). Protamine is an inhibitor of angiogenesis. *Nature*, **297**, 307–312

179. Maione, T. E., Gray, G. S., Petro, J., Hunt, A. J., Donner, A. L., Bauer, S. I., Carson, H. F. and Sharpe, R. J. (1990). Inhibition of angiogenesis by a recombinant human platelet factor-4 and related peptides. *Science*, **247**, 77–79

180. Sharpe, R. J., Byers, H. R., Scott, C. F., Bauer, S.I. and Maione, T. E. (1990). Growth inhibition of murine melanoma and human colon carcinoma by recombinant human platelet factor 4. *J. Natl. Cancer Inst.*, **82**, 848–853

181. Rastinejad, F., Polverini, P. J. and Bouck, N. P. (1989). Regulation of the activity of a new inhibitor of angiogenesis by a cancer suppressor gene. *Cell*, **56**, 345–355

182. Good, D. J., Polverini, P. J., Rastinejad, F., Le Beau, M. M., Lemons, R. S., Frazier, W. A. and Bouck, N. P. (1990). A tumor suppressor-dependent inhibitor of angiogenesis is immunologically and functionally indistinguishable from a fragment of thrombospondin. *Proc. Natl. Acad. Sci. USA*, **87**, 6624–6628

183. Taraboletti, G., Roberts, D., Liotta, L. A. and Giauazzi, R. (1990). Platelet thrombospondin modulates endothelial cell adhesion, motility, and growth: A potential angiogenesis regulatory factor. *J. Cell Biol.*, **111**, 765–772

184. Bouck, N. (1990). Tumor angiogenesis: the role of oncogenes and tumor suppressor genes. *Cancer Cells*, **2**, 179–185

185. Grant, D. S., Kleinman, H. K. and Martin, G. R. (1990). The role of basement membranes in vascular development. *Ann. NY Acad. Sci.*, **588**, 61–72

186. Form, D. M., Pratt, B. M. and Madri, J. A. (1986). Endothelial cell proliferation during angiogenesis. Modulation by basement membrane components. *Lab. Invest.*, **55**, 521–530

187. Martinez-Hernandez, A. (1988). The extracellular matrix and neoplasia. *Lab. Invest.*, **58**, 609–612

188. Maragoudakis, M. E., Sarmonika, M. and Panoutsacopoulou, M. (1988). Inhibition of basement membrane biosynthesis prevents angiogenesis. *J. Pharmacol. Exp. Ther.*, **244**, 729–733

189. Maragoudakis, M. E., Missirlis, E., Sarmonika, M., Panoutsacopoulou, M. and Karakiulakis, G. (1990). Basement membrane biosynthesis as a target to tumor therapy. *J. Pharmacol. Exp. Ther.*, **252**, 753–757

190. Grant, D. S., Lelkes, P. I., Fukuda, K. and Kleinman, H. K. (1991). Intracellular mechanisms involved in basement membrane induced blood vessel differentiation *in vitro*. *In Vitro Cell. Devel. Biol.*, **27A**, 327–336

191. Graf, J., Iwamoto, Y., Sasaki, M., Martin, G. R., Kleinman, H. K., Robey, F. A. and Yamada, Y. (1987). Identification of an amino acid sequence in laminin mediating cell attachment, chemotaxis, and receptor binding. *Cell*, **48**, 989–996

192. Iwamoto, Y., Robey, F. A., Graf, J., Sasaki, M., Kleinman, H. K., Yamada, Y. and Martin, G. R. (1987). YIGSR, a synthetic laminin pentapeptide, inhibits experimental metastasis formation. *Science*, **238**, 1132–1134

193. Kubota, Y., Kleinman, H. K., Martin, G. R. and Lawley, T. J. (1988). Role of laminin and basement membrane in morphological differentiation of human endothelial cells into capillary-like structures. *J. Cell Biol.*, **107**, 1589–1598

194. Grant, D. S., Tashiro, K., Segui–Real, B., Yamada, Y., Martin, G. R. and Kleinman, H. K. (1989). Two different laminin domains mediate the differentiation of human endothelial cells into capillary-like structures *in vitro*. *Cell*, **58**, 933–943

195. Sakamoto, N., Iwahana, M., Tanaka, N. G. and Osada, Y. (1991). Inhibition of angiogenesis and tumor growth by a synthetic laminin peptide, CDPGYIGSR-NH$_2$. *Cancer Res.*, **51**, 903–906

196. Nicosia, R. F. and Bonanno, E. (1991). Inhibition of tumor angiogenesis *in vitro* by Arg-Gly-Asp-containing synthetic peptide. *Am. J. Pathol.*, **138**, 829-833

197. Brem, H. and Folkman, J. (1975). Inhibition of tumor angiogenesis mediated by cartilage. *J. Exp. Med.*, **141**, 427–439

198. Langer, R., Brem, H., Falterman, K., Klien, M. and Folkman, J. (1976). Isolation of a cartilage factor that inhibits tumor neovascularisation. *Science*, **193**, 70–72

199. Sorgente, N. and Dorey, C. K. (1980). Inhibition of endothelial cell growth by a factor isolated from cartilage. *Exp. Cell Res.*, **128**, 63–71

200. Takigawa, M., Shirai, E., Enomoto, M., Hiraki, Y., Fukuya, M. et al. (1985). Cartilage-derived anti-tumor factor (CATF) inhibits the proliferation of endothelial cells in culture. *Cell Biol. Int. Rep.*, **9**, 619–625

201. Moses, M. A., Sudhalter, J. and Langer, R. (1990). Identification of an inhibitor of neo-vascularisation from cartilage. *Science*, **248**, 1408–1410

202. Docherty, A. J. P., Lyons, A., Smith, B. J., Wright, E. M., Stephens, P. E., Harris, T. J. R., Murphy, G. and Reynolds, J. J. (1985). Sequence of human tissue inhibitor of metallopro-teinases and its identity to erythroid-potentiating activity. *Nature*, **318**, 66–69

203. Carmichael, D. F., Sommer, A., Thompson, R. C., Anderson, D., Smith, C. G., Welgus, H. G. and Stricklin, G. P. (1986). Primary structure of cDNA cloning of human fibroblast collagenase inhibitor. *Proc. Natl. Acad. Sci. USA*, **83**, 2407–2411

204. Stetler-Stevenson, W. G., Krutzsch, H. C. and Liotta, L. A. (1989). Tissue inhibitor of metalloproteinase (TIMP-2). A new member of the metalloproteinase inhibitor family. *J. Biol. Chem.*, **264**, 17374–17378

205. Khokha, R., Waterhouse, P., Yagel, S., Lala, P. K., Overall, G. M., Norton, G. and Denhardt, D. T. (1989) Antisense RNA-induced reduction in murine TIMP levels confers oncogenicity in Swiss 3T3 cells. *Science*, **243**, 849–850

206. Liotta, L. A., Steeg, P. S. and Stetler-Stevenson, W. G. (1991). Cancer metastasis and angiogenesis: An imbalance of positive and negative regulation. *Cell*, **64**, 327–336

207. Brem. S., Preis, I., Langer, R., Folkman, J. and Patz, A. (1977). Inhibition of neovascular-ization by an extract derived from vitreous. *Am. J. Ophthalmol.*, **84**, 323–328

208. Raymond, L. and Jacobson, B. (1982). Isolation and identification of stimulatory and inhibitory cell growth factors in bovine vitreous. *Exp. Eye Res.*, **34**, 267–286

209. Taylor, C. M. and Weiss, J. B. (1985). Partial purification of a 5.7 K glycoprotein from bovine vitreous which inhibits both angiogenesis and collagenase activity. *Biochem. Biophys. Res. Commun.*, **133**, 911–916

210. Taylor, C. M., Thompson, J. M. and Weiss, J. B. (1991). Matrix integrity and the control of angiogenesis. *Int. J. Radiat. Biol.*, **60**, 61–64

211. Sjolund, M. and Thyberg, J. (1989). Suramin inhibits binding and degradation of platelet-derived growth factor in arterial smooth muscle cells but does not interfere with autocrine stimulation of DNA synthesis. *Cell Tissue Res.*, **256**, 35–43

212. Ono, K., Nakane, H. and Fukushima, M. (1988). Differential inhibition of various deoxyribonucleic and ribonucleic acids by suramin. *Eur. J. Biochem.*, **172**, 349–353

213. Stein, C. A., LaRocca, R. V., Thomas, R., McAtree, N. and Myers, C. E. (1989). Suramin: an anticancer drug with a unique mechanism of action. *J. Clin. Oncol.*, **7**, 499–508

214. Fantini, J., Guo, T.-J., Marvaldi, J., Rougon, G. (1990). Suramin inhibits proliferation of rat glioma cells and alters N-chorioallantoic membrane cell surface expression. *Int. J. Cancer*, **45**, 554–561

215. Plouet, J. and Moukadari, H. (1990). Characterization of the receptor to vasculotropin on bovine adrenal cortex-derived capillary endothelial cells. *J. Biol. Chem.*, **265**, 22071–22074

222

216. Yayon, A. and Klagsbrun, M. (1990). Autocrine transformation by chimeric signal peptide-basic fibroblast growth factor: Reversal by suramin. *Proc. Natl. Acad, Sci. USA*, **87**, 5346–5350

217. Betzholtz, C., Johnsson, A., Heldin, C.-H. and Westermark, B. (1986). Efficient reversion of Simian sarcoma virus-transformation and inhibition of growth factor-induced mitogenesis by suramin. *Proc. Natl. Acad. Sci. USA*, **83**, 6440–6444

218. Wilks, J. W., Scott, P. S.,Vrba, L. K. and Cocozza, J. M. (1991). Inhibition of angiogenesis with combination treatment of angiostatic steriods and suramin. *Int. J. Radiat. Biol.*, **60**, 73–77

219. Ciomei, M., Pesenti, E., Sola, F., Pastori, W., Mariani, M., Grandi, M. and Spreafico, F. (1991). Antagonistic effect of suramin on bFGF: *in vitro* and *in vivo* results. *Int. J. Radiat. Biol.*, **60**, 78

220. LaRocca, R. V., Cooper, M. R., Uhrich, M., Danesi, R., Walther, M. M., Linehan, W. M. and Myers, C. E. (1991). Use of suramin in treatment of prostatic carcinoma refractory to conventional hormonal manipulation. *Urol. Clin. N. Am.*, **18**, 123–129

221. LaRocca, R. V., Stein, C. A., Danesi, R., Cooper, M. R., Uhrich, M. and Myers, C. E. (1991). A pilot study of suramin in the treatment of metastatic renal carcinoma. *Cancer*, **67**, 1509–1513

222. Mariani, M., Piao, A., Ciomei, M., Pastori, W., Franzetti, C., Melegaro, G., Grandi, M. and Mongelli, N. (1992). *In vitro* activity of novel sulphonic derivatives of distamycin A. In Steiner, R., Weisz, P. B. and Langer, R. (eds.) *Angiogenesis. Key Principles – Science – Technology – Medicine.* pp. 455–458. (Basel: Birkhäuser Verlag AG)

223. Sola, F., Biasoli, G., Pesenti, E., Farao, M., Della Torre, P., Mongelli, N. and Grandi, M. (1992). *In vivo* activity of novel sulphonic derivatives of distamycin A. In Steiner, R., Weisz, P.B. and Langer, R. (eds.) *Angiogenesis. Key Principles – Science – Technology – Medicine.* pp. 459–462. (Basel: Birkhäuser Verlag AG)

224. Matsubara, T. and Ziff, M. (1987). Inhibition of human endothelial cell proliferation by gold compounds. *J. Clin. Invest.*, **79**, 1440–1446

225. Koch, A. E., Cho, M., Burrows, J., Leibovich, S. J. and Polverini, P. J. (1988). Inhibition of production of macrophage-derived angiogenic activity by the anti-rheumatic agents gold sodium thiomalate and auranofin. *Biochem. Biophys. Res. Commun.*, **154**, 205–212

226. Matsubara, T., Saura, R., Hirohata, K. and Ziff, M. (1989). Inhibition of human endothelial cell proliferation *in vitro* and neovascularisation *in vivo* by D-penicillamine. *J. Clin. Invest.*, **83**, 158–167

227. Francois, J., Cambie, E. and Feher, J. (1973). Collagenase inhibition with penicillamine. *Ophthalmologica*, **166**, 222–225

228. Shapiro, R. and Vallee,, B. L. (1987). Human placental ribonuclease inhibitor abolishes both angiogenic and ribonucleolytic activities of angiogenin. *Proc. Natl. Acad. Sci. USA*, **84**, 2238–2241

229. Folkman, J. (1989). Successful treatment of an angiogenic disease. *N. Engl. J. Med.*, **320**, 1211–1212

230. Salahuddin, S. Z., Nakamura, S., Bibeerfeld, P., Kaplan M. H., Markham, P. D., Larsson, L. and Gallo, R. C. (1988). Angiogenic properties of Kaposi's sarcoma-derived cells after long-term culture *in vitro*. *Science*, **242**, 430–432

231. Ensoli, B., Nakamura, S., Salahuddin, S. Z., Biberfeld, P., Larsson, L., Beaver, B., Wong-Staal, F. and Gallo, R. C. (1989). AIDS–Kaposi's sarcoma-derived cells express cytokines with autocrine and paracrine growth effects. *Science*, **243**, 223–226

232. Shing, Y. (1991). Biaffinity chromatography of fibroblast growth factor. *Meth. Enzymol.*, **198**, 91–95

233. Ruff, M. R. and Gifford, G. E. (1985). Tumor necrosis factor. *Lymphokine Rep.*, **2**, 137–272

234. Rej., R. N., Holme, K. R. and Perlin, A. S. (1990). Marked stereo selectivity in the binding of copper ions: Contrast with the binding of gadolinium calcium ions. *Carbohyd. Res.*, **207**, 143–152

235. Gullino, P. M. (1986). Considerations of the mechanisms of the angiogenic response. *Anticancer Res.*, **6**, 153–158

236. Rowe, J. M., Kasper, S., Shiv, R. F. C. and Friesen, H. G. (1986). Purification and characterization of a human tumor-derived growth factor. *Cancer Res.*, **46**, 1408–1412

237. McAuslan, B. R. and Reilly, W. (1980). Endothelial cell phagokinesis in response to specific metal ions. *Exp. Cell Res.*, **130**, 147–157

238. Shymko, R. M. and Glass, L. (1976). Cellular and geometric control of tissue growth and mitotic instability. *J. Theoret. Biol.*, **63**, 355–374

239. Fajardo, L. F., Prionas, S. D., Kowalski, J. and Kwan, H. (1988). Hyperthermia inhibits angiogenesis. *Radiat. Res.*, **114**, 297–306
240. Leuning, M., Goetz, A. E., Dellian, M., Zetterer, G., Gamarra, F., Jain, R. and Messmer, K. (1992). Interstitial fluid pressure in solid tumors following hyperthermia. Possible correlation with therapeutic response. *Cancer Res.*, **52**, 487–490
241. Burchenal, J. H. (1976). Adjuvant therapy-theory, practice, and potential. *Cancer*, **37**, 46–56
242. DeVita, V. T. Jr. (1983). The relationship between tumor mass and resistance to chemotherapy: Implications for surgical adjuvant treatment of cancer. *Cancer*, **51**, 1209–1220
243. Kerbel, R. S. (1991). Inhibition of tumor angiogenesis as a strategy to circumvent acquired resistance to anti-cancer therapeutic agents. *Bio-Essays*, **13**, 31–36
244. Tsanaclis, A. M. C., Brem, S. S., Gately, S., Schipper, H. M. and Wang, E. (1991). Statin immunolocalization in human brain tumors: Detection of noncycling cells using a novel marker of cell quiescence. *Cancer*, **68**, 786–792
245. Maciag, T. (1990). Molecular and cellular mechanisms of angiogenesis. In DeVita, V. T. Jr., Hellman, S. and Rosenberg, S.A. (eds.) *Important Advances in Oncology.*, pp. 85–98. (Philadelphia: Lippincott)
246. Nagashima, T., Hoshino, T. and Cho, K. G. (1987). Proliferative potential of vascular components in human glioblastoma multiforme. *Acta Neuropathol. (Berl.)*, **73**, 301–305
247. Stenn, K. S., Fernandez, L. A. and Tirrell, S. J. (1988). The angiogenic properties of the rat vibrissa hair follicle associated with the bulb. *J. Invest. Dermatol.*, **90**, 409–411
248. Gospodarowicz, D. and Thakral, K. (1978). Production of a corpus luteum angiogenic factor responsible for proliferation of capillaries and neovascularization of the corpus luteum. *Proc. Natl. Acad. Sci. USA*, **75**, 847–851
249. Denekamp, J. (1984). Vasculature as a target for tumour therapy. *Prog. Appl. Microcirc.*, **4**, 28–38
250. Deane, B. R., Greenwood, J., Lantos, P. L. and Pratt, O. E. (1984). The vasculature of experimental brain tumors: Part 4. The quantification of vascular permeability. *J. Neurol. Sci.*, **65**, 59–68
251. Tanaka, N. G., Sakamoto, N., Korenaaga, H., Inoue, K., Ogawa, H. and Osada, Y. (1991). The combination of a bacterial polysaccharide and tamoxifen inhibits angiogenesis and tumour growth. *Int. J. Radiat. Biol.*, **60**, 79–83
252. Denekamp, J. (1991). The current status of targeting tumour vasculature as a means of cancer therapy: an overview. *Int. J. Radiat. Biol.*, **60**, 401–408
253. Murray, J. C. (1991). Coagulation and cancer. *Br. J. Cancer*, **64**, 422–424
254. Murray, J. C., Smith. K. A. and Thurston, G. (1989). Flavone acetic acid induces a coagulopathy in mice. *Br. J. Cancer*, **60**, 729–733
255. Mahadevan, V., Malik, S. T. A., Meager, A., Fiers, W., Lewis, G. P. and Hart, I. R. (1990). Role of tumor necrosis factor in flavone acetic acid-induced tumor vasculature shutdown. *Cancer Res.*, **50**, 5537–5542
256. Murray, J. C., Smith, K. A. and Stern, D. (1991). Flavone acetic acid and TNF-α act synergistically to promote endothelial procoagulant activity *in vitro* and inhibit tumour growth *in vivo*. *Int. J. Radiat. Biol.*, **60**, 278
257. Nichol, C. A. (1977). Pharmacokinetics: selectivity of action related to physicochemical properties and kinetic patterns of anticancer drugs. *Cancer*, **40**, 519–528
258. Brem, H., Mahaley, M. S. Jr., Vick, N. A., Black, K. L., Schold, S. C., Burger, P. C., Friedman, A. H., Ciric, I. S., Eller, T. W., Cozzens, J. W. and Kenealy, J. N. (1991). Interstitial chemotherapy with drug polymer implants for the treatment of recurrent glioma. *J. Neurosurg.*, **74**, 441–446
259. Folkman, J. (1990). How the field of controlled-release technology began, and its central role in the development of angiogenesis research. *Biomaterials*, **11**, 615–618
260. Tamargo, R. J., Leong, K. W. and Brem, H. (1990). Growth inhibition of the 9L glioma using polymers to release heparin and cortisone acetate. *J. Neuro-Oncol.*, **9**, 131–138
261. Langer, R. (1992). Delivery systems for angiogenesis stimulators and inhibitors. In Steiner, R., Weisz, P. B. and Langer, R. (eds.) *Angiogenesis. Key Principles – Science – Technology – Medicine.* pp. 327–330. (Basel: Birkhäuser Verlag AG)
262. Madarnas, P., Benrezzak, O. and Nigam, V. N. (1989). Prophylactic antiangiogenic tumor treatment. *Anticancer Res.*, **9**, 897–901
263. Peterson, H.-L. (1986). Tumor angiogenesis inhibition by prostaglandin synthetase inhibitors. *Anticancer Res.*, **6**, 251–254

264. Folkman, J. and Klagsbrun, M. (1987). A family of angiogenic peptides. *Nature*, **329**, 671–672.
265. Merwin, J. R., Newman, W., Beall, L. D., Tucker, A. and Madri, J. (1991). Vascular cells respond differentially to transforming growth factor-beta$_1$ and factor-beta$_2$ *in vitro*. *Am. J. Pathol.*, **138**, 37–51
266. Folkman, J. and Brem, H. (1992). Angiogenesis and inflammation. In Gallin, J. I., Goldstein, I. M. and Snyderman, R. (eds) *Inflammation: Basic Principles and Clinical Correlates* (New York: Raven Press). (in press)
267. Kerr, D. J., Maughan, T., Newlands, E., Rustin, G., Bleehen, N. M., Lewis, C. and Kaye, S. B. (1989). Phase II trials of flavone acetic acid in advanced malignant melanoma and colorectal carcinoma. *Br. J. Cancer*, **60**, 104–106
268. Brien, S. E., Zagzag, D. and Brem, S. (1989). Rapid in situ cellular kinetics of intracerebral tumor angiogenesis using a monoclonal antibody to bromodeoxyuridine. *Neurosurgery*, **25**, 715–719
269. Watanabe, H., Hori, A., Seno, M., Kozai, Y., Igarashi, K., Ichimori, Y. and Kondo, K. (1991). A sensitive enzyme immunoassay for human basic fibroblast growth factor. *Biochem. Biophys. Res. Commun.*, **175**, 229–235
270. Fujimoto K., Ichimori, Y., Kakizoe, T., Okajima, E., Sakamoto, H., Sugimura, T. and Terada, M. (1991). Increased serum levels of basic fibroblast growth factor in patients with renal cell carcinoma. *Biochem. Biophys. Res. Commun.*, **180**, 386–392
271. Minniti, C. P., Maggi, M. and Helman, L. J. (1992). Suramin inhibits the growth of human rhabdomyosarcoma by interrupting the insulin-like growth factor II pathway. *Cancer Res.*, **52**, 1830–1835
272. Eisenberger, M. A. and Fontana, J. A. (1992). Suramin, an active nonhormonal cytotoxic drug for treatment of prostate cancer: Compelling reasons for testing in patients with hormone refractory breast cancer. *J. Natl. Cancer Inst.*, **84**, 3–5
273. Scher, H. I., Jodrell, D. I., Iversen, J. M., Curley, T., Tong, W., Egorin, M. J. and Forrest, A. (1992). Use of adaptive control with feedback to individualize suramin dosing. *Cancer Res.*, **52**, 64–70
274. Cardinelli, M., Sartor, O. and Robbins, K.-C. (1992). Suramin, an experimental chemotherapeutic drug, activates the receptor for epidermal growth factor and promotes the growth of certain malignant cells. *J. Clin. Invest.*, **89**, 1242–1247
275. Isacchi, A., Statuto, M., Chiesa, R., Bergonzoni, L., Rusnati, M., Sarmientos, P., Ragnotti, G. and Presta, M. (1991). A six-amino acid deletion in basic fibroblast growth factor dissociates its mitogenic activity from its plasminogen activator-inducing capacity. *Proc. Natl. Acad. Sci. USA*, **88**, 2628–2632
276. Hannum, C. H., Wilcox, C. J., Arend, W. P., Joslin, F. G., Dripps, D. J., Heimdal, P. L., Armes, L. G., Sommer, A., Eisenberg, S. P. and Thompson, R. C. (1990). Interleukin-1 receptor antagonist activity of a human interleukin-1 inhibitor. *Nature*, **343**, 336–340
277. Dalsgaard, C.-J., Hultgardh–Nilsson, A., Haegerstrand, A. and Nilsson, J. (1989). Neuropeptides as growth factors. Possible roles in human diseases. *Regul. Pept.*, **25**, 1–9
278. Woll, P. J. (1991). Neuropeptide growth factors and cancer. *Br. J. Cancer*, **63**, 469–475
279. Cuttitta, F., Carney, D. N., Mulshine, J., Moody, T. W., Fedorko, J., Fischler, A. and Minna, J. D. (1985). Bombesin-like peptides can function as autocrine growth factors in human small-cell lung cancer. *Nature*, **316**, 823–826
280. Woll, P. and Rozengurt, E. (1988). [D-Arg^1,D-Phe^5,D-Trp^{7,9},Leu^{11}]-substance P, a potent bombesin antagonist in Swiss 3T3 cells, inhibits the growth of human small cell lung cancer cells *in vitro*. *Proc. Natl. Acad. Sci. USA*, **85**, 1859–1863
281. Avis, F. P., Maneckjee, R., Cuttitta, F., Nakanishi, Y., Mulshine, J. and Avis, I. (1988). The role of gastrin releasing peptide in a pancreatic tumor cell line (CAPAN). *Proc. Am. Assoc. Cancer Res.*, **29**, 54
282. Szepeshazi, K., Schally, A. V., Cai, R.-Z., Radulovic, S., Milovanovic, S. and Szoke, B. (1991). Inhibitory effect of bombesin/gastrin-releasing peptide antagonist RC-3095 and high dose of somatostatin analogue RC–160 on nitrosamine-induced pancreatic cancers in hamsters. *Cancer Res.*, **51**, 6980–5986
283. Beitz, J. G., Davol, P., Clark, J. W., Kato, L., Medina, M., Frackelton, R. A. Jr., Lappi, D. A., Baird, A. and Calabresi, P. (1992). Antitumor activity of basic fibroblast growth factor-saporin mitotoxin *in vitro* and *in vivo*. *Cancer Res.*, **52**, 227–230
284. Hori, A., Sasada, R., Matsutani, E., Naito, K., Sakura, Y., Fujita, T. and Kozai, Y. (1991). Suppression of solid tumor growth by immunoneutralizing monoclonal antibody against human fibroblast growth factor. *Cancer Res.*, **151**, 6180–6184

285. Chiang, M.-Y., Chan, H., Zounes, M. A., Freier, S. M., Lima, W. F. and Bennet, C. F. (1991). Antisense oligonucleotides inhibit intercellular adhesion molecule 1 expression by two distinct mechanisms. *J. Biol. Chem.*, **266**, 18162–18171

286. Morrison, R. S. (1991). Suppression of basic fibroblast growth factor expression by antisense oligodeoxynucleotides inhibits the growth of transformed astrocytes. *J. Biol. Chem.*, **266**, 728–734

287. Denekamp, J. (1982). Endothelial cell proliferation as a novel approach to targeting tumour therapy. *Br. J. Cancer*, **45**, 136–139

288. Denekamp, J., Hill, S. and Hobson, B. (1983). Vascular occlusion and tumour cell death. *Eur. J. Cancer Clin. Oncol.*, **19**, 271–275

289. West, C. M. L., West, D. C., Kumar, S. and Moore, J. V. (1990). A comparison of the sensitivity to photodynamic treatment of endothelial and tumour cells in different proliferative states. *Int. J. Radiat. Biol.*, **58**, 145–156

290. Reinhold, H. S. and Endrich, B. (1986). Tumour microcirculation as a target for hyperthermia. *Int. J. Hyperthermia*, **2**, 111–137

291. Denekamp, J. (1992). Anti-angiogenic versus anti-vascular approaches to cancer therapy. In Maragoudakis, M. E. (ed.) *Angiogenesis in Health and Diseases*, pp. 303–306. (New York: Plenum)

292. Denekamp, J. (1990). Vascular attack as a therapeutic strategy or cancer. *Cancer Metastasis Rev.*, **9**, 267–282

293. Denekamp, J. (1989). Induced vascular collapse in tumours: a way of increasing the therapeutic gain in cancer therapy. *Br. J. Radiol. Rep.*, **19**, 63–70

294. Hart, M. N., DeBault, L. E., Sadewasser, K. L., Cancilla, P. A. and Henriques, E. M. (1981). Morphologic effects of antibody to mouse brain endothelium *in vivo*. *J. Neuropathol. Exp. Neurol.*, **40**, 84–91

295. Caldwell, P. R. B., Wigger, H. J., Butler, P. B. Jr. and Gigli, I. (1982). In Nossel, H. L. and Vogel, H. J. (eds.) Pulmonary endothelial cell injury induced by antibody fragments to angiotensin converting enzyme. *Pathobiology of the Endothelial Cell*, pp. 425–430. (New York: Academic Press)

296. Clarke, M. S. F. and West, D. C. (1991). The identification of proliferation and tumour-induced proteins in human endothelial cells: possible target for tumour therapy. *Electrophoresis*, **12**, 500–508

297. Wang, J. M., Hunter, R. D. and Kumar, S. (1992). A monoclonal antibody (E-9) binds preferentially to the vasculatures of human tumours, embryonic and regenerating tissues. In Steiner, R., Weisz, P. B. and Langer, R. (eds.) *Angiogenesis. Key Principles – Science – Technology – Medicine*. pp. 266–271. (Basel: Birkhauser Verlag AG).

298. Muzykantov, V. R. and Danilov, S. M. (1991). Glucose oxidase-conjugated with anti-endothelial monoclonal antibodies: *in vitro* and *in vivo* studies. *Int. J. Radiat. Biol.*, **60**, 11–15

299. Thorpe, P. E., Wallace, P. M., Knyba, R. E., Watson, G. J., Mahadevan, V. A., Land, H., Yerganian, G. and Brown, P. J. (1991). Selective killing of proliferating vascular endothelial cells by anti-fibronectin receptor immunotoxin. *Int. J. Radiat. Biol.*, **60**, 24

300. Bagshawe, K. D., Springer, C. J., Searle, F., Antoniw, P., Sharma, S. K., Melton, R. G., and Sherwood, R. F. (1988). A cytotoxic agent can be generated selectively at cancer sites. *Br. J. Cancer*, **58**, 700–703

301. Auerbach, R. (1991). Vascular endothelial cell differentiation: organ-specificity and selective affinities as the basis for developing anti-cancer strategies. *Int. J. Radiat. Biol.*, **60**, 1–10

302. Pauli, B. U. and Lee, C.-L. (1988). Organ preference of metastasis. The role of organ-specifically modulated endothelial cells. *Lab. Invest.*, **58**, 379–387

303. Auerbach, R. (1988). Patterns of tumor metastasis: organ selectivity in the spread of cancer cells. *Lab. Invest.*, **58**, 361–364

304. Nicolson, G. L. (1988). Organ specificity of tumor metastasis: role of preferential adhesion, invasion and growth of malignant cells at specific secondary sites. *Cancer Metastasis Rev.*, **7**, 143–188

305. McCarthy, S. A., Kuzu, I., Gatter, K. C. and Bicknell, R. (1991). Heterogeneity of the endothelial cell and its role in organ preference of tumour metastasis. *Trends Pharmacol. Sci.*, **12**, 462–467

306. Hepner, G. H. and Miller, B. E. (1983). Tumor heterogeneity: biological implications and therapeutic consequences. *Cancer Metastasis Rev.*, **2**, 5–2

307. Rupnick, M. A., Carey, A. and Williams, S. K. (1988). Phenotypic diversity in cultured cerebral microvascular endothelial cells. *In Vitro Cell Devel. Biol.*, **24**, 435–444

308. Aaronson, S. A. (1991). Growth factors and cancer. *Science*, **254**, 1146–1153.

309. Yaish, P., Gazit, A., Gilon, C. and Levitzki, A. (1988). Blocking of EGF-dependent cell proliferation by EGF receptor kinase inhibitors. *Science*, **242**, 933–93

310. Nishizuka, Y, (1984). The role of protein kinase C in cell surface signal transduction and tumour promotion. *Nature*, **308**, 693–69

311. Doctrow, S. R. and Folkman, J. (1987). Protein kinase C activators suppress stimulation of capillary endothelial cell growth by angiogenic endothelial mitogens. *J. Cell Biol.*, **104**, 679–687

312. Montesano, R. and Orci, L. (1985). Tumor-promoting phorbol esters induce angiogenesis *in vitro*. *Cell*, **42**, 469–477

313. Morris, P. B., Hida, T., Blackshear, P. J., Klintworth, G. K. and Swain, J. L. (1988). Tumor-promoting phorbol esters induce angiogenesis in vivo. *Am. J. Physiol.*, **254**, C318–C322

314. Brem, S., Medina, D. and Gullino, P. M. (1977). Angiogenesis: A marker for experimental neoplastic transformation of mammary hyperplasia. *Science*, **195**, 880–882

315. Brem, S., Jensen, H. M. and Gullino, P. M. (1978). Angiogenesis as a marker of preneoplastic lesions of the human breast. *Cancer*, **41**, 239–244

316. Gullino, P. M. (1981). Angiogenesis and neoplasia. *N. Engl. J. Med.*, **305**, 884–88

317. Ross, R. (1989). Successful growth of tumours. *Nature*, **339**, 16–17

318. Polverini, P. J. and DiPietro, L. A. (1992). Role of macrophages in angiogenesis. In Maragoudakis, M. E. (ed.) *Angiogenesis in Health and Diseases*, NATO-ASI Series, pp. 43–54. (New York: Plenum)

319. Nabel, E. G., Plautz, G., Boyce, F. M., Stanley, J. C. and Nabel, G. J. (1989). Recombinant gene expression *in vivo* within endothelial cells of the arterial wall. *Science*, **244**, 1342–1344

320. Wilson, J. M., Birinyi, L. K., Salomon, R. N., Libby, P., Callow, A. D. and Mulligan, R. C. (1989). Implantation of vascular grafts lined with genetically modified endothelial cells. *Science*, **244**, 1344–1346

321. Zwiebel, J. A., Freeman, S. M., Kantoff, P. W., Cornetta, K., Ryan, U. S. and Anderson, W. F. (1989). High-level recombinant gene expression in rabbit endothelial cells transduced by retroviral vectors. *Science*, **243**, 220–222

322. Gullino, P. M. and Grantham, F. H. (1961). Studies on the exchange of fluids between host and tumor. II. The blood flow of hepatomas and other tumors in rats and mice. *J. Natl. Cancer Inst.*, **27**, 1465–1491

323. Gospodarowicz, D., Ferrara, N., Schweigerer, L. and Neufield, G. (1987). Structural characterization and biological functions of fibroblast growth factor. *Endocrine Rev.*, **8**, 95–114

324. Vaisman, N., Gospodarowicz, D. and Neufield, G. (1990). Characterization of the receptors for vascular endothelial growth factor. *J. Biol. Chem.*, **265**, 19461–19466

325. Schulze-Osthoff, K., Risau, W., Vollmer, E. and Sorg, C. (1990). *In situ* detection of basic fibroblast growth factor by highly specific antibodies. *Am. J. Pathol.*, **137**, 85–92

326. Patz, A., Brem, S., Finkelstein, D., Chen, C.-H., Lutty, G., Bennett, A., Goughlin, W. R. and Gardener, J. (1978). A new approach to the problem of retinal neovascularization. *Ophthalmology*, **85**, 626–637

327. Peacock, D. J., Banquerigo, M. L. and Brahn, E. (1992). Angiogenesis inhibition suppresses collagen arthritis. *J. Exp. Med.*, **175**, 1135–1138

328. Folkman, J. (1972). Angiogenesis in psoriasis: Therapeutic implications. *J. Invest. Dermatol.*, **59**, 40–43

329. Kumar, S. and West, D. C. (1990). Psoriasis, angiogenesis, and hyaluronic acid. *Lab. Invest.*, **62**, 664–665

330. Brem, S. (1992). The development of therapeutic angiosuppression: problems and progress. In Maragoudakis, M. (ed.) *Angiogenesis in Health and Disease*, NATO-ASI Series. pp. 295–302. (New York: Plenum Press)

8
Preclinical evaluation and phase I trials

I. R. JUDSON

DRUG ACQUISITION AND SCREENING

The discovery of new anticancer agents has occurred, variously, by a mixture of screening, analogue development, rational design and serendipity. Until quite recently, the majority of potential new agents were tested initially *in vivo* in mice against rapidly growing leukaemias, such as the P388 and L1210. However, experience with the National Cancer Institute, USA (NCI) *in vivo* tumour panel as a screening tool has been relatively disappointing because the majority of agents thus identified are inactive against slowly growing solid tumours[1]. The major challenge for the development of new treatments for cancer is to identify new agents with activity against the common solid tumours, such as colon and non-small-cell lung cancer (NSCLC). This has led to the establishment at NCI of an *in vitro* testing system based on human tumour cell lines[2]. While the predictive ability of this model is unknown, it is demonstrating the ability to confirm the pattern of activity of established drugs[3]. Moreover, there have been some examples of new compounds which exhibit tissue-determined selectivity and unusual patterns of cytotoxicity. Nevertheless, *in vitro* screens, as currently employed, are ill-designed to demonstrate activity with drugs which require metabolic activation, drugs acting via the immune system and drugs with bell-shaped dose–response curves. A more detailed discussion of *in vitro* testing is to be found in Chapter 3.

In parallel with *in vitro* cell lines, many human tumours can also be grown as xenografts in immune-deprived or nude mice. It is hoped that these will provide better models for human solid tumours to confirm activity seen *in vitro* and assist the development of drugs which can overcome the intrinsic or acquired resistance characteristics of many solid tumours[4]. However tempting it may be to extrapolate from activity against such tumours to potential clinical activity in the same tumour types, one must be a little cautious. Because of the heterogeneity of human malignancy, it is essential to employ a number of different examples of each tumour in order to provide a spectrum of responsiveness. Furthermore, it is by no means certain that drug resistance *in vitro* provides a good model for investigating clinical drug resistance. For example, by continuously exposing tumour cells to gradually increasing drug concentrations, it is possible to produce several orders of magnitude of resistance to certain agents. In contrast, given the poor therapeutic index of most anticancer agents, two- to three-fold resistance may render a drug clinically inactive. Nevertheless, tumour panels do exist in which good agreement has been demonstrated between the clinical response of the original tumours and their subsequent sensitivity to treatment as xenografts[5]. Such information may be very helpful, not only in identifying new agents, but also in guiding their subsequent clinical evaluation.

PRECLINICAL EVALUATION

Toxicology and determination of safe starting dose

Before a new agent can be tested against human malignancy, its toxicity must first be investigated rigorously in animals. This has two purposes; the identification of specific toxic side-effects and the determination of a maximum tolerated dose (MTD). For the majority of antiproliferative agents in current use, the dose-limiting toxicity in rodents is directly related to the inhibition of cell division in the bone marrow or gut. As a result, there is a good correlation between the MTD for acute administration in mice and the MTD in man. However, rodents are not such good models for predicting organ-specific damage, such as pulmonary, cardiac or neurotoxicity, and, since rodents do not vomit, they do not predict for emetic potential, a major side-effect of anticancer drugs.

Freireich et al., and other investigators, studied the relationships between human and animal toxicity for anticancer agents[6] in a variety of species, showing that the MTD, expressed in mg/m^2, was approximately equivalent between species. The mouse was second only to the rhesus monkey in terms of the accurate prediction of human toxicity[6]. Although a good correlation exists between small-animal and human toxicity, the variations remain quite large and thus it is unsafe to commence the testing of drugs in man at doses which are toxic to rodents. A margin of error is required which will allow the starting dose to be totally safe, yet not so low that large numbers of patients are required during the dose escalation phase.

A number of different ways have been devised for determining a safe starting dose based on retrospective studies of phase I trials[7]. For example, if the starting dose were taken as 1/10 the dose (mg/m^2) producing 10% lethality, LD_{10}, in dogs, the likelihood of exceeding the MTD would be around 1%. However, the dog is more sensitive to certain types of toxicity, e.g. to the gut; hence reliance on dog toxicology would be likely to lead to too low a starting dose in man. Having reviewed the data from mice, dogs and monkeys, the National Cancer Institute of the USA concluded that 1/10 the LD_{10} in mice is a safe starting dose, provided this is tolerated in the dog. An alternative approach is to use 1/6 of the mouse LD_{10} or 1/3 of the dose causing minimal reversible toxicity in the dog, sometimes referred to as the 'toxic dose low', whichever is the lower.

Regulatory differences exist between Europe and the USA concerning the toxicity studies required for a new anticancer agent. Dog toxicology is still required in the USA but is not mandatory in Europe[8]. A joint committee of the

European Organisation for Research and Treatment of Cancer (EORTC) and the Cancer Research Campaign (CRC) of the UK recently published guidelines for preclinical toxicology testing of new anticancer agents, which is usually confined to mice and rats[9]. This is based on the principle that the safe starting dose in man will be defined as 1/10 the LD_{10} in the mouse, expressed in mg/m^2. In brief, this entails: the determination of the LD_{10} and LD_{50} doses for single administration in the mouse using intravenous and intraperitoneal routes; histopathology; a single-dose study for identification of acute toxicity, especially to the bone marrow, using a dose close to the LD_{10}; repeat-dose studies in mice; and, finally, a chronic-dose study in rats at 1/10 the mouse LD_{10}, i.e. the potential starting dose, which must be shown to be non-toxic. There may be special requirements for antiendocrine agents[10] or those which will be administered orally. Ideally, the drug should be tested using a formulation identical to that which will be employed in the clinical studies.

Although the dog may overpredict for toxicity in man, the dog may provide useful data concerning organ-specific toxicities[8]. Occasionally there may be a specific requirement for toxicology in larger animals. For example, in the case of inhibitors of the enzyme, thymidylate synthase (TS), dog toxicology is likely to be helpful since rodents seriously underpredict for toxicity owing to their higher circulating plasma thymidine concentration[11]. Thymidine can be salvaged via thymidine kinase, thus circumventing the toxic and antitumour effects of TS inhibition.

Pharmacokinetics

The study of pharmacokinetics is a vital part of preclinical development in helping to define optimum dose schedules, therapeutic index and possibly even mechanism of action. Collins et al. made a major contribution to anticancer drug development by demonstrating the potential value of preclinical pharmacokinetic data in expediting dose escalation in phase I trials[12]. He emphasized the serious consequences of choosing too low a starting dose in that a much larger number of dose escalation steps is required. This results in a prolonged, more expensive study in which more patients receive suboptimal doses with little possibility of therapeutic benefit. He showed that, for certain drugs, the area under the concentration × time curve (AUC) at the mouse LD_{10} correlated much more closely with the AUC at the human MTD than did the mouse LD_{10} (mg/m^2) with the human MTD, i.e. the ratio of the AUC's was closer to unity than the dose ratio. In cases such as doxorubicin, this can be readily explained by a much higher clearance in man, while the AUC's at toxic doses in mouse and man are equivalent.

In order to exploit this approach, one must first establish that the drug displays a linear pharmacokinetic profile in the mouse, i.e. elimination is not dependent on a saturable mechanism which can lead to a very rapid increase in plasma concentration above a certain dose threshold. An example of a good correlation between dose and AUC is given in Figure 8.1.

This must be confirmed in man, requiring constant vigilance during the escalation process. There must be an assay of sufficient sensitivity to measure

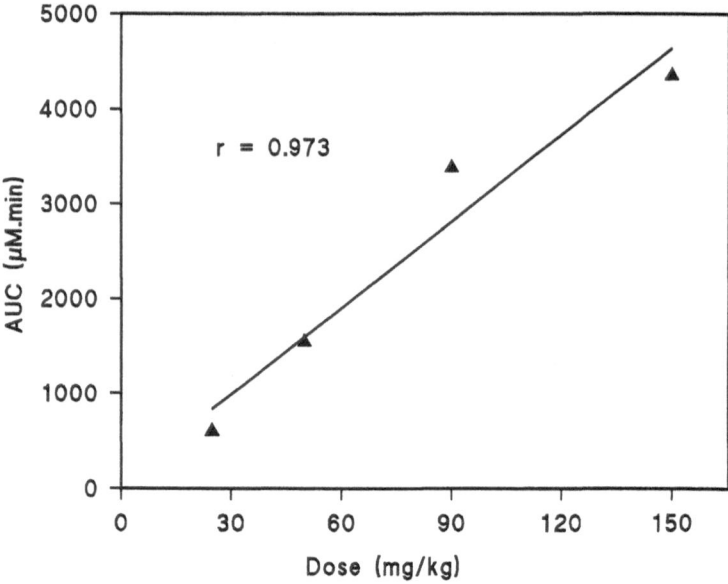

Figure 8.1 Correlation between dose and AUC for Trimelamol in the mouse

plasma levels accurately at the starting dose in man, i.e. 1/10 the mouse LD_{10}. There must be a direct relationship between toxicity and plasma concentration, which might not hold for an antimetabolite where maintenance of the plasma concentration above an inhibitory threshold for a certain period of time is more important than the AUC[13].

Antimetabolites are also a problem in that a number of drugs, typically nucleic acid analogues, require activation. Differences in target cell levels of activating and inactivating enzymes, as well as extracellular levels of nucleic acid precursors, may have a major effect on efficacy. For example, genetic variations in levels of thiopurine methyltransferase, an enzyme which inactivates 6-mercaptopurine, may be responsible for large variations in the efficacy of this drug[14]. Conversely, there may be species differences in metabolic activation via cytochrome P450-dependent processes, which may have been responsible for the poor clinical activity of pentamethylmelamine[15] (see Figure 8.2).

Where an active metabolite is responsible for antitumour activity, as in the case of cyclophosphamide, pentamethylmelamine, dacarbazine (DTIC) and other agents, this should be measured and interspecies comparisons made of the extent of activation. If the active metabolite is only to be found intracellularly, plasma concentrations will be unhelpful, as in the case of cytosine arabinoside (ara-C) where plasma levels bear little relationship to intracellular levels of the phosphorylated metabolite, ara-CTP[13]. Species differences in plasma protein binding could lead to differences in levels of free drug, hence activity. Once more, when major differences are observed, it may be more appropriate to extrapolate on the basis of the free drug AUC[16]. Major species differences in target cell sensitivity might also cause serious problems.

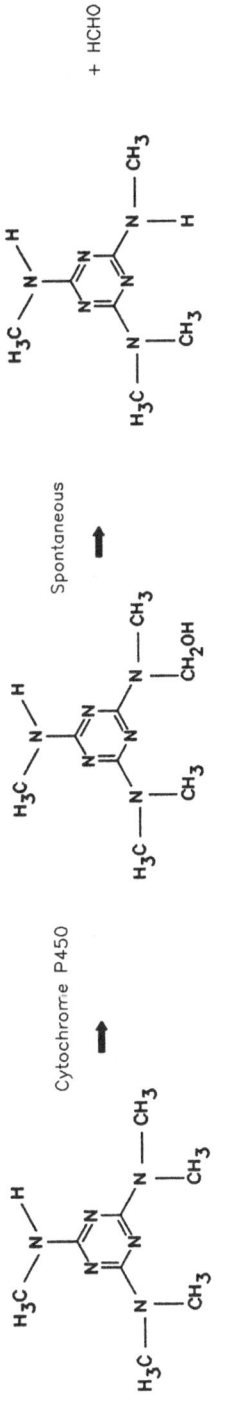

Figure 8.2 Proposed mechanism for metabolic activation of N-methylmelamines, such as pentamethylmelamine shown here, by stepwise oxidative N-demethylation. The hydroxymethyl intermediate is thought to be the active metabolite. Failure to activate this drug was thought to be responsible for its disappointing activity in man[15]

Determination of optimum schedule

Another important aspect of preclinical investigation which is sometimes not explored adequately is that of schedule-dependent activity and/or toxicity. Cytosine arabinoside was nearly abandoned because the schedule dependency of the drug's cytotoxic effect was not appreciated until the superiority of administration by continuous infusion was demonstrated[17]. Similarly, the degree of schedule dependency of etoposide was not fully recognized at the time of its introduction to clinical practice, in spite of preclinical evidence that fractionated dose schedules were superior. The benefit of prolonged exposure was unequivocally demonstrated in a randomized study in small-cell lung cancer[18]. Continuous infusion protocols have also been employed as a means of reducing drug toxicity where this is associated with peak plasma concentration, e.g. the cardiotoxicity of doxorubicin appears to be reduced by prolonged infusion[19].

CLINICAL EVALUATION

Aims of phase I trials

A phase I study is performed to discover the side-effects and maximum tolerated dose of a new drug in man and to recommend a dose and schedule for testing in specific tumour types. However, it is not appropriate to approach this merely as a toxicology exercise. It is important to conduct the study in such a way that patients are given the maximum chance of deriving therapeutic benefit. Although the majority of phase I trials do not produce responses[7], this is not sufficient reason to discount the possibility entirely. As already discussed, preclinical investigations will have established an appropriate starting dose, usually based on the LD_{10} in mice, and ideally the optimum schedule will have been determined in at least one tumour model. There may be indications of organ-specific toxicity which will need to be assessed prospectively. Pharmacokinetics will have been performed to investigate metabolism and excretion. It may be apparent that any reduction in renal or hepatic function could lead to increased toxicity due to drug retention; hence there is a need to monitor these particularly carefully. It may be appropriate to attempt to use pharmacokinetics to expedite dose escalation, provided the necessary preconditions are met.

Ethical problems and patient selection

Phase I studies pose two conflicting ethical problems for the investigator. Patients treated at too low a dose have no chance of therapeutic benefit, while those treated near the MTD may suffer serious, even fatal, toxicity. Therefore, there is a need both to expedite dose escalation and to avoid unnecessary toxicity.

In selecting appropriate patients for phase I studies, there are two main considerations. Firstly, patients with a very poor immediate prognosis are not only unlikely to respond but may not survive long enough to yield much in the way of useful information concerning the side-effects of the new drug. From the ethical point of view, this is clearly unacceptable since the last few weeks of such a patient's life will be marred by the side-effects of a drug which is unlikely to ameliorate his/her symptoms. Secondly, because of their increased susceptibility to toxicity, such patients will bias the determination of dose-limiting toxicity, leading to an underestimation of the MTD[7]. If care is not taken to prevent this source of error, it could lead to the conduct of phase II studies at too low a dose, perhaps resulting in a drug being falsely labelled inactive.

It is well known that older patients, those with a poor performance status and those with more extensive disease progression are likely to tolerate chemotherapy relatively poorly. In separate phase I studies of methyl-CCNU, a dose of 150 mg/m² was recommended on the basis of experience in a population of heavily treated patients[20], whereas 290 mg/m² was found to be a suitable starting dose for patients with untreated brain tumours[21]. Both extensive prior treatment with drugs, such as mitomycin C and chloroethylnitrosoureas, which are bone marrow stem cell poisons, and radiotherapy to the spine and pelvis, are likely to increase the severity and duration of myelosuppression by diminishing bone marrow reserve.

However remote the chance of therapeutic benefit in phase I, signs of activity should nevertheless be sought, especially if the drug under test is an analogue of a known active drug. In this situation, it will be apparent which tumours are likely to respond and some attempt should be made to recruit such patients. For example, in the phase I trial of Trimelamol, an analogue of hexamethylmelamine, a drug which is used in the treatment of ovarian cancer, the majority of patients treated had refractory or recurrent ovarian cancer. This recruitment bias was rewarded in that responses were observed in ovarian cancer and Hodgkin's disease[22]. It is worth nothing that, in addition to the possibility of direct benefit, patients with refractory cancer may derive considerable comfort from the knowledge that their participation may benefit others in the future. This must not be used as means of persuasion but may give patients a sense of purpose in the terminal phase of their illness.

Pharmacokinetics and pharmacodynamics

Pharmacokinetics is the study of the relationship between drug (or metabolite) concentration versus time, whereas pharmacodynamics is the study of dose versus response (effect). Both need to be taken into account during the investigation of a new drug, especially if there is reason to believe that activity may be dependent on the schedule of administration.

As discussed above, the work of Collins et al.[12] suggests the possibility of using pharmacokinetics to expedite dose escalation by relating mouse pharmacokinetics to toxicity and allowing rapid dose escalation in man until the plasma concentrations associated with that toxicity are approached. For example, one such protocol allows for doubling of the dose until the AUC is 40% that of the AUC at the mouse LD_{10}. Further escalations then follow a conventional scheme. The retrospective analysis of data from phase I clinical trials may lend support to this concept by indicating the large number of escalation steps which could have been saved, but there are some important caveats. A number of such analyses have been carried out, including a comprehensive review by the Pharmacology and Metabolism Group of the EORTC[16].

Several phase I studies have been performed in which an attempt has been made to exploit these concepts. Serious practical problems have been encountered, such as insufficient assay sensitivity at the starting dose in the case of amphethinile and oxantrazole[23,24] and excessive interpatient variation in AUC at the first dose levels with the anthrapyrazole, CI941, which prevented accurate dose escalation based on AUC[25]. In a phase I trial of the anthracycline, iodo-doxorubicin, dose escalation had to be performed based on the sum of the parent drug and active metabolite concentrations[26]. However, there is some evidence that phase I trials can indeed be made more efficient by the appropriate use of preclinical pharmacokinetic data, as shown by the development of deoxyspergualin[27]. This drug caused acute peak-level toxicity but toxicity was reduced and efficacy against the L1210 tumour improved by the use of a continuous infusion. This information was used to raise the entry dose 25-fold compared with the dose suggested by single intravenous bolus toxicity. As a result, the number of escalation steps was reduced from 21 to 9, with a likely saving of 70 patients and years duration of the study.

The preclinical study of toxicity, antitumour activity, optimum schedule of administration, drug disposition and elimination will help to guide clinical trials, but it is important to confirm that the drug is behaving in a similar fashion in man. In addition to its potential use in dose escalation, an adequate pharmacokinetic assay must be available in order to allow toxicity to be correlated with plasma and tissue levels and to examine interpatient variability. It is known that drug clearance may vary widely between patients[28]. A summary of reasons for variable drug clearance is given in Table 8.1. For drugs which undergo extensive metabolic alteration, particularly to active species, it is necessary to investigate their metabolism as part of the phase I study. Poor metabolic activation in man compared with experimental animals may result in a lack of antitumour activity, as was the case with pentamethylmelamine[15].

Sometimes the reasons for variations in clearance are apparent and can be allowed for, such as impairment of liver or renal function. For example, it is well known that jaundiced patients require a large reduction in the dose of doxorubicin. However, the dose modifications which are required in such a

Table 8.1 Reasons for interpatient variability in pharmacokinetics

---

Distribution
    Differences in body fat component (lipophilic drugs)
    Ascites or pleural effusion (phase-specific agents, e.g. methotrexate)
    Hypoalbuminaemia (highly protein-bound drugs)

Elimination
    Liver impairment (doxorubicin)
    Kidney impairment (methotrexate, carboplatin, cisplatin, melphalan)

Bioavailability (oral drugs)
    Nausea and vomiting
    Effect of antiemetics on gastric emptying and transit time

---

situation remain empirical[29]. Recent work with the isomer, epirubicin, suggests that dose modifications based on alanine transaminase levels may be a means of delivering these agents safely to patients with impaired liver function[30]. Carboplatin is largely excreted unchanged in the urine; hence, there is a good correlation between glomerular filtration rate (GFR) and carboplatin clearance. This has led to the development of dosage formulae based on GFR which give a much more accurate prediction of subsequent drug exposure (AUC) than dosage based on surface area[31,32]. The use of such formulae should have the effect of both reducing excessive toxicity in patients with impaired renal function and preventing suboptimal dosage in patients with above-average clearance. Horwich et al.[33] showed that patients receiving carboplatin for the treatment of testicular tumours were more likely to relapse if the calculated carboplatin AUC, based on the formula: dose (mg) = AUC(GFR (ml/min + 25), was <4 mg/ml.min.

If we now look at the relationship between pharmacokinetics and drug effect, i.e. pharmacodynamics, we must ask the question: what pharmacokinetic parameter is likely to be most important for an individual drug? This may be peak plasma concentration, AUC or steady state concentration during continuous infusion. For example, Evans and colleagues[34], at the St Jude Children's Hospital, Memphis, investigating the use of high-dose methotrexate (MTX) for the treatment of acute lymphoblastic leukaemia (ALL), showed that children with a steady state MTX concentration $<16 \mu$mol/L were three times more likely to relapse than those with higher concentrations. Individualized treatment for childhood ALL, which takes into account variations in methotrexate clearance, is now being tested prospectively in comparison with standard dosage methods.

Different criteria apply to alkylating agents, including platinum complexes, and Egorin et al.[31] showed a clear relationship between exposure to carboplatin as defined by the AUC and the subsequent percentage fall in platelet count. A recent analysis appears to show that, in the case of ovarian cancer, a drug exposure/response relationship exists up to an AUC of between 5 and 7 mg/ml.min, beyond which no further increase in response rate is observed but toxicity continues to increase[35].

In a phase I study of teniposide, pharmacokinetic monitoring showed that variations in plasma clearance were such that certain patients treated at lower doses actually received a higher systemic exposure. There was a poor correlation between dose and toxicity but a good correlation between drug exposure (AUC) and both toxicity and response[36]. Pharmacokinetic studies with etoposide have helped to clarify the relationship between the threshold concentrations required for efficacy and toxicity and also confirmed that the benefits of dose fractionation were not due to drug accumulation, since the total AUC for a dose of 500 mg/m² was the same whether this was given by a single 24-hour infusion or as 5×100 mg/m² daily[18].

When testing a new drug, if the appropriate pharmacokinetic parameter determining toxicity is known, whether this is the AUC or duration of time a critical plasma concentration is exceeded, this might lead to a definition of 'maximum tolerated systemic exposure' as an end point for the phase I trial rather than MTD, as suggested by Evans[37]. The acknowledgement that the dosage of certain agents needs to be individualized in order to achieve the desired biological effect has led to the development of computer programs which assist the determination of the appropriate dose based on the pharmacokinetics of the previous dose, so-called 'adaptive control'[38]. This is particularly useful in the case of a drug with a long half-life which is being given intermittently.

Although pharmacokinetics are informative, plasma concentrations may not always reflect accurately intracellular concentrations, which may lead to a poor correlation between plasma concentrations and drug effect. Measurement of intracellular concentrations might be more appropriate. For example, Plunkett *et al.*[39] have shown a strong positive correlation between a trough concentration of the phosphorylated metabolite ara-CTP of $\geq 75\,\mu$mol/L in leukaemic cells and the likelihood of subsequent remission. This information has been used to develop a pharmacologically guided dosage schedule. Correlations have also been made between DNA adduct formation in peripheral blood cells in patients with ovarian cancer treated with cisplatin which demonstrate a good correlation between median adduct levels and response to treatment[40]. Changes in tumour metabolism subsequent to drug exposure can be studied using non-invasive techniques, such as nuclear magnetic resonance spectroscopy[41].

Definition of the maximum tolerated dose (MTD) and dose escalation strategies

Since a phase I study must try to avoid serious and irreversible toxicity, definition of the MTD may sometimes be very difficult. For drugs with a clear relationship between dose and the degree of myelosuppression, it should not be necessary to escalate to a dose which causes serious, potentially fatal, toxicity. Predictable grade III granulocytopenia, for example, could be regarded as defining the MTD whereas production of grade IV toxicity ($<0.5 \times 10^9$/L) would be hazardous because of the significant risk of potentially fatal infection. Such an end-point may be readily quantified, but emesis, neuropathy and mucositis are all more difficult to define and may vary more widely between patients. Where toxicities are cumulative or delayed, this problem becomes especially difficult. The working definition of MTD used by the Cancer Research Campaign Phase I Committee suggests the "highest safely tolerable dose", i.e. WHO grade III of any of the following: myelosuppression, diarrhoea, mucositis, skin toxicity, or WHO grade II–III hepatic, renal, pulmonary, cardiac or neurological toxicity. An approximate description of WHO grades I–IV would be mild, moderate, severe and potentially life-threatening, respectively, although, of course, the latter only applies to the bone marrow or essential organs, not hair loss. A summary of some of the more common criteria for defining the MTD is given in Table 8.2.

A variety of methods have been used for dose escalation, most commonly a modification of the Fibonacci series using large initial escalations, reducing to 33% (in the true series, $U_{n+1} = U_n + U_{n-1}$, the recurring increment is 61%)(see Table 8.3). More aggressive methods have been employed, e.g. 100% increments until the first signs of biological effect, reducing to 50% increments until major biological effects are observed, then small 20–25% steps up to the MTD, at which dose a larger number of patients are treated to establish this with

Table 8.2 Definition of the maximum tolerated dose (MTD): the highest dose causing none of these toxicities

Origin	MTD
Bone marrow	Granulocytes <0.5×10^9/L, platelets <50×10^9/L, severe haemolytic anaemia
Gut	Diarrhoea requiring iv fluid replacement, severe mucositis preventing oral intake
Liver	Bilirubin >45μmol/L, ALT >100 iu/L
Kidney	Creatinine >300μmol/L, or irreversible progressive dose-related decrease in glomerular filtration rate
Heart	Left ventricular failure, life-threatening arrhythmias
Central nervous system	Paralysis, mental deterioration, fits, coma
Skin	Severe exfoliative dermatitis

Table 8.3 Dose escalation strategies

Fibonacci		'Modified Fibonacci'		Geometric
$U_{n+1} = U_n + U_{n-1}$				Constant percentage,
1	—	1	—	e.g. 40%
2	100%	2	100%	– smaller increments
3	50%	3.3	65%	may be used
5	67%	5	52%	
8	60%	7	40%	
13	62%	9	29%	
22	69%	12	33%	
35	59%	16	33%	

greater confidence[9]. Such methods appear to be safe, but, at each step, the toxicity observed will depend on patient selection, and the rapidity with which the MTD will be reached depends on its distance from the starting dose. The slope of the dose–response curve will also be important. The use of pharmacokinetics in expediting dose escalation has been discussed above.

If sporadic toxicities are observed, possibly due to predisposing factors, such as unsuspected bone marrow infiltration, it is important to treat a larger number of patients at that dose level. If the toxicity does not recur, then dose escalation should proceed as planned. Escalation in the same patient may sometimes be allowed. This has the advantage, for any individual patient, of increasing the likelihood of therapeutic benefit but makes it more difficult to identify cumulative toxicity. Generally, if such escalations are permitted, they are usually limited to one per patient and discontinued once significant toxicities are observed.

A prime purpose of the phase I study is to select a dose for phase II trial. Therefore, once the MTD has been established, a larger number of patients, e.g. a minimum of 6, are treated at that dose to study the degree of interpatient variability and to ensure that a suitable dose for phase II can be recommended. Too high a dose will lead to excessive toxicity, but too low a dose may result in a drug failing to show activity in phase II, especially if the dose–response curve is steep and the therapeutic index low. Recommendations to titrate the dose against the patient's white blood count are often not followed owing to the weight given to other side-effects, such as emesis. As suggested by Evans[37], it may be worth considering a pharmacological end-point rather than a fixed dose for drugs with extremely variable kinetics.

Toxicity grading

There is general agreement concerning how the toxicity of anticancer treatment should be graded and reported. However, differences still exist between the guidelines used by different cooperative groups[42]. The WHO scheme is widely accepted[43] and, with certain exceptions, such as nausea and vomiting, for which the WHO scale is not ideal, there is broad agreement between WHO toxicity grades and those of other schemes. However, it would be preferable if one scheme was in universal use. An alternative is available, called the Common Toxicity Criteria, which is superior to the WHO scheme in a number of important areas. There are plans to introduce the Common Toxicity Criteria scales into studies conducted by the Early Clinical Trials Group of the EORTC and the Phase I/II Committee of the CRC. These scales are now in widespread use in the USA where they have been adopted by the National Cancer Institute and many cooperative groups. It seems likely that they will soon become the international standard. Difficulties may arise over recording toxicity duration if one is relying on the patient's recall of events. The use of some form of diary card may be helpful. This method may also be used for assessing quality of life[44].

Early clinical evaluation of cytokines

Particular problems have been encountered with the early clinical study of certain cytokines or immunomodulators which require separate consideration. Unlike cytotoxic agents, protein cell regulators, or cytokines, such as α-interferon, interleukin-2 (IL-2) and tumour necrosis factor (TNF), exhibit species specificity to a variable degree. However, since these agents are now generally produced in bacteria, using recombinant DNA technology, it is possible to administer the pure human protein. When investigating antitumour activity, one can test human cytokines, such as interferons, against human tumour xenografts in the nude mouse. Nevertheless, there is still a problem concerning preclinical evaluation. Given the known species specificity, is it appropriate to test the human cytokine for toxicity in the mouse rather than the mouse-specific protein?

How should the starting dose be determined and what methods are appropriate for dose escalation? For example, in a phase I trial of human recombinant TNF at the Royal Marsden Hospital, a starting dose was chosen 100-fold lower than the LD_{10} in mice[45]. If this had not been done, the starting dose would have been toxic since the mouse LD_{10} was actually equivalent to the human MTD. In addition, it has been shown that a bell-shaped dose–response curve is sometimes observed, i.e. the maximum therapeutic effect is achieved below the MTD, further dose escalations not merely increasing toxicity but actually reducing the chance of benefit[46]. Thus, agents such as these require the development of new strategies for clinical evaluation which take into account the inadequacy of current preclinical models and the need to define different end-points based on biological activity rather than MTD[47].

How can these problems be overcome? Firstly, it is vital to measure the immunological changes which accompany treatment in order to try to determine the maximum effective dose in biological terms. Such measurements may also be used to help identify the most appropriate schedule. It has taken many years to discover the most appropriate schedules of administration for the interferons, but a more rational approach with an integral study of the appropriate biological changes should speed up the development of new agents[48]. Similar problems might arise with new agents which act by interfering with the cell signalling cascade, such as protein kinase C inhibitors. Certain of these drugs may also exhibit bell-shaped dose–response curves and act as stimulators or inhibitors depending on the concentration and target cell. For example, bryostatin 1 causes maximum inhibition of leukaemic cell growth at low concentrations, higher concentrations reducing the effect, while similar concentrations have the capacity to stimulate normal bone marrow precursors[49]. These issues are dealt with in more detail in Chapter 9.

CONCLUSIONS

The development of new anticancer agents requires an integrated and detailed study of mechanism, toxicology, pharmacokinetics and pharmacodynamics both in preclinical models and in man. Owing to advances in analytical methodology, it is usually possible to perform accurate measurements of drug concentration in blood and other tissues and to examine the correlation between systemic exposure and drug effect. Pharmacokinetics may be used to expedite dose escalation and may provide more appropriate end-points in the case of drugs with extremely variable clearance. Non-invasive techniques, such as positron emission tomography and magnetic resonance spectroscopy, are being developed which should make it possible to study the changes in tumour metabolism which follow drug administration. The introduction of agents which may be optimally active below the MTD, such as the interferons, offers a challenge to develop new strategies for phase I clinical evaluation in which biological effect, rather than toxicity, forms the basis for defining the phase II dose. Wherever possible, this should also be applied to antiproliferative agents. This should ensure that new drugs are given a fair test and that patients will receive the best possible chance of benefiting as a result.

References

1. Driscoll, J. (1984). The preclinical new drug research program of the National Cancer Institute. *Cancer Treat. Rep.*, **68**, 63–76

2. Alley, M., Scudiero, D., Monks, A., Hursey, M., Czerwinski, M., Fine, D., Abbott, B., Mayo, J., Shoemaker, R. and Boyd, M. (1988). Feasibility of drug screening with panels of human tumor cell lines using a microculture tetrazolium assay. *Cancer Res.*, **48**, 589–601

3. Paull, K., Shoemaker, R., Hodes, L., Monks, A., Scudiero, D., Rubinstein, L., Plowman, J. and Boyd, M. (1989). Display and analysis of patterns of differential activity of drugs against human tumor cell lines: Development of Mean Graph and COMPARE algorithm. *J. Natl. Cancer Inst.*, **81**, 1088–1092

4. Young, R. (1990). Mechanisms to improve chemotherapy effectiveness. *Cancer*, **65**, 815–822

5. Harrap, K., Jones, M., Siracky, J., Pollard, L. and Kelland, L. (1990). The establishment, characterisation and calibration of human ovarian carcinoma xenografts for the evaluation of novel platinum anticancer drugs. *Ann. Oncol.*, **1**, 65–76

6. Freireich, E., Gehan, E., Rall, D., Schmidt, L. and Skipper, H. (1966). Quantitative comparison of toxicity of anticancer agents in mouse, rat, hamster, dog, monkey and man. *Cancer Chemother. Rep.*, **50**, 219–245

7. Bodey, G. and Legha S. (1987). The phase I study: general objectives, methods, and evaluation. *Dev. Oncol.*, **46**, 153–174

8. Grieshaber, C. and Marsoni, S. (1986). Relation of preclinical toxicology to findings in early clinical trials. *Cancer Treat. Rep.*, **70**, 65–73

9. Joint Steering Committee of the EORTC and the CRC (1989). General guidelines for the preclinical toxicology of new cytotoxic anticancer agents in Europe. *Eur. J. Cancer*, **26**, 411–414

10. Judson, I. (1989). New endocrine agents, guidelines for future development. *Br. J. Cancer*, **60**, 153–154

11. Jackman, A., Taylor, G., Calvert, A. and Harrap K. (1984). Modulation of anti-metabolite effects: Effects of thymidine on the efficacy of the quinazoline-based thymidylate synthetase inhibitor, CB3717. *Biochem. Pharmacol.*, **33**, 3269–3275

12. Collins, J., Zaharko, D., Dedrick, R. and Chabner, B. (1986). Potential roles for preclinical pharmacology in phase I clinical trials. *Cancer Treat. Rep.*, **70**, 73–80

13. Riva, C., Rustum, Y. and Preisler, H. (1985). Pharmacokinetics and cellular determinates of response to 1-B-D-arabinofuranosylcytosine. *Semin. Oncol.*, **12**, 1–8

14 Lennard, L., Lillyman, J., Van Loon, J. and Weinshilboum, R. (1990). Genetic variation in response to 6-mercaptopurine for childhood acute lymphoblastic leukaemia. *Lancet*, **336**, 225–229

15 Rutty, C., Newell, D., Muindi, J. and Harrap, K. (1982). The comparative pharmacokinetics of pentamethylmelamine in man, rat and mouse. *Cancer Chemother. Pharmacol.*, **8**, 105–111

16. EORTC PAM Group (1987). Pharmacokinetically guided dose escalation in phase I clinical trials. Commentary and proposed guidelines. *Eur. J. Cancer Clin. Oncol.*, **7**, 1083–1087

17. Schein, P., Davis, R., Carter, S., Newman, J., Schein, D. and Rall, D. (1970). The evaluation of anticancer drugs in dogs and monkeys for the prediction of qualitative toxicities in man. *Clin. Pharmacol. Ther.*, **11**, 3–40

18. Slevin, M., Clark, P., Joel, S., Malik, S., Osborne, R., Gregory, W., Lowe, D., Reznek, R. and Wrigley, P. (1989). A randomized trial to evaluate the effect of schedule on the activity of etoposide in small-cell lung cancer. *J. Clin. Oncol.*, **9**, 1333–1340

19. Legha, S., Benjamin, R., Mackay, R., Yap, H., Wallace, S., Ewer, M., Blumenschein, G. and Bodey, G. (1982). Adriamycin therapy by continuous intravenous infusion in patients with metastatic breast cancer. *Cancer*, **49**, 1762–1766

20. Kutcher, J. and Gailani, S. (1972). Phase I study of 1-(2-chloroethyl)-3-(4-methylcyclohexyl)-1-nitrosourea (Me-CCNU) in cancer patients. *Clin. Res.*, **20**, 568

21. Young, R., Walder, M., Canello, G., Schein, P., Chabner, B. and DeVita, V. (1973). Initial clinical trials with methyl-CCNU 1-(2-chlorethyl-3-(4-methylcyclohexyl)-1-nitrosourea (Me-CCNU). *Cancer*, **31**, 1164–1169

22. Judson, I., Calvert, A., Rutty, C., Abel, G., Gumbrell, L., Graham, M., Evans, B., Wilman, D., Ashley, S. and Cairnduff, F. (1989). Phase I trial and pharmacokinetics of Trimelamol (N^2,N^4,N^6-trihydroxymethyl-N^2,N^4,N^6-trimethylmelamine). *Cancer Res.*, **49**, 5475–5479

23. Smith, D., Ewen, C., Mackintosh, J., Fox, B., Thatcher, N., Scarffe, J., Vezin, R. and Crowther, D. (1988). A phase I and pharmacokinetic study of amphethinile. *Br. J. Cancer*, **57**, 623

24. Hantel, A., Donehower, R., Rowinsky, E., Vance, E., Clarke, B., McGuire, W., Ettinger, D., Noe, D. and Grochow, L. (1990). Phase I study and pharmacodynamics of piroxantrone (NSC 349174), a new anthrapyrazole. *Cancer Res.*, **50**, 3284–3288

25. Foster, B., Graham, M., Newell, D., Gumbrell, L. and Calvert, A. (1988). Phase I study of the anthrapyrazole CI941 with pharmacokinetically guided dose escalation. *Proc. Am. Soc. Clin. Oncol.*, **7**, 64

26. Gianni, L., Surbone, A., Vigano, L., Gambetta, A. and Bonadonna, G. (1989). The pharmacokinetics guidelines for phase I dose escalations: the case of 4'dehydroxy-4'-iodo-doxorubicin (I-Dox). Proceedings of the 6th NCI-EORTC *Symposium on New Drugs in Cancer Therapy*, p. 297 (Amsterdam:NCI/EORTC)

27. Collins, J., Grieshaber, C. and Chabner, B. (1990). Pharmacologically guided phase I clinical trials based upon preclinical drug development. *J. Natl. Cancer Inst.*, **82**, 1321–1326

28. Rowland, M. (1985). Models to identify sources of pharmacokinetic variability. In Rowland, M., Sheiner, L. Steiner, J.-L. (eds.) *Variability in Drug Therapy*, pp. 11–28. (New York, NY; Raven Press)

29. Sulkes, A. and Collins, J. (1987). Reappraisal of some dosage adjustment guidelines. *Cancer Treat. Rep.*, **71**, 229–233

30. Twelves, C. J., Dobbs, N. A., Gregory, W. M., Summers, L. A., Rubens, R. D. and Richards, M. A. (1991). A dosage nomogram for epirubicin (Epi) based on liver biochemistry tests. *Br. J. Cancer*, **63** (Suppl. XIII), 54

31. Egorin, M., Van Echo, D., Tipping, S., Olman, E., Whitacre, M., Thompson, B. and Aisner, J. (1984). Pharmacokinetics and dosage reduction of *cis*-diammine(1,1-cyclobutane-dicarboxylato)platinum in patients with impaired renal function. *Cancer Res.*, **44**, 5432

32. Calvert, A., Newell, D., Gumbrell, L., O'Reilly, S., Burnell, M., Boxall, F., Siddik, Z., Judson, I., Gore, M. and Wiltshaw, E. (1989). Carboplatin dosage: prospective evaluation of a simple formula based on renal function. *J. Clin. Oncol.*, **11**, 1748–1756

33. Horwich, A., Dearnaley, D. P., Nicholls, J., Jay, G., Mason, M., Harland, S., Peckham M. J. and Hendry, W. F. (1991). Effectiveness of carboplatin, etoposide, and bleomycin combination chemotherapy in good-prognosis metastatic testicular nonseminomatous germ cell tumours. *J. Clin. Oncol.*, **9**, 62–69

34. Evans, W. E., Crom, W. R., Abromowitch, M., Dodge, R., Look, A. T., Bowman, W. P., George, S. L. and Pui, C.-H. (1986). Clinical pharmacodynamics of high-dose methotrexate in acute lymphocytic leukaemia. *N. Engl. J. Med.*, **314**, 471–477

35. Egorin, M., Jodrell, D., Canetta, R., Langenburg, P., Goldbloom, E., Burroughs, J., Goodlow, J., Tan, S. and Wiltshaw, E. (1991). Tumor response and toxicity in ovarian cancer correlates with carboplatin (CBDCA) area under the curve (AUC). *Proc. Am. Soc. Clin. Oncol*, **10**, 184

36. Rodman, J., Abromowitch, M., Sinkule, J., Rivera, G. and Evans, W. (1987). Clinical pharmacodynamics of continuous infusion teniposide: Systemic exposure as a determinant of response in a phase I trial. *J. Clin. Oncol.*, **5**, 1007–1014

37. Evans, W. (1988). Clinical pharmacodynamics of anticancer drugs: a basis for extending the concept of dose-intensity. *Blut*, **56**, 241–248

38. Conley, B., Forrest, A., Egorin, M., Zuhowski, E., Sinibaldi, V. and Van Echo, D. (1989). Phase I trial using adaptive control dosing of hexamethylene bisacetimide (NSC 95580). *Cancer Res.*, **49**, 3436–3440

39. Plunkett, W., Iacoboni, S., Estey, E., Danhauser, L., Liliemark, J. and Keating, M. (1985). Pharmacologically directed ara-C therapy for refractory leukemia. *Semin. Oncol.*, **12**, 20–30

40. Reed, E., Ozols, R., Tarone, R., Yuspa, S. and Poirier, M. (1987). Platinum-DNA adducts in leukocyte DNA correlate with disease response in ovarian cancer patients receiving platinum-based chemotherapy. *Proc. Natl. Acad. Sci. USA*, **84**, 5024–5028

41. Stubbs, M., Rodrigues, L., Gusterson, B. and Griffiths, J. (1990). ^{31}PMRS of tumours. Monitoring tumour growth and regression by ^{31}P magnetic resonance spectroscopy. *Adv. Enz. Regul.*, **30**, 217–230

42. Vietti, T. J. (1980). Evaluation of toxicity: clinical issues. *Cancer Treat. Rep.*, **64**, 457–461

43. WHO (1979). *WHO Handbook for Reporting Results of Cancer Treatment. WHO Offset Publication*, **48**. (Geneva: WHO)

44. Fayers, P., Jones, D. and Girling, D. (1985). Measurement of quality of life in cancer clinical trials. *Cancer Treat. Symp.*, **2**, 25–30

45. Selby, P., Hobbs, S., Viner, C., Jackson, E., Jones, A., Newell, D., Calvert, A., McElwain, T., Fearon, K., Humphreys, J, and Shiga, T. (1987). Tumour necrosis factor in man: Clinical and biological observations. *Br. J. Cancer*, **56**, 803–808

46. Talmadge, J., Tribble, H., Pennington, R., Philips, H. and Wiltrout, R. (1987). Immuno-modulatory and immunotherapeutic properties of recombinant gamma interferon and recombinant tumour necrosis factor in mice. *Cancer Res.*, **47**, 2563–2570

47. Herberman, R. (1985). Design of clinical trials with biological response modifiers. *Cancer Treat. Rep.*, **69**, 1161–1164

48. Talmadge, J. (1989). Development of immunotherapeutic strategies for the treatment of malignant neoplasia. *Pathol. Immunopathol. Res.*, **8**, 250–275

49. Jones, R., Sharkis, S., Miller, C., Rowinsky, E., Burke, P. and May, W. (1990). Bryostatin 1, a unique biological response modifier: anti-leukaemic activity *in vitro*. *Blood*, **75**, 1319–1323

9
Evaluation: how should a new treatment be evaluated?

J. G. McVIE

The testing of new therapies in patients is a major challenge. The clinical trial has to be conducted to the highest ethical standards, yet it has to be designed to give the maximum chance of detecting a therapeutic effect whilst protecting patients from unnecessary exposure to an ineffective drug or unacceptable toxicity. This chapter will consider conventional cytotoxic drugs and some new molecules emerging from the laboratory which present new problems for clinical assessment.

CYTOTOXIC DRUGS

Toxicology protocols in the mouse for drugs which have myelotoxicity as their principal side-effect have been well tried and tested (see Chapter 8). In human phase I trials, starting doses based on the maximum tolerated dose in rodents[1] have proved a safe strategy, and escalation either by a modified Fibonacci scheme or, more recently, based on the area under the plasma concentration–time curve has led to efficient and speedy attainment of appropriate doses for phase II trials[2]. Problems with certain drugs have often been those associated with non-bone-marrow toxicity. End-points, such as neurotoxicity (central or peripheral), gastrointestinal and liver toxicity have been difficult to define, and late toxicity, such as the pulmonary toxicity associated with bleomycin, mitomycin and busulphan and the cardiotoxicity associated with the anthracyclines, was totally missed in preclinical toxicology studies. Phase II trials of cytotoxic drugs have usually been successful in that inactive drugs have been rapidly discarded. Generally six or so signal tumour types have been chosen and a given number of patients in each category treated with each test drug. Statistical models have differed but generally around 20 patients eligible and evaluable for trial have been included with each tumour type. Whenever possible, allowance has been made for previous exposure to chemotherapy and radiotherapy, and drugs have not been discarded until tested in a reasonable number of chemotherapy-naive patients. Until recently, colon cancer was widely regarded as chemoresistant, and therefore patients with metastatic colorectal tumours who had not received

245

previous chemotherapy were included in either phase I or phase II trials. Patients with malignant melanoma and renal carcinoma have also been used in this way. Patients with small cell lung cancer, Hodgkin disease or teratoma, however, have almost always received a battery of conventional cytotoxic drugs before being tested with a new anticancer drug. Because of this, potent drugs, such as etoposide, were slow to be recognized in any of these cancers. Yet etoposide is probably one of the most active drugs in small cell cancer when given to a chemotherapy-naive patient. It produces almost no responses, however, when tested in patients previously treated with conventional combination chemotherapy, such as cyclophosphamide, doxorubicin and vincristine[3].

Analogue development has dominated new drug discovery over the last 15 years. It has therefore been possible, for instance, to compare two anthracyclines directly with each other in a randomized phase II trial. Thus, in one European Organization for Research on Treatment of Cancer (EORTC) trial, randomized patients with metastatic breast cancer received carminomycin or 4'-epidoxorubicin[4]. Although, strictly speaking, one cannot compare response rates or survival in a phase II trial, the two arms of the trial can be analysed separately as two distinct phase II trials and the response rates reported. Similarly, the toxicity spectrum is of interest because, unlike conventional non-randomized phase II trials, selection bias has been dealt with by the randomization step and toxicity recording is, in theory at least, equal for both cohorts of patients. In this particular example, there were no responses in 20 patients treated with carminomycin and 7 patients treated with epidoxorubicin. Carminomycin produced deep and unpredictable granulopenia, whereas epirubicin mimicked the toxicity spectrum expected from its parent compound, doxorubicin. It was further developed and carminomycin was abandoned. Other uses of this model have been in comparing two formulations of the same drug. For instance, recently, oral and intravenous ifosfamide have been compared with one another in lung cancer by the EORTC[5]. The intravenous drug has been available for several years; the oral formulation was the test compound and was rumoured to be associated with a higher incidence of cerebellar toxicity.

Very few of these analogues have been accepted for registration purposes by the US Food and Drugs Administration (FDA). This body has required phase III evaluation of new drugs and a proven survival benefit. Trials have therefore been designed to test the new drug in a head-on comparison with the parent compound, sometimes as single agents (for instance epidoxorubicin versus doxorubicin or cyclophosphamide versus ifosfamide, both in soft tissue sarcoma) but more often in combination (e.g. cyclophosphamide, epirubicin, 5-fluorouracil versus cyclophosphamide, doxorubicin, 5-fluorouracil in breast cancer). Considerable debate has ensued over whether these drugs should be compared at equimolar concentrations or equitoxic concentrations and, in general, the latter approach has been favoured. The only interesting information to emerge from the trial of the two oxazosphorines in soft tissue sarcoma was that, whereas they were equivalent in terms of response rate and survival, there was a cross-over advantage for ifosfamide[6]. In other words, several patients who had failed to respond to cyclophosphamide went on to respond to ifosfamide. The opposite did not occur. In trials of anthracyclines with cross-over design, no lack of cross-resistance has been shown for any of the doxorubicin analogues.

When mitoxantrone (an anthracene dione) was compared with doxorubicin, there were a handful of patients who responded to doxorubicin after failing to respond to mitoxantrone[7]. Only rarely did the opposite occur.

It requires over a thousand patients to rule out a clear survival advantage for one element of a combination of chemotherapeutic drugs compared with another, and most trials submitted for registration purposes have been too small. This has, perhaps, been one reason for the lack of acceptance by the FDA. More recently, the FDA has conceded that quality of life perhaps might also be a measurable end point, but no hint has been given of how quality of life should be measured. What is clear is that quality of life, when it has been measured, for instance in lung cancer trials, has been shown *not* to be equivalent to ECOG or Karnofsky performance status, nor equivalent to side-effects of therapy. Quality of life must be measured in terms of degree of anxiety, depression, well-being, dependence or independence, self-confidence, interpersonal relationships, etc.[8] It therefore deserves to be measured as a separate end point. It is particularly important that this concept be properly defined because of the explosion of claims from pharmaceutical companies that their product is associated with increased 'quality of life'. The number of studies which have actually used appropriate quality-of-life measures to prove such claims is infinitesimal.

In the absence of novel cytotoxic drugs, clinical research has explored other strategies for overcoming the problem of drug resistance, namely high-dose chemotherapy or altered scheduling of cytotoxic drugs. Thus, with the help of autologous bone-marrow reinfusion (and more recently haemopoietic growth factors, such as G-CSF and GM-CSF), patients resistant to conventional doses of therapy have been treated with higher doses of the same drugs. Increased response rates have been reported in breast cancer, small cell lung cancer, teratoma, melanoma, ovarian cancer and glycoma. Far too few randomized studies have tested high-dose therapy, and those studies which have tested it have been negative except in leukaemia in children, adult lymphoma and, perhaps, lately, in myeloma where an impact on survival has been suggested by this strategy. Non-bone-marrow toxicity has become dose limiting and new growth factors for lung, liver and gastrointestinal tract are needed.

Splitting the dose of etoposide over five days instead of administering the total all in one day leads to a dramatic increase in response rate in small cell lung cancer. Three trials have now demonstrated this in randomized comparisons, and the same strategy is now being tested for schedules of etoposide spread out over longer time periods, up to 21 days. The mechanism for this alteration of resistance spectrum is not clear, but it is certainly not pharmacokinetic.

A very important part of one of these trials was the measurement of the area under the plasma concentration–time curve (AUC) in patients treated in both arms of the trial[9]. Exactly the same AUC was shown in both sets of patients. Building such pharmacological monitoring into the trial was thus extremely important in ruling out one possible explanation for the result. Clearly, had appropriate assays been available for etoposide–topoisomerase cleavable complex formation and subsequent DNA strand breakage in tumour cells in both sets of patients, the study would have been even more revealing. It is possible that the etoposide topoisomerase II interaction is the key to this schedule dependence. If so, then this could be appropriately extended to other drugs which act predominantly via topoisomerases, such as amsacrine, ellipticinium, doxorubicin and teniposide. Monitoring of intracellular events at or near the site of action of any anticancer drug should be the rule in all early clinical trials. Further randomization of doses, schedules and indeed drugs in early phase II trials, leading where appropriate to phase III, is recommended at an earlier stage of new drug development.

NON-CYTOTOXIC COMPOUNDS

Excitement generated by the increased accent on discovery of non-cytotoxic compounds, partly reflected by the chapter headings of this book, had led to a rethink of methodology for testing these compounds. The kinds of compounds in question are listed in Table 9.1.

Table 9.1

Hormones	Chemoprevention agents
Growth factors	Antimetastatic compounds
Interferons/interleukins	Angiogenesis compounds
Monoclonal antibodies	Radioprotectors
Modulators of resistance	Chemoprotectors
Differentiation modifiers	Antigrowth factors

Hormones and growth factors

Table 9.1 is not exhaustive and some of the problems are common to more than one of the listed agents. For instance, the approach to testing a hormone might not be very different from that required to test a growth factor. Hormones are classically tested in patients whose cancer cells bear the relevant receptors. Breast cancer patients who have responded to a first-line hormone will often respond to a second. This is an excellent example of identifying the relevant subpopulation of patients for optimal test of a new substance directed at a given receptor or target[10]. The appropriate dose is found by escalation, not to the maximum tolerable dose, but to a dose which provides saturation of the relevant receptors.

The revolution in molecular biology which has led to optimism about the discovery of new kinds of molecules for anticancer therapy has also delivered the possible probes which might best be used to select patients for study and for monitoring the effects of other novel methods of intervention. Thus, the recognition of epidermal growth factor (EGF) is particularly interesting because some cancer cells show increased EGF receptors as a result of an oncogene amplification. This opens up the possibility for blocking those receptors with an EGF look-alike molecule. It is clearly logical to try such a strategy in patients who have been identified as having either the amplified oncogene or the increased expression of the EGF receptor. It is also obvious that the effect of a new drug intended either to switch off the oncogene expression or to block the EGF receptor, thus switching off the fuel to the fire, could be monitored given the appropriate probes for the oncogene, the relevant mRNA or an assay for the growth factor or its receptor.

Interferons and interleukins

The best example of inappropriate development of a new class of anticancer agents has been the interferons; these potentially exciting compounds were developed in early trials as if they were cytotoxic drugs with the accent on maximum tolerated dose and little thought was given to their mode of action and the possibility that this might be optimal at a non-toxic dosage. Similarly, investigation of optimal schedules for delivery of interferons (and other biological response modifiers or immune modulators) has been delayed several years after the start of phase I trials. Interferon α was notoriously unsuccessful as an agent which visibly shrank cancers in the relevant time period of observation. There is some evidence, however, that interferon, where it has had an antitumour effect, for instance in the indolent lymphomas, has only worked some months after the start of treatment[11]. This contrasts with the expected prompt tumour shrinkage which would be associated with an effective cytotoxic drug. Early on in the development of the interferons, it was clear that, although the substances were native to the body, they could still produce extraordinary and novel toxicity for which the current toxicity grading systems, for instance the WHO system, were inappropriate. The capillary leak syndrome, almost lethal in some cases, was totally unexpected in the early trials of interleukin-2 and also posed a problem in terms of grading.

It now appears that the most interesting results from the use of interferons to treat cancer will be seen in trials of patients who have minimal residual disease. In retrospect, this is not entirely surprising; it was predicted in the very earliest days of immunotherapy with BCG and other non-specific passive immunotherapeutic agents. The design of trials to test interferon α in an adjuvant setting would appear to be an excellent model for several other substances in Table 9.1. Thus, in recent studies, patients with small cell lung cancer who have achieved complete remission by any chemotherapy, plus or minus local radiation, have been randomized to receive interferon or no therapy[12]. Typical end points of this study are time to relapse (which is almost inevitable in small cell lung cancer) and survival. The argument is that, if interferon is to have an effect on restoring immune function, it is most likely to do so when the tumour burden is at its smallest, that is in a patient who is in clinically complete remission. It is unlikely that interferon as a single agent will have a large effect in such a trial. Therefore, the number of patients required will be thousands rather than hundreds. As only patients who are in complete remission are relevant, the number of patients to be treated prior to randomization is two or three times greater. Very large numbers of patients are therefore required to answer these simple questions, particularly given the number of candidate compounds which are either in the clinic already or in preclinical development.

Interleukin-2 (IL-2) was initially thought to be ineffective as a single agent in melanoma and renal cell carcinoma but greatly potentiated the effect when administered together with lymphocyte activated killer (LAK) cells. LAK cells added greatly to the above-mentioned toxicity of IL-2 but impressive response rates were seen in the early phase II trials in both diseases. Particularly notable were the handful of complete remissions achieved – around 10% of the total – because these remissions have proved to be extremely durable. Some patients with renal cell carcinoma are still in remission four years or more after one single cycle treatment of IL-2 and LAK cells. The randomized trials which compared IL-2 with and without LAK cells in larger numbers of patients have been recently reported, however, and the results are similar for both arms[13]; therefore, only toxicity is associated with LAK cells and they could be abandoned. It appears now that tumour-infiltrating lymphocytes constitute the relevant subpopulation of the soup known as LAK cells and, although more difficult to concentrate, identify and isolate, these cells are now going into combination study with IL-2. A randomized trial will once again be needed to evaluate the combination versus IL-2 alone.

Monoclonal antibodies

After the first wave of enthusiasm which accompanied the description of complete response associated with an anti-idiotypic antibody against a B-cell lymphoma, it has become clear that this was an exceptional case and that this intellectually appealing concept has in fact severe practical limitations[14]. Early clinical trials of anti-idiotypic antibodies were simple to carry out. There were few problems with allergic responses or any other toxicity associated with the antibodies *per se*. Adequate targeting was demonstrated by direct aspiration of cells from lymphomatous lymph nodes, spleen, liver and bone marrow, and, because several patients included in the early trials had lymphomatous cells easily identifiable in the systemic circulation, efficient targeting was proven and the first end point of the study was positive in most patients. Disappearance of targeted lymphoma cells, however, was quite another matter and, in the vast majority of patients, any minor responses which were seen were extremely short-lived.

Monoclonal antibody therapy is easy to monitor, as most monoclonals can be tagged without difficulty to radioisotopes and imaged with conventional gamma camera or SPECT scanning. Antibodies against monoclonal antibodies used therapeutically can be monitored easily in plasma, and antitumour effect need only be monitored using the usual parameters of tumour size. The next generation of studies involves sophisticated monoclonal antibodies conjugated to toxins, cytotoxic drugs or enzymes, and this creates a new difficulty in terms of monitoring. Although it is simple to check that the antibody has indeed reached its target effectively, frequently plasma or tissue enzymes have rapidly split the bond which held the conjugate together. Therefore, seeing the γ-camera picture of antibody in tumour does not necessarily mean that the 'warhead' is still bound to the monoclonal and had been delivered as planned. Double labelling techniques, whereby the business end of the conjugate and the monoclonal are separately labelled with different isotopes, should get round this problem but double labelling adds to the expense of the experiment and, at the end of the day, the clinical response is the bottom line.

Modulators of resistance

The discovery of the phenomenon known as multidrug resistance (MDR) has been important in planning drug trials. Cancer cells maintained in culture can be made resistant to naturally occurring anticancer drugs. What is interesting is that the cells which have been made resistant to one naturally occurring substance are often found, on testing, to have become resistant to all naturally occurring compounds[15]. This phenomenon is accompanied by amplification of the relevant gene leading to increased concentration at the cell membrane of an exit pump called the P glycoprotein which has a molecular weight of 170000. This pump is the efflux mediator for a number of noxious natural substances and the over-expression of the gene responsible for its production leads to superefficient despatch of any naturally occurring anticancer drug which breaches the cell membrane. Of considerable interest has been the finding that the pump can be inhibited directly or competitively by a number of seemingly unrelated compounds, such as cyclosporin, calcium channel blockers, tamoxifen and tetracycline. Even more interesting is the finding, by application of monoclonal antibodies, that the P glycoprotein is over-expressed in certain primary tumours and in certain other tumours which have been exposed and become resistant to cytotoxic drugs. It may therefore be a relevant mechanism for clinical resistance. Assuming that one can thereby identify patients who have primary tumours expressing the P glycoprotein, the following strategies provide possible ways of testing new drugs designed to circumvent the exit pump. Colon cancer is resistant to doxorubicin, vincristine or etoposide, or any naturally occurring compound. Any of these could be administered to colon cancer patients, together with the MDR-targeted drug in a phase II trial and any response at all would of course be due to the combination. The other possibility is to take a group of patients who are known to respond to chemotherapy, for instance soft tissue sarcoma patients, and randomize them between doxorubicin (probably the best single agent for this cancer) and doxorubicin plus the MDR-targeted drug. A direct comparison first in phase II to check that toxicity was not increased by the MDR pump agent would be appropriate. There is no reason to think that the MDR mechanism is solely restricted to cancer cells. It may indeed be a mechanism whereby normal cells protect themselves from noxious substances, and, indeed, it has been shown to be present in association with chemotherapy-resistant malaria. A phase III trial would be required to allow true comparison and the end point would be either increased duration of response or increased survival. Large numbers of patients would be needed to show a small but nevertheless potentially useful clinical impact.

There are several cancers which respond promptly and dramatically to conventional cytotoxic drugs. Small cell lung cancer is a good example. Others are ovarian cancer and head and neck cancer. Sadly, equally typical of these diseases is their almost invariable tendency to recur, frequently in chemotherapy-resistant form. Assuming that a population of MDR-positive patients could be identified from such previously treated individuals, then the same chemotherapy could be re-initiated with the MDR-targeted drug. If the latter were given at a concentration high enough to allow the exit pump to be bypassed or inactivated, then, all other things being equal, the initial therapy should be successful in inducing a response again. A substance identified in this way would then be appropriately tested in phase III, together with the same combination of drugs in first-line chemotherapy in the hope that it might prevent the emergence of clinical drug resistance.

The intense activity of research into drug resistance mechanisms during the last two years is now yielding other clues similar to the MDR phenomenon. It is possible, for instance, that intracellular glutathione levels may explain some of the resistance to alkylating agents. Also, a membrane protein has been associated with methotrexate resistance, and yet another protein has been associated with resistance to cisplatin. As none of these three classes of compounds are involved in the multidrug resistance mechanism, these are exciting developments which suggest that selection of patient groups and strategy for testing putative intervention agents could conceivably be modelled on the MDR situation discussed above.

Differentiation modifiers

It has been proved that many lymphomas are characterized by a differentiation block and pile up of clonogenic cells all bearing the same differentiation markers. It has also been known for many years that a number of different substances, such as phorbol esters and retinoids, are successful in overcoming such a block *in vitro*. HL60 is a promyelomonocytic leukaemia model much studied in the laboratory. It can be encouraged to differentiate into polymorph leukocyte or monocyte lines according to the nature of the applied stimulant. An exciting clinical counterpart has recently been reported, first in China and then confirmed in France[16]. Several patients with acute promyelomonocytic leukaemia have achieved complete remission after administration of *trans*-retinoic acid as a single agent. Remissions have lasted only for a few months but the fact that they have occurred at all is quite extraordinary and has generated a rekindling of interest in this field of therapeutics. Design of clinical trials to test potentially active retinoids should, in theory, be straightforward, and the acute promyelomonocytic leukaemia example is a good one. The end point is simple, namely re-attainment of the differentiation capacity of the cells themselves; moreover, the duration of effect is also measurable. It is not so simple, however, in non-leukaemic tumours which are inaccessible for tumour cell sampling and study. Retinoids have been applied topically to early skin cancers with only temporary effects. More meaningful, particularly if taken in the context of eventual chemopreventive strategies, has been the use of retinoids in pre-malignant lesions, such as leucoplakia. This is a common condition associated in the Far East with betel nut chewing and, if not treated, leucoplakia leads inexorably to carcinoma of the oral cavity. The effect of retinoids applied locally or systemically can be measured easily by visual inspection and confirmed by a simple superficial biopsy for histological assessment. Not all cancers are likely to be candidates for differentiation strategies but it is likely that the most useful effects would be seen when applied to early stages of the malignant process. Further discussion of intermediate biomarkers as end points is dealt with under *Chemoprevention agents*.

Chemoprevention agents

The concept of using systemic or local therapy with a drug to prevent cancer is becoming more real as we understand more of the underlying mechanisms of the cancer process. The identification of oncogenes, tumour suppressor genes and the possibility of measuring carcinogen-DNA adducts has made the identification of high-risk groups a reality. Using the same technology, intermediate markers can be identified to monitor the course of a chemopreventive strategy, and can indeed be used to predict outcome. It has been known for many years that certain cancer-prone conditions, such as familial polyposis coli, xeroderma pigmentosum and ataxia telangiectasia, are genetic, although none of the genes have been cloned for these three examples. High-risk groups can be identified by family history alone, screened and invited to participate in intervention trials. The absence of tumour-suppressor genes, such as the retinoblastoma and p53 genes, in certain cancers opens up much wider horizons for focusing on potential cancer patients. In colon cancer, there are at least five possible genetic markers, such as *ras*, 5q allelic deletion, 17q, 18q and p53, which are found in increasing numbers in parallel with the degree of progression of the colon cancer[17]. It is likely that the order of occurrence of these mutations is important, as well as the actual number which occur inside one cell. Given that appropriate probes for these intermediate markers are rapidly becoming available for routine use, the stage is set for intervention with appropriate drugs.

The drugs tested in the past have been predominantly the retinoids, either vitamin A in various forms, β-carotene or other analogues. Vitamin C has also been tested, as has vitamin E in patients with familial polyposis coli, and now the National Cancer Institute has over a hundred potential compounds in its *in vitro* screen and just under a hundred in the *in vivo* screen. There are five new compounds undergoing toxicology studies and ten in phase I clinical trial. Details of the screening trials *in vitro* and *in vivo* are given elsewhere.

The steps for designing a chemoprevention study are to define the intervention, the dose of drug and the schedule. Early trials at phase I and phase II levels are aimed at assessing tolerance and measuring the pharmacokinetics of the drug. End points for dose escalation are not toxicity but rather attainment of the relevant drug concentration at the target site. The appropriate population has to be defined according to the genetic or familial parameters outlined above. The intermediate markers which might be measured or used as end points should be clearly delineated before starting, and the phase II study should be directed to measuring the efficacy and the feasibility of using the planned intermediate markers as end points. Possible biomarkers which might be used for phase II trial could be differentiation markers gained from cytology or histology, or evidence of DNA ploidy or cytogenetic markers. They might also be: growth factors or their receptors; tumour suppressor genes or the proteins they code for; DNA repair enzymes or DNA adducts.

Appropriate end points for phase III trials would be cancer incidence, a reduction in mortality in existing cancer, or the prevention of new lesions, such as in xeroderma pigmentosum, prevention of new lesions in high-risk groups, for instance contralateral breast cancer in patients who have already had one cancer[18], or appearance of a second smoking-related cancer in the aero-digestive tract after successful eradication of a lung or head–neck primary cancer; or simply reversal of precursor lesions assessed by histology. Scale-up to millions of people has to be kept in mind and any intervention has to be cost-effective. It has been known for some time, for instance, that vitamin A is effective in reversing leucoplakia in Indians who cannot give up the betel nut habit. The high cost of vitamin A, however, makes this an inappropriate remedy for intervention in Third World countries. Testing of an easily derived natural source of vitamin A, such as red palm oil, is a much more attractive alternative.

Antimetastatic compounds

A number of new insights have been gained recently into the mechanisms of metastatic growth. It is known, for instance, that certain tumour cells can invade through natural restrictive membranes common in tissue compartments by producing local burrowing enzymes. There is a model protein (TIMP-2) now available which inhibits such tumour cell enzymes. Targeting such an enzyme inhibitor to the site of a local primary tumour would be important to test its usefulness in specifically preventing metastasis. There are no good methodological techniques which are better than a randomized trial to test such an intervention. Clearly, a tumour that metastasizes dependably and fast would be useful in order to secure rapid screening results of potential analogues of such a protein, and the only end point of relevance would be the appearance of metastasis. Not many such models exist because clinical cancer which was locally eradicated would only cause death by metastasis if metastasis had already occurred at the time of local intervention. It would clearly be unethical to leave a clinically diagnosed cancer *in situ* while applying an antimetastatic device and thus delaying potentially curative local regional therapy. As several cytotoxic drugs are sometimes used preoperatively to increase operability of a primary tumour, for instance in osteosarcoma, this might be a relevant model in which to test an antimetastatic strategy. Again, however, a randomized design would be required so that a patient received either conventional cytotoxic therapy or the same plus the metastatic device. All patients would then be treated locally and the end point of the study would be appearance of distant metastasis and/or eventual death. A simpler but methodologically more suspect model would be limited small cell lung cancer where metastasis outside the chest is the rule rather than the exception. All patients in this category would conventionally receive combination chemotherapy, assuming they were fit, and this could be randomized against the same chemotherapy plus an antimetastatic drug. Two trials have already reported that the anticoagulant, warfarin, is effective in exactly this model. Overall survival was improved but not the cure rate[19].

There is a tumour suppressor gene, called NM-23, which is normally an inhibitor of metastasis and which has been shown to be a useful prognostic factor in breast cancer. This might be a legitimate target for developing antimetastatic gene therapy; or, at the minimum, serve as a way of stratifying subgroups appropriate for antimetastasis trials.

Angiogenesis compounds

One of the key properties of the growing metastasis is that it attracts new capillary growth into its midst. Interference with angiogenesis, therefore, has long been a potential target for inhibition of growth of metastasis, and, for that matter, inhibition of growth of local primary tumours (see Chapter 7). A number of candidate angiogenesis inhibitory substances are now emerging from preclinical testing and clinicians are confronted again with the problem of how best to assess these in early clinical trials. The logical end point of anti-angiogenesis would be the inhibition of neovascularization. A sensitive technique to monitor this process is urgently required. It is highly likely that the new generation of Doppler colour ultrasound machines will prove a useful tool in this respect. As this machine is sensitive enough to visualize the neovascularization occurring with the development of a single ovum in the human ovary, it is likely to prove of considerable value in the clinical research situation. Other non-invasive techniques which might prove useful would be magnetic resonance spectroscopy or PET scanning, both of which would be likely to require the assistance of vascular probes. At the end of the day, drugs which successfully inhibit neovascularization would have to be tested in the same kind of adjuvant trials as outlined above.

Radioprotectors, chemoprotectors and (anti)growth factors

Each of these categories can be looked on as part and parcel of supportive care and might be tested in the same way as a prophylactic antibiotic. Each, in its own way, can add to the positive side of the therapeutic ratio by decreasing side-effects, thus allowing higher effective doses to be delivered in conformity with the antitumour strategy. Several drugs in each category have been tested. WR-2721 has been claimed to protect from the radiation damage and bone marrow toxicity associated with some cytotoxic drugs, such as cyclophosphamide[20]; and GMCSF and GCSF have undergone extensive clinical trials as chemoprotectors. The early trials have concentrated correctly on establishing appropriate dosage, route of administration and, most importantly, duration and timing of therapy in relation to the toxic insult, be that radiotherapy or chemotherapy. End points in the haemopoietic growth factor studies have commonly been depth of nadir of platelet and white cell counts and rate of recovery. The number of intercurrent infections is also useful.

Antigrowth factors for normal tissues are now in preclinical trial and require intercalation with conventional cytotoxic regimes. An effective inhibitor of haemopoietic stem cells could replace the need for autologous bone marrow transplants.

Randomized studies are essential for absolute proof that these new and frequently expensive factors or chemicals are indeed capable of producing a positive cost–benefit ratio.

The main message to be gleaned from this discussion is that new technology has given birth to new opportunities for different kinds of therapeutic modulation in cancer. These new developments are different from conventional cytotoxic drugs and different from each other. They require tailor-made clinical trial protocols which clearly earmark the appropriate patient population, usually using the appropriate molecular biological probe. Each intervention must be tested for feasibility and efficacy, not necessarily by dose escalation to achieve toxicity. Rather more use should be made of intermediate biomarkers, such as changes in differentiation, growth factor receptor status, presence or absence of resistance associated proteins, etc. A switch to randomized trials will have to be made very much earlier with these new compounds because the real end points will only be realized by randomized study design. Ideally, they will most commonly be tested as adjuvants to conventional therapy and therefore large numbers of patients will be required to ensure that small but clinically meaningful advantages are not missed.

References

1. Rozencweig, M., Staquet, M., Pinedo, H. M., *et al.* (1985). EORTC Guidelines for Phase I Trials with Single Agents in Adults. *Eur. J. Cancer Clin. Oncol.,* **21,** 1005–1007
2. EORTC Pharmacokinetics and Metabolism Group (1987). Pharmacokinetically-guided dose escalation in phase I clinical trials. *Eur. J. Cancer Clin. Oncol.,* **23,** 1083–1087
3. Wolff, S. N., Johnson, D. H., Hande, K. R., *et al.* (1983). High dose etoposide as single-agent chemotherapy for small cell carcinoma of the lung. *Cancer Treat. Rep.,* **67,** 957–958
4. Rozencweig, M., Ten Bokkel Huinink, W., Cavalli, F., *et al.* (1984). Randomized phase II trial of carminomycin versus 4'-epiodoxorubicin in advanced breast cancer (Early Clinical Trials Group of the European Organization for Research on Treatment of Cancer). *J. Clin. Oncol.* **2,** 275–281
5. Lind, M. J., Margison, J. M., Cerny, T., *et al.* (1989). Comparative pharmacokinetics and alkylating activity of fractionated intravenous and oral ifosfamide in patients with bronchogenic carcinoma. *Cancer Res.,* **49,** 753–757
6. Bramwell, V. H. C., Mouridsen, H. T., Santoro, A., *et al.* (1986). Cyclophosphamide versus ifosfamide: Preliminary report of a randomized phase II trial in adult soft tissue sarcomas. *Cancer Chemother. Pharmacol.,* **18** (Suppl. 2), S13–S16
7. Henderson, I. C., Allegra, J. C., Woodcock, T., *et al.* (1989). Randomized clinical trial comparing mitoxantrone with doxorubicin in previously treated patients with metastatic breast cancer. *J. Clin. Oncol.,* **17** (5), 560–571
8. Van Dam F. S. A. M., Linnsen, A. C. G., Couzijn, A. L. (1988). Evaluating quality of life: Behavioural measures in clinical cancer trials. In Staquet, M., Sylvester, R., Buyse, M. (eds.) *The Practice of Clinical Trials.* Oxford University Press
9. Slevin, M. L., Clark, P. I., Joel, S. P., *et al.* (1989). A randomized trial to evaluate the effect of schedule on the activity of etoposide in small-cell lung cancer. *J. Clin. Oncol.,* **7** (9), 1333–40
10. Joint Committee: Cancer Research Campaign Headquarters, 2 Carlton House Terrace, London SW1, UK (1989). Operation manual for control of selection, production, preclinical toxicology and phase I trials of endocrine agents for patients with cancer. *Br. J. Cancer,* **60,** 265–269

11. Merigan, T. C. (1988). Human interferon as a therapeutic agent. *N. Engl, J. Med.*, **318**, 1458–1460
12. Mattson, K., Niiranen, A., Holsti, L., *et al.* (1989). Low dose natural α interferon as maintenance therapy for small cell lung cancer (SCLC). A phase III study. *Proc. ASCO*, **8**, 227
13. Bajorin, D. F., Sell, K. W., Richards, J. M., *et al.* (1990). A randomized trial of interleukin-2 plus lymphokine activated killer cells versus interleukin-2 alone in renal cell carcinoma. *Am. Assoc. Cancer Res. Proc.*, **31**, 186
14. Rankin, E. M., Hekman, A., Vyth Dreese, F. A., *et al.* (1983). Monoclonal antibodies against B-cell non-Hodgkin lymphomas (NHL). *Br. J. Cancer*, **48,** 147–148
15. Kartner, N., Riordan, J. R. and Ling, V. (1983). Cell surface P-glycoprotein associated with multidrug resistance in mammalian cell lines. *Science*, **221**, 1285–1287
16. Degos, C., Chomienne, P., Ballerini, M. E., *et al.* (1990). All-trans retinoic acid: A novel differentiation therapy for acute promyelocytic leukemia. *Am. Soc. Clin. Oncol. Prog. Proc.*, **9**, 207
17. Vogelstein, B., Eric, R. F., Stanley, R., *et al.* (1989). Genetic alterations during colorectal tumorigenesis. *Am. Assoc. Cancer Res. Proc.*, **30**, 634–635
18. Waun, K., Scott, M. L., Loretta, M. I., *et al.* (1990). Prevention of second primary tumours with isotretinoin in squamous-cell carcinoma of the head and neck. *N. Engl. J. Med.*, **323**, 795–800
19. Zacharski, L. R., Henderson, W. G., Rickles, F. R., *et al.* (1981). Effect of warfarin on survival in small cell carcinoma of the lung. *J. Am. Med. Assoc.*, **245**, 831
20. Glover, D., Glick, J. H., Weiler, C., *et al.* (1986). WR-2721 protects against the hematologic toxicity of cyclophosphamide: A controlled phase II trial. *J. Clin. Oncol.* **41**, 584–588

10
Oncogene-targeted antisense oligonucleotides: tools for genetic analysis or new anticancer drugs?

E. SAISON-BEHMOARAS and C. HÉLÈNE

During the last decade, a large number of cellular genes, called proto-oncogenes, have been discovered. The inappropriate expression of the proto-oncogenes can lead to malignant transformation. New oncogenes are continually reported and it is reasonable to expect that 200–300 will be identified over the next few years. Although a clear picture of oncogene proteins as signal transducing elements has emerged, their respective roles in normal cell proliferation or differentiation remain largely unknown. The data that are accumulating will eventually elucidate the pathways by which signals are transmitted from plasma membrane receptors to the nucleus and will allow us to understand the molecular mechanisms by which oncogenes regulate gene expression. The more recent discovery of anti-oncogenes or tumour-suppressing genes should also help to decipher the pathways controlling cell growth and differentiation. It is not unreasonable to suggest that our growing understanding of oncogene action will provide a molecular description of events leading to malignancy. A more speculative consideration is whether our understanding of cellular regulatory pathways can be exploited as a basis for the development of new strategies for cancer treatment.

A novel approach to inhibit specifically the production of cellular oncoproteins lies in the use of antisense oligonucleotides. The first example of the utilization of a short DNA fragment to inhibit selectively the translation of a messenger RNA was described in 1977–78 by Paterson et al.[1] and Hastie and Held[2]. The basic idea to target an oligonucleotide to a nucleic acid was based on a very simple assumption: hybridization of an oligonucleotide to a nucleic acid should disturb the normal function of the latter. Indeed, these authors showed that hybrid-arrest of translation by DNA fragments complementary to messenger RNA could be used for the analysis of mRNA populations. At the same time, Taniguchi and Weissman[3] and Eckardt and Lührmann[4] targeted short oligoribonucleotides to the 3' end of 16 S ribosomal RNA from *E. coli* in order to prevent the formation of the 70 S ribosomal unit. The first utilization of a synthetic oligodeoxyribonucleotide in order to inhibit selectively the expression of a gene was reported by Zamecnik and Stephenson[5]. They targeted a tridecamer to the 3' and 5' reiterated terminal sequences of Rous sarcoma virus RNA. Addition of the tridecamer to chick embryo fibroblast tissue cultures infected with Rous sarcoma virus resulted in inhibition of virus production. The tridecamer was able to inhibit the translation of proteins specified by the viral RNA in the wheat germ embryo cell free system[6]. Although this work showed the possible use of an oligodeoxynucleotide to inhibit virus production, with the potential to target oligodeoxynucleotides to RNA and DNA oncogenic viruses as well as to specific cell oncogenes, it did not trigger many investigations at that time. The dogma that only proteins were involved in gene regulation was well established; consequently, the use of nucleic acids to regulate gene expression was considered a laboratory curiosity.

Around 1981, Tomizawa and Itoh described the involvement of an RNA.RNA hybrid in the regulation of plasmid Col E1 replication and the control of plasmid copy number in bacteria[7]. The synthesis of the RNA primer used by the replication machinery was shown to be controlled by a smaller complementary RNA. After that, many examples of the involvement of regulatory RNAs in procaryotes were reported[8,9]. Recently, such a mechanism for the control of gene expression in eucaryotes has been described. A post-transcriptional down-regulation of p53 mRNA is governed by the induced synthesis of a counter-transcript[10].

The discovery of the involvement of small RNAs in gene regulation constituted the starting point for the development of the 'anti-sense' strategy to control gene expression artificially in living cells in culture[11,12], in transgenic plants[13] or in animals[14]. The first strategy that was developed consisted of inserting, downstream of an inducible promoter, part of a DNA sequence coding for the protein to be regulated in a reverse orientation compared with that of the gene itself. Association between anti-sense transcript and messenger RNA was expected physically to prevent the translation of the mRNA. The association between these two RNAs could also interfere with other processes, like splicing of the mRNA or transport from the nucleus to the cytoplasm[15].

Anti-sense sequences can also be made in the form of synthetic oligoribo- or oligodeoxyribonucleotides. Recent improvements in chemical synthesis and modifications of oligodeoxynucleotides have led to intense investigation, during the past 5 years, of anti-sense nucleic acids as tools to control artificially a single gene inside cells. Anti-sense oligodeoxynucleotides and their modified analogues that display increased resistance to DNases readily appeared good candidates, as they could be very powerful agents for specifically inhibiting viral genes inside infected cells. Such agents could be important in the treatment of viral diseases. In tissue culture, anti-sense oligonucleotides have inhibited infections by Rous sarcoma virus[5]; influenza virus[16]; vesicular stomatitis virus[17,18]; herpes simplex virus[19,20]; human immunodeficiency virus[21-29]; and simian virus SV40[30]. All these studies have demonstrated the discriminating power of the anti-sense oligonucleotides. For example, a modified oligonucleotide targeted to the intron–exon splice acceptor site of an immediate early gene of herpes simplex virus type 1 inhibited HSV 1 proliferation without affecting the proliferation of HSV 2, which possesses a different sequence at the intron–exon junction. The cytopathic effect of influenza virus type A was inhibited using a heptanucleotide covalently attached to an intercalating agent. This heptanucleotide, targeted to part of the 3'-terminal sequence which is common to the eight RNAs of the type A virus, had no effect on a type B virus bearing a different sequence at the 3' end of its eight RNAs.

Anti-sense oligonucleotides have also been used to inhibit endogenous genes of cells in culture in a specific way. Oncogenes have constituted one of the major targets for anti-sense oligonucleotides. The major challenge is to make anti-sense agents that will inactivate the mutated or translocated oncogene but not its normal precursor or proto-oncogene which is generally essential to cell survival.

WHAT HAS BEEN DONE WITH ANTI-SENSE OLIGONUCLEOTIDES S TARGETED TO AN ONCOGENE?

myc

The c-myc proto-oncogene has been highly conserved during evolution: it is found in all vertebrates and expressed in most normal dividing cells throughout the cell cycle[31]. The c-myc gene codes for a 49 kDa polypeptide and expresses a nuclear protein[32]. Amplification, translocation, overexpression, or abnormal regulation of the proto-oncogene c-myc has been observed in a wide variety of human leukaemias and solid tumours[31-33].

The specific role (or roles) of the c-myc gene in lymphocyte mitogenesis was initially unknown. However, it was shown that inducing T lymphocytes to proliferate by addition of mitogen leads to a rapid accumulation of c-myc mRNA when lymphocytes enter the cell cycle, suggesting the importance of myc in the G_0 to G_1 transition[34,35]. On the other hand, DNA synthesis may be suppressed by antibodies against c-myc protein, which suggests also that the c-myc protein may be required for entry into S phase[36]. However, accumulation of c-myc transcripts is not by itself sufficient to induce T-lymphocyte proliferation[37-39]. Heikkila *et al.*[40] have addressed the question of whether c-myc induction is required for proliferation of T lymphocytes by attempting to inhibit c-myc protein expression with anti-sense oligomers. An oligodeoxyribonucleotide complementary to the first five codons of human c-myc messenger RNA, added to fresh peripheral blood lymphocytes (G_0) four hours before addition of the mitogen, inhibited c-myc protein synthesis. Thirty μmol/L of anti-sense oligomer was sufficient to decrease 90% of myc expression six hours after mitogen treatment. The authors studied the effects of inhibition of c-myc protein expression on entry into the cell cycle and reported that anti-sense treatment did not inhibit G_0 to G_1 traversal as assessed by morphological blast transformation, but it did prevent entry into S phase. This work was the first example of the use of anti-sense oligomers to determine one of the functions of an oncogene. Later Harel-Bellan *et al.*[41], using the same oligonucleotide, showed that the 15 mer penetrates T lymphocytes without any treatment in a time-dependent manner, a plateau being reached after 3 hours of incubation. The entry into S phase was blocked by the 15 mer in a dose-dependent manner. These effects were ascribed to the specific inhibition of c-myc protein synthesis as shown by two-dimensional gel electrophoresis of proteins extracted from peripheral T cells treated for two hours with anti-sense prior to mitogen (PHA) stimulation for three hours.

HL-60 cells are leukaemia cells that are arrested in the promyelocytic stage of myeloid development with a proliferative capacity but an inability to differentiate in the absence of inducing agents[42,43]. They differentiate along the granulocytic pathway when treated with dimethyl sulphoxide[42] or retinoic acid[44] and along the monocytic pathway when treated with phorbol ester[45] or vitamin D analogues[46]. A decrease in c-myc expression is associated with the induction of differentiation. The malignant phenotype of HL-60 may be related in part to an 8- to 30-fold amplification of the c-myc gene. Holt et al.[47] have addressed the following question: could anti-sense inhibition of myc affect HL-60 proliferation and differentiation? Using the same 15-mer as Heikkila et al., they showed that, as early as four hours after incubation with 4 μmol/L of anti-sense oligomer, the steady-state level of c-myc protein decreased about 90% compared with control HL-60 cells or cells grown in the presence of 4 μmol/L sense oligomer. They also showed that the decrease in c-myc expression was associated with a decrease in HL-60 proliferation rate. A 50% decrease in the growth rate of HL-60 cells, treated with anti-sense oligomer, was observed over a 5-day period. HL-60 cells, treated for 5 days with 4 μmol/L of anti-sense oligomer, showed significant changes in morphology and the authors observed a large number of differentiated cells. By using the anti-sense approach, this study demonstrated that, although c-myc expression is normally influenced by extracellular factors, direct inhibition of c-myc expression can bypass surface events and influence cell proliferation and differentiation directly. Amplification of the c-myc gene has been found in several types of human tumours, such as lung, breast and colon carcinomas[48-51]. In addition, a correlation between high tissue-specific expression of c-myc and cancer has been demonstrated by constructing trangenic mice carrying a c-myc gene under the control of a hormonally inducible MMTV promoter. These transgenic mice developed mammary adenocarcinomas[52].

Anti-sense oligonucleotides have been shown to inhibit myc expression selectively in T lymphocytes and promyelocytic leukaemia HL-60 cells. This anti-sense strategy could therefore be used in principle, to modulate expression of the c-myc gene in cancer treatment. But, beside all the problems to be solved before therapeutic application is possible, an inherent disadvantage of the myc system is that normal cells require this proto-oncogene to grow, so subsequently normal cells will be affected along with tumour cells. In several tumours, however, the genetic lesions result in the generation of aberrant messenger RNA molecules which are not present in normal cells. For example, in mouse plasmacytomas and in human Burkitt's lymphoma coding sequences from the c-myc gene are translocated from their normal chromosomal position into an active immunoglobulin locus on another chromosome[53,54]. Burkitt's lymphoma is a very aggressive B-cell neoplasm and the majority of such tumours carry chromosome 8q24 translocation breakpoints which are located at the site of the c-myc proto-oncogene. The breakpoints on chromosome 8 involve sequences both upstream and downstream of c-myc, in the immediate 5' flanking region and within the gene itself. However, the c-myc gene involved in the translocation is always the allele that is transcribed. When the breakpoints are located downstream from the normally used promoter, transcription is initiated from cryptic promoters in the first intron. In these cases, intron sequences downstream from the cryptic promoter are not subject to splicing since the consensus donor splice sequence at the 5' end is lost. Therefore c-myc transcripts in such tumours contain 5' intron sequences not present in normal cells. It is evident that Burkitt's lymphomas containing such aberrant transcripts provide an excellent opportunity to test the potential of the anti-sense approach to tumour-specific therapy. Indeed McManaway et al.[55] targeted a 21-mer anti-sense oligonucleotide to the first intron of the translocated c-myc gene. They obtained an almost total growth inhibition of Burkitt's lymphoma cell lines treated for four days with 100μmol/L of 21-mer. The anti-sense oligonucleotide had no effect on proliferation of control cells bearing a breakpoint at the 3' end of the c-myc gene. This paper provides the first example of the successful use of an anti-sense oligonucleotide targeted to a genetic lesion in a tumour that can differentiate tumour cells from normal cells. This strategy is not limited to Burkitt's lymphomas and could be used with all pathologically relevant aberrant mRNA molecules.

myb

The proto-oncogene, c-myb, is the normal cellular homologue of the avian myeloblastosis virus transforming gene, v-myb[56]. Experimental evidence has suggested that the proto-oncogene, c-myb, plays a major role in the regulation of haematopoiesis in vitro[57]. C-myb is preferentially expressed in primitive haematopoietic cell tissues and haematopoietic tumour cell lines of several species[58]. Using an 18 mer targeted to a region starting from the second codon of c-myb mRNA, Gewirtz and Calabretta[59] demonstrated that exposure of partially purified human haematopoietic progenitor cells to the oligomer inhibited the formation of erythroid, myeloid and megakaryocytic colonies in a semi-solid culture medium. They observed the reduction in the number of colonies four days after plating cells with 14μmol/L of the 18-mer anti-sense oligonucleotide. These results suggested that c-myb anti-sense inhibited the proliferation of early haematopoietic progenitor cells. To determine if the c-myb anti-sense oligomer preferentially arrested proliferation at a specific stage of development, Anfossi et al.[60] treated four human myeloid leukaemia cells lines (HL-60, ML-3, KG-1 and KG-1a), each blocked at different stages of differentiation. Treatment for five days with 10μmol/L of c-myb anti-sense 18-mer resulted in a significant decrease in cell proliferation in all of the lines, with a larger effect on HL-60 cells. The effect of the c-myb anti-sense oligomer on the proliferation of HL-60 cells was more dramatic than that of c-myc anti-sense oligomer, but differentiated cells were not detected, suggesting that c-myc and c-myb regulate cell proliferation in the myeloid lineage by independent mechanisms. In HL-60 cells, the c-myc gene is amplified 10- to 30-fold and is highly expressed[61,62] whereas the c-myb proto-oncogene is preferentially expressed in haematopoietic tissues[1,2]. It is possible, therefore, to target anti-sense oligomers simultaneously to myc and myb proto-oncogenes in order to provide the rationale for an anti-sense-based therapy of leukaemia.

ras

In mammalian species, the *ras* family of proto-oncogenes consists of three functional *ras* genes, designated H (Harvey) *ras*-1, K (Kirsten)-*ras*-2 and N-*ras*[63]. These *ras* genes code for very similar 21 kDa proteins (p21 *ras*). Both H- and K-*ras* genes have genetic counterparts in the Harvey and Kirsten strains of the acutely transforming rat sarcoma retroviruses. To date, no viral homologue of N-*ras* has been identified. The *ras* genes have been highly conserved throughout evolution and are found in such diverse organisms as man[64-66], chicken[67], insects[68] and yeast[69,70]. There are two main regions of the *ras* genes where a base change can result in oncogenic activation[71-73]; the first is located around codon 12. *In vitro* mutagenesis studies of the H-*ras* gene at codon 12 have shown that the substitution of any amino acid, with the exception of glycine and proline, results in oncogenic activation[73]. The second region for *ras* activation has been localized around codon 61[74]. Substitution of glutamine at position 61 by amino acids other than proline or glutamic acid leads to onco-genic activation[75]. At amino acid 59, a threonine substitution for alanine also results in transforming activity[73]. Based on the NIH3T3 transfection assay, mutations in the *ras* genes were originally estimated to occur in 10–30% of human cancers[76]. With the recent use of sensitive DNA hybridization technology, the frequency of *ras* gene mutations in human tumours appears to be even higher. Usually a single member of the *ras* proto-oncogene family is mutated in a defined cancer. For example, H-*ras* mutation has been reported in human bladder and urinary tract carcinomas[71,72,77], while mutant K-*ras* genes are more common in lung and colon carcinomas[78,79]. In studies of colorectal cancer, 40% have been found to contain mutated K-*ras* genes[80,81]. In this case, a high incidence of glycine to aspartic acid substitutions at codon 12 has been observed. Recent studies have shown that mutations in K-*ras* genes are also found in about 95% of primary pancreatic carcinomas[82]. Melanomas and haematopoietic malignancies contain activated N-*ras*[83,84] which is detected also in 60% of patients with acute myeloid leukaemia[85]. An activated N-*ras* gene with a single nucleotide substitution in codon 13 was detected in three of eight patients with myelodysplastic syndrome. All three patients have progressed to a true leukaemia within one year[86]. In addition to the mutational activation of *ras* proto-oncogenes in human cancers, a number of reports have implicated a link between overexpression of the normal *ras* gene and neoplastic transfor-mation[87,88]. Elevated levels of p21 have been reported in primary colon tumours[89], in both prostate and bladder carcinomas[87,90] as well as in human glioblastomas[91]. Therefore, overexpression of p21 *ras* seems to provide an alternative mechanism to explain the activation of *ras* proto-oncogene functions in human cancers, although at a lower frequency than mutations. The functions of p21 *ras* proteins in normal cells have not yet been elucidated. They play a regulatory role in signal transduction, in cell growth and in the maintenance of differentiation. Microinjection of high concentrations of the normal *ras* protein into NIH3T3 fibroblasts causes both morphological transformation and initiation of DNA synthesis in the absence of added serum[92]. Co-injection of the *ras*-specific monoclonal antibody, Y13-259, has been reported to neutralize the transforming ability of p21. Normal NIH3T3 cells induced to enter the resting stage of the cell cycle by incubation at low serum concentrations, then stimulated by the addition of serum, were blocked from entering S phase after microinjection with antibody Y13-259[93,94]. No inhibition of S phase was observed if Y13-259 was injected 22 hours after serum stimulation. Microinjection experiments have also indicated the role of p21 *ras* proteins in differentiation. Pheochromocytoma (PC 12) cells differentiate into non-replicating, sympathetic neuron-like cells upon exposure to nerve growth factor (NGF). Microinjection of Y13-259 into PC12 cells before NGF treatment inhibited neurite formation and resulted in the temporary regression of partially extended neurites. Microinjection of oncogenic H-*ras* proteins into PC12 cells resulted in cessation of cell division and promoted their morphological differentiation into neuron-like cells[95].

Since many tumour cells contain a mutated allele of only one of the *ras* genes, we have addressed the question as to whether it is possible to make anti-sense agents that will inactivate the mutated oncogene without altering the proto-oncogene expression which might be essential for cell survival. In other words, we have sought to design an oligonucleotide which will be very strongly bound to the mutated mRNA and yet be unstable in association with the wild-type mRNA. The first condition requires the use of a short anti-sense oligomer since a long one will form stable complexes with both targets under physiological conditions (37° C, salt conditions and pH prevailing inside cells). But it is expected that too short an oligomer will not be able to form a sufficiently stable complex with the target sequence (at 37°C) to elicit a biological response. In order to increase oligomer affinity, we chose to link an intercalating agent covalently to one end of the oligomer. If the linker between the oligonucleotide and the intercalator is appropriately chosen, intercalation can occur into the mini double helix formed when the oligonucleotide is bound to its complementary sequence. Stabilization of the complexes was observed when 2-methoxy-6-chloro-9-amino acridine (Acr) was linked to an oligomer[96,97].

If the target sequence of the oligonucleotide is mutated in such a way that the last base pair of the oligonucleotide–RNA hybrid cannot form, then intercalation should be lost and the hybrid strongly destabilized. We chose to target a modified 9-mer to the H-*ras* gene of a bladder carcinoma cell line (T24/EJ) which is activated by virtue of a G→T transversion in the 12th codon. The anti-sense oligonucleotide sequence was chosen to be complementary to the mRNA sequence downstream of the mutation, with the last base pair formed with U on the mutated mRNA so that an A.G mismatch should be present when the oligonucleotide binds to the proto-oncogene. We found that the single nucleotide change from G to T at the 12th amino acid codon in the *ras* gene was indeed sufficient to allow discrimination between the two mRNAs by the 9-mer oligonucleotide. Studies *in vitro* established that the acridine-linked 9-mer preferentially inhibited the synthesis of the mutated *ras* p21 protein[98]. Further substitution of the oligonucleotide by a dodecanol chain enhanced the inhibitory effect without affecting selectivity. We demonstrated that addition of this oligonucleotide to the culture medium of T24 cells containing only the activated H-*ras* inhibited their proliferation whereas the proliferation of human mammary cells containing normal H-*ras* was unaffected[98].

WHAT DO WE KNOW ABOUT THE MECHANISM OF ACTION OF ANTI-SENSE OLIGONUCLEOTIDES?

Several mechanisms can potentially be involved in the inhibition of oncogene expression by anti-sense oligodeoxynucleotides, such as:

(1) Translation arrest.
(2) Specific blockage of mRNA transport.
(3) Enhanced mRNA degradation through a mechanism involving RNase H.
(4) Inhibition of initiation or elongation processes in transcription.

In vitro studies have shown that an enzyme (RNase H) which recognizes RNA–DNA hybrids and cleaves the RNA strand is involved in anti-sense-mediated inhibition of translation[99,100]. Such studies have led to the conclusion that, in the absence of RNase H activity, only 5' non-coding sequences or sequences in the vicinity of the AUG start codon could be chosen as targets of anti-sense oligonucleotides, whereas coding sequences could be chosen only if RNase H activity were present. In cells in culture there is no clear demonstration of the involvement of RNase H activity. Gewirtz *et al.*[101] have shown that the decrease in myb gene product synthesis in anti-sense-treated cells was due to greatly decreased c-myb mRNA levels. By selective amplification of c-myb cDNA sequences using the polymerase chain reaction technique after reverse transcription of the total RNA of untreated and anti-sense-treated cells, they showed that c-myb mRNA was virtually undetectable in PHA-stimulated peripheral blood mononuclear cells treated with an anti-sense oligo-nucleotide[101]. Harel-Bellan *et al.*[102] have also shown that the steady-state level of lymphokine mRNA is decreased in cells treated with IL-2 or IL-4 anti-sense oligodeoxynucleotides. Although a likely hypothesis is that messages are degraded by an RNase H activity, the lower level of detectable message could also result from a feedback effect due to the disappearance of the protein or blockage of mRNA transport. Holt *et al.*[47] have detected an S1 nuclease-resistant duplex in HL-60 cells following incubation with 5' end-labelled anti-myc oligomer. They determined that 30% of c-myc mRNA was complexed with the anti-sense oligomer after four hours of incubation. These results rather suggest that all the anti-sense–RNA duplex was not degraded in the cytoplasm by RNase H. Recently, Becker *et al.*[103] reported that anti-sense oligonucleotides complementary to codon 60, the first splice donor-acceptor site, or codon 94 and 95 (second splice donor-acceptor site) of the basic fibroblast growth factor mRNA were as effective as an oligonucleotide complementary to the initiation codon as regards inhibiting melanoma cell proliferation. The former oligodeoxynucleotides can bind only after bFGF pre-mRNA has been spliced. This study indicated that anti-sense oligonucleotides can act on mature RNAs. However, all other oligonucleotides tested so far in similar studies could hybridize to both pre-mRNA and mature mRNA. Obviously, several mechanisms can contribute to the success of the anti-sense strategy. The different contributions of various mechanisms will probably depend on the cell line, as well as the localization of the target sequence of the mRNA. It is, however, very important to investigate the mechanism of action of anti-sense oligonucleotides inside cells in order to establish the best target sequences in mRNA.

OLIGONUCLEOTIDE SURVIVAL AND UPTAKE

The rates of nucleolytic degradation and cell uptake are two factors that will limit the use of anti-sense oligonucleotides in therapeutic applications. To the first question – How can we make oligonucleotides resistant to nucleases? – the chemists have devoted a huge amount of work. Indeed, several possibilities have been described which introduce modifications to the phosphodiester backbone: methylphosphonates[18,19,26,104–106], phosphorothioates[27,29,107], phosphoroselenoates[108], phosphoroamidates[109] and phosphorodithioates[110]. All these substitutions increase the resistance of oligonucleotides to degradation by nucleases.

Another approach to improving nuclease resistance consists of changing the anomeric configuration of the nucleoside. In synthetic [α] anomers, the base is on the same side as the 3' OH group (instead of the 5' OH group in natural [β] anomers) with respect to the main sugar plane. [α]-Oligomers hybridize well to complementary sequences but bind in an opposite orientation with respect to [β]-oligomers. They form parallel-stranded structures and are poor substrates for nucleases[111,112]. Modifications of the phosphodiester backbone lead to two diastereoisomers per linkage except for the phosphorodithioates. Therefore, an oligonucleotide with n units is in fact a mixture of 2^{n-1} compounds which can bind to the target with different affinities. However, all substitutions lead to oligomers which bind to complementary sequences. [α]-Oligodeoxynucleotides and methyl phosphonates do not render their target RNA susceptible to RNase-cleavage[107], whereas phosphorothioates, selenoates and dithioates do.

Deoxyoligonucleoside methylphosphonates (MP) and phosphorothioates (PS) have been used to inhibit the *ras* oncogene and B-cell lymphoma/leukaemia-2 (BCL2) gene. Using rabbit reticulocyte lysate as cell free translation system, Yu *et al.*[113] have shown that an 8-mer MP complementary to eight nucleotides spanning the twelfth amino acid codon of human c-Ha-*ras* inhibited *ras* expression at 200 μmol/L. They also showed[114] that an 11-mer MP targeted to the start codon and downstream of murine *ras* mRNA also inhibited p21 synthesis *in vitro* at 200 μmol/L. These high concentrations are required because MP oligonucleotides exhibit reduced hybridization compared with normal phosphodiesters and probably do not induce RNase H cleavage. Oligonucleotide MP are relatively poorly soluble in aqueous media since they have no polar terminal phosphate or phosphodiester groups. However, a reduction of *ras* p21 by over 90% occurred after a total of 60 hours' treatment of transformed NIH 3T3 cells overexpressing p21, using 50 μmol/L of an 11-mer MP complementary to the initiation codon region of murine *ras* mRNA[115]. Reed *et al.* used 20-mer anti-sense oligodeoxynucleotides specific for sequences in mRNAs from the B-cell lymphoma/leukaemia 2 (BCL 2) gene and inhibited the growth in culture of a human leukaemia cell line[116]. They compared normal phosphodiester (PO) and nuclease-resistant phosphorothioate (PS) oligonucleotides with regard to specificity, potency and kinetics. An anti-sense BCL2 PS oligonucleotide was a more potent inhibitor of 697 leukaemia cell growth than its normal oxygen-based counterpart. PS anti-sense oligodeoxynucleotides reduced cellular proliferation by 50% at concentrations of approximately 15–25 μmol/L whereas the normal oligodeoxynucleotide only achieved 50% inhibition at 125–250 μmol/L. Both PO and PS anti-sense oligodeoxynucleotides suppressed the proliferation of leukaemia cells through non-cytotoxic mechanisms. A comparison of inhibition kinetics by PO and PS oligo-deoxynucleotides revealed that the latter compounds have a slower onset of action. Maximal inhibition of leukaemia cell proliferation by PO anti-sense oligomers occurred 2–3 days after initiation of cultures, whereas PS oligodeoxynucleotides required 4–7 days to achieve maximal inhibition. These results are in good agreement with a previous report where 5'-linked acridine oligodeoxynucleotides were used to investigate the kinetics of entry of PO and PS oligodeoxynucleotides into HL-60 leukaemia cells[117]. Although the rate and magnitude of entry varied with the length of the oligodeoxynucleotide, in general, PO oligodeoxynucleotides attained their final intracellular concen-trations within 48 hours. In contrast, PS oligodeoxynucleotides reached comparable levels only after 4–5 days. Taken together, these results suggest that phosphorothioates are more potent than phosphodiesters with half maximal inhibition of leukaemic cell growth occurring at concentrations 5–10 times lower.

The mechanism or mechanisms whereby polyanionic oligonucleotides and their phosphorothioate analogues become internalized is (or are) complex. Saturable uptake kinetics and an 80 kDa cell-surface protein with specific nucleic acid binding properties that may mediate this process have been described[118,119]. Phosphorothioates are excellent competitive inhibitors of acridine-labelled oligodeoxynucleotide uptake. Thus, it appears that the ionic character of the oligonucleotide backbone may be critical for utilization of this uptake mechanism by oligodeoxynucleotides. Methylphosphonates which lack ionizable groups were found not to inhibit acridine-labelled oligo-deoxynucleotide uptake, suggesting that the increased hydrophobicity of methylphosphonates allows them to be passively transported across the cell membrane. Whether the 80 kDa surface protein is involved in oligode-oxynucleotide transport is not yet known. Knowledge of the properties of the uptake process will allow us to design oligodeoxynucleotides that are transported more efficiently and are more resistant to degradation.

ANTI-SENSE OLIGODEOXYNUCLEOTIDES: TOOLS FOR GENETIC ANALYSIS OR NEW ANTI-CANCER DRUGS?

In procaryotes, much genetic analysis has been successful using a variety of mutants or thermolabile mutants that do not express a particular gene. In mammalian cells, anti-sense oligonucleotides could offer a method for selective blockage of gene expression. This decade has seen an explosion in the discovery of cellular genes which function abnormally during oncogenic transformation. Many different approaches have led to the identification of cellular gene sequences which could function as oncogenes. At least 50 proto-oncogenes have been identified in the human genome but only eight of them (c-Ha-ras-1, c-Ki-ras-2, N-ras, c-erbB1, c-erbB2, c Myc, N-myc, L-myc and c-abl) have been clearly shown to be involved in human cancer. With the exceptions of bcr-abl in chronic myeloid leukaemia and of c-myc in Burkitt's lymphoma, particular oncogenes appear to be involved in only a fraction of the tumours belonging to a given type of malignancy. Much epidemiological and experimental evidence argues that multiple genetic alterations are responsible for malignant change. Indeed, several lines of evidence suggest that changes in more than one proto-oncogene are involved in tumours. Although about 50 genes termed oncogenes have already been described, it is estimated that at least 200–300 will eventually be identified. The generation of oncogenes from their non-transforming homologues (proto-oncogenes) can occur in different ways[120]:

(1) Proto-oncogenes can become activated following chromosomal translocation, the well-known examples being the reciprocal translocation of the human c-abl proto-oncogene from chromosome 9 to 22 observed in over 95% of patients with chronic myelogenous leukaemia (CML), and translocations of the c-myc gene in Burkitt's lymphoma and plasmacytomas. Myc genes are rearranged by recombination with the immunoglobulin loci.

(2) Oncogenes can be generated by mutations within coding regions, the paradigm being the human *ras* oncogene in which a single point mutation is sufficient to produce a transforming protein. Point mutations have also been identified in growth factor receptors such as 'neu' and CSF-1 which are sufficient to activate the intrinsic protein-tyrosine kinase activity of the receptor and its transforming ability.

(3) Spontaneous gene amplification may lead to an increased concentration of proto-oncogene product as in the case of the neu proto-oncogene which is amplified in approximately 30% of human breast carcinomas.

Definition of the precise role of oncogenes in the multi-step process of carcinogenesis awaits further investigation. Briefly, we should seek answers to the questions :

(1) What are the exact roles of oncogenes in the regulation of cell proliferation?

(2) What are their roles in the discrete stages of tumorigenesis?

Despite all the efforts aimed at answering these two questions, they still remain a challenge. One of the best examples is to be seen in the intensive *ras* oncogene studies undertaken in a number of laboratories following the finding in 1982 of cellular *ras* oncogene activation in human tumours. Since then, roughly four hundred reports have been published, but the biological function of Harvey-*ras*, Kirsten *ras* and N-*ras* remains unclear. The anti-sense approach might prove very useful in answering questions about the function of *ras* proto and oncogenes, since it is possible to inhibit selectively one of the *ras* species and follow the consequences as regards cell behaviour. One of the latest examples

269

showing the value of anti-sense oligonucleotides in genetic analysis has been provided by Rosolen et al.[121]. Some neuroblastomas have been demonstrated to display in vitro two different morphologies which can 'transdifferentiate' between each other: epithelial-like cells which are contact-inhibited and are not tumorigenic in nude mice (called 'S') and round neurotic ones which are not contact-inhibited and are tumorigenic (called 'N'). In an N-myc amplified neuroblastoma, N-myc is preferentially expressed in 'N' but not in 'S' cell subclones. In order to determine whether specific inhibition of a low level of N-myc expression could alter cell biology, the authors utilized anti-sense oligonucleotides to inhibit specifically N-myc protein expression in the transdifferentiating neuroepithelioma cell line exhibiting elevated c-myc expression but a very low level of N-myc expression from unamplified N-myc alleles. They reported that exposure of these cells to N-myc anti-sense oligomer led to a decrease in N-myc protein, DNA synthesis and cell growth rate without any concomitant decrease in c-myc protein. Since N-myc anti-sense oligomer treatment appeared to alter the proportions of N and S cells, such that treated CHP 100 cultures consisted predominantly of large S-like cells, the authors suggested that N-myc anti-sense oligomer-treated cultures may have lost the N component of wild-type cultures, resulting in slower growth of the remaining cells for reasons other than a direct effect on proliferative capacity[121]. They have now tested the anti-sense approach in vivo. They are utilizing implantable microinfusion pumps to deliver anti-sense oligomers at a constant rate to nude mice given injections of human tumour cells and have demonstrated a reduction in tumor size.

Different strategies have been described for augmenting cell association and enhancing both the resistance to degradation of oligomers and their entry into cells. One of them is the encapsulation of anti-sense oligonucleotides in liposomes which, by virtue of their limited permeability, restrict access to the suspending medium and protect the anti-sense oligomer against enzymatic degradation. Liposomes may in turn be coupled to various ligands, including monoclonal antibodies or protein A, that permit their targeting to specific cell populations. Depending on the target molecule and cell, the liposomes are taken up and release the encapsulated product intracellularly. Leonetti et al.[123] have encapsulated a 15-mer targeted to the 5'-end region of the mRNA coding the N protein of vesicular stomatitis virus (VSV). They showed that oligomers encapsulated in liposomes resist DNase attack and are active at concentrations 1–2 orders of magnitude lower than those reported for unencapsulated oligomer sequences. Coupling of lipophilic membrane anchoring groups, such as cholesterol or phenazinium residues, to oligonucleotides can also facilitate their delivery into mammalian cells[124]. Further investigations aimed at improving the potency, stability and targeting of oligodeoxynucleotides are required before these substances can be applied to situations in vivo.

Our growing understanding of oncogenes can surely be exploited as a basis for development of new strategies for cancer treatment. Because of the importance of proto-oncogenes in normal cell physiology, useful therapeutic agents would have to interfere specifically with oncogene but not proto-oncogene function. Most oncogenes are only slightly different from the homologous proto-oncogenes. The anti-sense approach offers the first rational means to design chemotherapeutic agents which have explicit potential to interfere selectively with the function of oncogenes.

This review has been mainly devoted to anti-sense action of oligonucleotides which involves targeting them to mRNA. Binding of an oligonucleotide to its target is a reversible process, and complete inhibition of any biological process will inevitably be difficult to achieve at low doses. The design of reactive oligonucleotide derivatives is aimed at developing substances which will form a specific tight complex with the target and react with it efficiently. Chemically and photochemically activatable reagents have been attached to oligonucleotides, and site-directed chemical and photochemical reactions have been achieved in various model systems[125,126]. Oligonucleotides can also be targeted to DNA where they can locally form triple helices[127]. Homopyrimidine and homopurine oligonucleotides might be used in such an 'antigene' strategy. Binding of a homopyrimidine oligonucleotide to the major groove of DNA can inhibit interaction with sequence-specific proteins. This has been shown for restriction endonucleases[128,129], methylases and a transcription-activating factor[128]. Recently, Cooney et al.[130] have shown that a triple helix-forming purine-rich 27-mer oligonucleotide reduced the transcription efficiency of the myc gene upon binding to one of the regulatory elements of the c-myc gene[130]. Reactive groups have also been attached to the end of homopyrimidine oligonucleotides to mediate irreversible reactions on the target sequences[131–134]. There is clearly still much to be learnt about the potential use of antigene oligonucleotides before any therapeutic application can be contemplated.

References

1. Paterson, B. M., Roberts, B. E. and Kuff, E. L. (1977). Structural gene identification and mapping by DNA-m RNA hybrid-arrested cell-free translation. *Proc. Natl. Acad. Sci. USA*, **74**, 4370–4374
2. Hastie, N. D. and Held, W. A. (1978). Analysis of mRNA populations by cDNA mRNA hybrid-mediated inhibition of cell-free protein synthesis. *Proc. Natl. Acad. Sci. USA*, **75**, 1217–1221
3. Taniguchi, T. and Weissmann, C. (1978). Inhibition of β RNA 70 S ribosome initiation complex formation by an oligonucleotide complementary to the 3' terminal region of E. coli 16 S ribosomal RNA. *Nature*, **275**, 770–772
4. Eckardt, H. and Lührmann, R. (1979). Blocking of the initiation of protein biosynthesis by a pentanucleotide complementary to the 3' end of Escherichia coli 16 S rRNA. *J. Biol. Chem.*, **254**, 11 185–11 188
5. Zamecnik, P. C. and Stephenson, M. L. (1978). Inhibition of Rous sarcoma virus replication and cell transformation by a specific oligodeoxynucleotide. *Proc. Natl. Acad. Sci. USA*, **75**, 280–284
6. Stephenson, M. L. and Zamecnik, P. C. (1978). Inhibition of Rous sarcoma viral RNA translation by a specific oligodeoxyribonucleotide. *Proc. Natl. Acad. Sci. USA*, **75**, 285–288
7. Tomizawa, J.-I. and Itoh, T. (1981). Plasmid ColE1 incompatibility determined by interaction of RNA I with primer transcript. *Proc. Natl. Acad. Sci. USA*, **78**, 6096–6100
8. Inouye, M. (1988). Antisense RNA: its function and applications in gene regulation – a review. *Gene*, **72**, 25–34
9. Inouye, M. and Delihas, N. (1988). Small RNAs in the prokaryotes: a growing list of diverse roles. *Cell*, **53**, 5–7
10. Khochbin, S. and Lawrence, J. J. (1989). An antisense RNA involved in p53 mRNA maturation in murine erythroleukemia cells induced to differentiate. *EMBO J.* **8**, 4107–4114
11. Izant, J. G. and Weintraub, H. (1984). Inhibition of thymidine kinase gene expression by antisense RNA: a molecular approach to genetic analysis. *Cell*, **36**, 1007–1015
12. Weintraub, H., Izant, J. G. and Harland, R. M. (1985). Anti-sense RNA as a molecular tool for genetic analysis. *Trends Genet.*, **1**, 22–25

13. Van Der Krol, Mol, J. N. M. and Stuitje, A. R. (1988). Antisense genes in plants: an overview. *Gene*, **72**, 45–50

14. Katsuki, M., Sato, M., Kimura, M., Yokohama, M., Kobayashi, K. and Nomura, T. (1988). Conversion of normal behaviour to Shiverer by myelin basic protein antisense cDNA in transgenic mice. *Science*, **241**, 593–595

15. Kim, S. K. and Wold, B. J. (1985). Stable reduction of thymidine kinase activity in cells expressing high levels of anti-sense RNA. *Cell*, **42**, 129–138

16. Zerial, A., Thuong, N. T. and Hélène, C. (1987). Selective inhibition of the cytopathic effect of type A influenza viruses by oligodeoxynucleotides covalently linked to an intercalating agent. *Nucleic Acids Res.*, **15**, 9909–9919

17. Lemaitre, M., Bayard, B. and Lebleu, B. (1987). Specific antiviral activity of a poly (L-Lysine) conjugated oligodeoxyribonucleotide sequence complementary to vesicular stomatitis virus N protein mRNA initiation site. *Proc. Natl. Acad. Sci. USA*, **84**, 648–652

18. Agris, C. H., Blake, K. R., Miller, P. S., Reddy, M. P. and Ts'o, P. O. P. (1986). Inhibition of vesicular stomatitis virus protein synthesis and infection by sequence-specific oligodeoxyribonucleoside methylphosphonates. *Biochemistry*, **25**, 6268–6275

19. Smith, C. C., Aurelian, L., Reddy, M. P., Miller, P. S. and Ts'o, P.O.P. (1986). Antiviral effect of an oligo (nucleoside methylphosphonate) complementary to the splice junction of herpes simplex virus type I immediate early pre-mRNAs 4 and 5. *Proc. Natl. Acad. Sci. USA*, **83**, 2787–2791

20. Kulka, M., Smith, C. C., Aurelian, L., Fishelevich, R., Meade, K., Miller, P. and Ts'o, P.O.P. (1989). Site specificity of inhibitory effects of oligo (nucleoside methylphosphonates) complementary to the acceptor splice junction of herpes simplex virus type 1 immediate early mRNA 4. *Proc. Natl. Acad. Sci. USA*, **86**, 6868–6873

21. Zamecnik, P. C., Goodchild, J., Taguchi, Y. and Sarin, P. S. (1986). Inhibition of replication and expression of human T-cell lymphotropic virus type III in cultured cells by exogenous synthetic oligonucleotides complementary to viral RNA. *Proc. Natl. Acad. Sci. USA*, **83**, 4143–4146

22. Matsukura, M., Shinokuza, K., Zon, G., Mitsuya, H., Reitz, M., Cohen, J. S. and Broder, S. (1987). Phosphorothioate analogues of oligodeoxynucleotides: inhibitors of replication and cytopathic effects of human immunodeficiency virus. *Proc. Natl. Acad. Sci. USA*, **84**, 7706–7710

23. Agrawal, S., Goodchild, J., Civeira, M. P., Thornton, A. H., Sarin, P. S. and Zamecnik, P. C. (1988). Oligodeoxynucleoside phosphoramidates and phosphorothioates as inhibitors of human immunodeficiency virus. *Proc. Natl. Acad. Sci. USA*, **85**, 7079–7083

24. Sarin, P. S., Agrawal, S., Civeira, M. P., Goodchild, J., Ikeuchi, T. and Zamecnik, P.C. (1988). Inhibition of acquired immunodeficiency syndrome virus by oligodeoxynucleoside methylphosphonates. *Proc. Natl. Acad. Sci. USA*, **85**, 7448–7451

25. Goodchild, J., Agrawal, S., Civeira, M. P., Sarin, P. S., Sun, D. and Zamecnik, P.C. (1988). Inhibition of human immunodeficiency virus replication by antisense oligodeoxynucleotides *Proc. Natl. Acad. Sci. USA*, **85**, 5507–5511

26. Zaia, J. A., Rossi, J. J., Murakawa, G. J., Spallone, P. A., Stephens, D. A., Kaplan, B. E., Eritja, R., Wallace, B. and Cantin, E.M. (1988). Inhibition of human immunodeficiency virus by using an oligonucleoside methylphosphonate targeted to the tat-3 gene. *J. Virol.*, **62**, 3914–3917

27. Agrawal, S., Ikeuchi, T., Sun, D., Sarin, P. S., Konopka, A., Maizel, J. and Zamecnik, P. C. (1989). Inhibition of human immunodeficiency virus in early infected and chronically infected cells by antisense oligodeoxynucleotides and their phosphorothioate analogues. *Proc. Natl. Acad. Sci. USA*, **86**, 7790–7794

28. Stevenson, M. and Iversen, P. L. (1989). Inhibition of human immunodeficiency virus type 1-mediated cytopathic effects by Poly (L–lysine) conjugated synthetic antisense oligodeoxynucleotides. *J. Gen. Virol.*, **70**, 2673–2682

29. Matsukura, M., Zon, G., Shinozuka, K., Robert-Guroff, M., Shimada, T., Stein, C. A., Mitsuya,H., Wong-Staal, F., Cohen, J. S. and Broder, S. (1989). Stepwise mechanism of HIV reverse transcriptase: Primer function of phosphorothioate oligodeoxynucleotide. *Proc. Natl. Acad. Sci. USA*, **86**, 4244–4248

30. Birg, F., Praseuth, D., Zerial, A., Thuong, N.T., Asseline, U., Le Doan, T. and Hélène, C. (1990). Inhibition of simian virus 40 DNA replication in CV-1 cells by an oligodeoxynucleotide covalently linked to an intercalating agent. *Nucleic Acids Res.*, **18**, 2901–2907

31. Bishop, J. M. (1987). The molecular genetics of cancer. *Science*, **235**, 305–311

32. Persson, H., Hennighausen, L., Taub, R., De Grado, W. and Leder, P. (1984). Antibodies to human c-myc oncogene product: evidence of an evolutionarily conserved protein induced during cell proliferation. *Science*, **225**, 687

33. Klein, G. and Klein, E. (1986). Conditioned tumorigenicity of activated oncogenes. *Cancer Res.*, **46**, 3211–3224

34. Kelly, K., Cochran, B. H., Stiles, C. D. and Leder, P. (1983). Cell-specific regulation of the c-myc gene by lymphocyte mitogens and platelet-derived growth factor. *Cell*, **35**, 603–610

35. Reed, J. C., Nowell, P. C. and Hoover, R. G. (1985). Regulation of c-myc mRNA levels in normal human lymphocytes by modulators of cell proliferation. *Proc. Natl. Acad. Sci. USA*, **82**, 4221–4224

36. Studzinski, G. P., Brelvi, Z. S., Feldman, S. C. and Watt, R. A. (1986). Participation of c-myc protein in DNA synthesis of human cells. *Science*, **234**, 467–470

37. Moore, J. P., Todd, J. A., Hesketh, R. and Metcale, J.C. (1986). c.fos and c-myc gene activation, ionic signals and DNA synthesis in thymocytes. *J. Biol. Chem.*, **261**, 8158–8162

38. Neckers, L. M., Bauer, S., McGlennen, R. C., Trepel, J. B., Rao, K. and Greese, W. C. (1986). Diltiazem inhibits transferrin preceptor expression and causes G1 arrest in normal and neoblastic T cells. *Mol. Cell. Biol.*, **6**, 4244–4250

39. Leder, A., Pattengale, P. K., Kuo, A., Stewart, T. A. and Leder, P. (1986). Consequences of widespread deregulation of the c-myc gene in transgenic mice: multiple neoplasms and normal development. *Cell*, **45**, 485–495

40. Heikkila, R., Schwab, G., Wickstrom, E., Loke, S. L., Pluznik, D. H., Watt, R. and Neckers, L.M. (1987). A c-myc antisense oligodeoxynucleotide inhibits entry into S phase but not progress from G_0 to G_1. *Nature*, **328**, 445–449

41. Harel-Bellan, A., Ferris, D. K., Vinocour, M., Holt, J. T. and Farrar, W. L. (1988). Specific inhibition of c-myc protein biosynthesis using an antisense synthetic deoxy-oligonucleotide in human T lymphocytes. *J. Immunol.*, **140**, 2431–2435

42. Collins, S. J., Ruscetti, F. W., Gallagher, R. E. and Gallo, R. C. (1978). Terminal differentiation of human promyelocytic leukemia cells induced by dimethylsulfoxide and other polar compounds. *Proc. Natl. Acad. Sci. USA*, **75**, 2458–2462

43. Gallengher, R., Collins, S., Trufillo, J., McCredie, K., Ahearn, M., Tsai, S., Metzgar, R., Aulakh, G., Ting, R., Ruscetti, F. and Gallo, R. (1979). Characterization of the continuous, differentiating myeloid cell line (HL 60) from a patient with acute promyelocytic leukemia. *Blood*, **54**, 713–733

44. Breitman, T. R., Selonick, S. E. and Collins, S. J. (1980). Induction of differentiation of the human promyelocytic leukemia cell line (HL 60) by retinoic acid. *Proc. Natl. Acad. Sci. USA*, **77**, 2936–2940

45. Rovera, G., O'Brian, T. G. and Diamond, L. (1979). Induction of differentiation in human promyelocytic leukemia cells by tumor promoters. *Science*, **204**, 868–870

46. Reitsma, P. H., Rothberg, P. G., Astrin, S. M., Trial, J., Bar-Shavit, Z., Hall, A., Teitelbaum, S.L. and Kahn, A. J. (1983). Regulation of myc gene expression in HL-60 leukemia cells by a vitamin D metabolite. *Nature (London)*, **306**, 492–495

47. Holt, J. T., Redner, R. L. and Nienhuis, A. W. (1988). An oligomer complementary to c-myc mRNA inhibits proliferation of HL-60 promyelocytic cells and induces differentiation. *Mol. Cell. Biol.*, **8**, 963–973

48. Little, C. D., Nau, M. M., Carney, D. N., Gazdar, A. F. and Minna, J. D. (1983). Amplification and expression of the c-myc oncogene in human lung cancer cell lines. *Nature*, **306**, 194–196

49. Alitalo, K., Schwab, M., Lin, C. C., Varmus, H. E. and Bishop, M. (1983). Homogeneously staining chromosomal regions contain amplified copies of an abundantly expressed cellular oncogene (c-myc) in malignant neuroendocrine cells from a human colon carcinoma. *Proc. Natl. Acad. Sci.*, **80**, 1701–1711

50. Schwab, M., Klempnauer, K. H., Alitalo, K., Varmus, H. and Bishop, M. (1986). Rearrangement at the 5′ end of an amplified c-myc in human COLO 320 cells is associated with abnormal transcription. *Mol. Cell. Biol.*, **6**, 2752–2755

51. Escot, C., Thiellet, C., Lidereau, R., Spyratos, F., Champeme, M., Gest, J. and Callahan, R. (1986). Genetic alteration of the c-myc proto-oncogene (MYC) in human primary breast carcinomas. *Proc. Natl. Acad. Sci. USA*, **83**, 4834–4838

52. Stewart, T. A., Pattengale, P. K. and Leder, P. (1984). Spontaneous mammary adenocarcinomas in transgenic mice that carry and express MMTV/myc fusion genes. *Cell*, **38**, 627–637

53. Adams, J., Gerondakis, S., Webb, E., Corcoran, L. M. and Cory, S. (1983). Cellular myc oncogene is altered by chromosome translocation to the immunoglobulin locus in murine plasmacytomas and is rearranged similarly in human Burkitt lymphomas. *Proc. Natl. Acad. Sci. USA*, **80**, 1982–1986

54. Crews, S., Boath, R., Hood, L., Prehn, J. and Calame, K. (1982). Mouse c-myc oncogene is located on chromosome 15 and translocated to chromosome 12 in plasmacytomas. *Science*, **218**, 1319–1321

55. McManaway, M. E., Neckers, L. M., Loke, S. L., Al Nasser, A. A., Redner, R. L., Shiramizu, B. T., Goldsmidts, W.L., Huber, B. E., Bhatia, K. and Magrath, I. T. (1990). Tumour-specific inhibition of lymphoma growth by an antisense oligodeoxynucleotide. *Lancet*, **335**, 808–811

56. Roussel, M., Saule, S., Lagnou, C., Rommens, C., Beug, T., Graf. T. and Stehelin, B. (1979). Three new types of viral oncogene of cellular origin specific for hematopoietic cell transformation. *Nature*, **281**, 452–455

57. Reddy, E. P. (1988). The myb oncogene. In Reddy, E. P., Skalka, A. M. and Curran, T. (eds.) *The Oncogene Handbook*, pp. 327–340. (Amsterdam: Elsevier)

58. Westin, E. W., Gallo, R. C., Arya, S. K., Eva, A., Souza, L. M., Bahuda, M. A., Aaronson, S. A. and Wong-Staal, F. (1982). Differential expression of the amv gene in human hematopoietic cells. *Proc. Natl. Acad. Sci. USA*, **79**, 2194–2198

59. Gewirtz, A. M. and Calabretta, B. (1988). A c-myb antisense oligodeoxynucleotide inhibits normal human hematopoiesis in vitro. *Science*, **242**, 1303–1306

60. Anfossi, G., Gewirtz, A. M. and Calabretta, B. (1989). An oligomer complementary to c-myc encoded mRNA inhibits proliferation of human myeloid leukemia cell lines. *Proc. Natl. Acad. Sci. USA*, **86**, 3379–3383

61. Collins, S. and Groudine, M. (1982). Amplification of endogenous Myc related DNA sequences in a human myeloid leukemia cell line. *Nature (London)*, **298**, 679–681

62. Dalla-Favera, R., Wong-staal, F. and Gallo, R. C. (1982). Oncogene amplification in promyelocytic leukemia cell line HL-60 and primary leukaemic cells of the same patient. *Nature (London)*, **299**, 61–63

63. Barbacid, M. (1987). Ras genes. *Annu. Rev. Biochem.*, **56**, 779–827

64. Shimizu, K., Birnbaum, D., Ruley, M. A., Fasano, O., Suard, Y., Edlund, L., Taparowsky, E., Goldfarb, M. and Wigler, M. (1983). Structure of the Ki-ras gene of the human lung carcinoma cell line calu-1. *Nature*, **304**, 497–500

65. Capon, D. J., Chen, E. Y., Levinson, A. D., Seeburg, P. H. and Goeddel, D. V. (1983). Complete nucleotide sequence of the T-24 human bladder carcinoma oncogene and its normal homologue. *Nature*, **302**, 33–37

66. Taparowsky, E., Shimizu, K., Goldfarb, M. and Wigler, M. (1983). Structure and activation of the human N-ras gene. *Cell*, **34**, 581–586

67. Westaway, Y. D., Papkoff, J., Moscovici, C. and Varmus, H. E. (1986). Identification of a provirally activated c-Ha-ras oncogene in an avian nephroblastoma via a novel procedure: cDNA cloning of a chimeric viral-host transcript. *EMBO J.*, **5**, 301–309

68. Silberderg, F. S., Schejter, E., Hoffman, F. M. and Shilo, B. Z. (1984). The Drosophila ras oncogenes: structure and nucleotide sequence. *Cell*, **37**, 1027–1033

69. De Feo-Jones, D., Scolnick, E. M., Koller, R. and Dhar, R. (1983). Ras related gene sequences indentified and isolated from Saccharomyces cerevisiae. *Nature*, **306**, 707–709

70. Fukui, Y. and Karizo, Y, (1985). Molecular cloning and sequence analysis of a ras gene from *Schizosaccharomyces pombe*. *EMBO J.*, **4**, 687–691

71. Reddy, E. P., Reynolds, R. K., Santos, E. and Barbacid, M. (1982). A single point mutation is responsible for the acquisition of transforming properties of the T24 bladder carcinoma oncogene. *Nature*, **300**, 149–151

72. Tabin, C., Bradley, S., Bargmann, C., Weinberg, R., Papageorge, A., Scolnick, E., Dhar, R., Lowy, D. and Chang, E. (1982). Mechanism of activation of a human oncogene. *Nature*, **300**, 143–149

73. Fasano, O., Aldrich, T., Tamanoi, F., Taparowski, E., Furth, M. and Wigler, M. (1984). Analysis of the transforming potential of the human H-ras gene by random mutagenesis. *Proc. Natl. Acad. Sci. USA*, **81**, 4008–4012

74. Yuasa, Y., Srivastava, S. K., Dunn, C. Y., Rhim, J. S., Reddy, E. P. and Aaronson, S. A. (1983). Acquisition of transforming properties by alternative point mutations within c-ras human proto-oncogene. *Nature*, **303**, 775–779

75. Der, C. J., Finkel, T. and Cooper, G. M. (1986). Biological and biochemical properties of human ras H genes mutated at codon 61. *Cell*, **44**, 167–176

76. Weinberg, R.A. (1984). Ras oncogenes and the molecular mechanisms of carcinogenesis. *Blood*, **64**, 1143–1145

77. Fujita, J., Oshida, O., Yuasa, Y., Rhim, J. S., Hatanaka, M. and Aaronson, S. A. (1984). Ha-ras oncogenes are activated by somatic alterations in human urinary tract tumors. *Nature*, **309**, 464–466

78. Mc Coy, M., Toole, J. J., Cunningham, J. M., Chang, E. H., Lowy, D. R. and Weinberg, R. A. (1983). Characterization of a human colon/lung carcinoma oncogene. *Nature*, **302**, 79–81

79. Santos, E., Martin-Zanca, D., Reddy, E. P., Pierotti, M. A., Della Porta, G. and Barbacid, M. (1984). Malignant activation of a K-ras oncogene in lung carcinoma but not in normal tissue of the same patient. *Science*, **223**, 661–664

80. Bos, J. L., Fearon, E. R., Hamilton, S. R., Verlaan-de Vries, M., van Boom, J. H., van der Eb, A. J. and Vogelstein, B. (1987). Prevalence of ras gene mutations in human colorectal cancers. *Nature*, **327**, 293–297

81. Forrester, K., Almoguera, C., Han, K., Grizzle, W. E. and Perucho, M. (1987). Detection of high incidence of K-ras oncogenes during human colon tumorigenesis. *Nature*, **327**, 298–303

82. Almoguera, C., Shibata, D., Forrester, K., Martin, J., Arnheim, N. and Perucho, M. (1988). Most human carcinomas of the exocrine pancreas contain mutant c-K-ras genes. *Cell*, **53**, 549–554

83. Albino, A. P., Le Strange, R., Oliff, A. I., Old, L. J. and Furth, M.E. (1984). Transforming ras genes from human melanoma: a manifestation of tumor heterogeneity. *Nature*, **308**, 69–72

84. Eva, A., Tronick, S. R., Gol, R. A., Pierce, J. H. and Aaronson, S. A. (1983). Transforming genes of human hematopoietic tumors: frequent detection of ras-related oncogenes whose activation appears to be independent of tumor. *Proc. Natl. Acad. Sci. USA*, **80**, 4926–4930

85. Bos, J. L., Toksoz, D., Marshall, C. J., Verlaan-de Vries, M., Veeneman, G. H., Van der Eb. A. J., Van Boom, J. H., Hanssen, J. W. G. and Steenvoorden, A. C. M. (1985). Amino-acid substitutions at codon 13 of the N-ras oncogene in human acute myeloid leukemia. *Nature*, **315**, 726–730

86. Hirai, H., Kobayashi, Y., Mano, H., Hagiwara, K., Maru, Y., Omine, M., Mizoguchi, H., Nishida, J. and Takaku, F. (1987). A point mutation of codon 13 of the N-ras oncogene in myelodysplastic syndrome. *Nature*, **327**, 430–432

87. Viola, M. V., Fromowitz, F., Oravez, S., Deb, S., Finkel, G., Lundy, J., Handi, P., Thor, A. and Schlom, J. (1986). Expression of ras oncogene p21 in prostate cancer. *N. Engl. J. Med.*, **314**, 133–137

88. Stewart, T. A., Pattengale, P. K. and Leder, P. (1984). Spontaneous mammary adenocarcinomas in transgenic mice that carry and express MMTV/myc fusion genes. *Cell*, **38**, 627–637

89. Gallick, G. E., Kurzrock, R., Kloetzer, W. S., Arlinghaus, R. B. and Gotterman, J. V. (1985). Expression of p21 ras in fresh primary and metastatic human colorectal tumors. *Proc. Natl. Acad. Sci. USA*, **82**, 1795–1799

90. Viola, M. V., Fromowitz, F., Oravez, S., Deb, S. and Schlom, J. (1985). Ras oncogene p21 expression is increased in premalignant lesions and high grade bladder carcinoma. *J. Exp. Med.*, **161**, 1213–1216

91. Gerosa, M. A., Tolarico, D., Fagnani, C., Raimondi, E., Calombatti, N., Tridente, G., De Carli, L. and Della Valle, G. (1989). Overexpression of N-ras oncogene and epidermal growth factor receptor gene in human glioblastoma. *J. Natl. Cancer Inst.*, **81**, 63–68

92. Stacey, D. W. and Kung, H. F. (1984). Transformation of NIH3T3 cells by microinjection of Ha-ras p21 protein. *Nature*, **310**, 508–511

93. Kung, H. F., Smith, M. R., Bekesi, E., Manne, V. and Stacey, D. W. (1986). Reversal of transformed phenotype by monoclonal antibodies against H-ras. *Exp. Cell. Res.*, **162**, 363–371

94. Mulcahy, L. S., Smith, M. R. and Stacey, D. W. (1985). Requirement for ras proto-oncogene function during serum-stimulated growth of NIH3T3 cells. *Nature*, **313**, 241–243

95. Bar-Sagi, D. and Feramisco, J. R. (1985). Microinjection of the ras oncogene protein into PC12 cells induces morphological differentiation. *Cell*, **42**, 841–848

96. Asseline, U., Delarue, M., Lancelot, G., Toulmé, F., Thuong, N. T., Montenay-Garestier, T. and Hélène, C. (1984). Nucleic acid-binding molecules with high affinity and base sequence specificity: Intercalating agents covalently linked to oligodeoxynucleotides. *Proc. Natl. Acad. Sci. USA*, **81**, 3297–3301

97. Toulmé, J. J., Krish, M. M., Loreau, N., Thuong, N. T. and Hélène, C. (1986). Specific inhibition of mRNA translation by complementary oligonucleotides covalently linked to intercalating agents. *Proc. Natl. Acad. Sci. USA*, **83**, 1227–1231

98. Saison-Behmoaras, T., Tocqué, B., Rey, I., Chassignol, M. Thuong, N. T. and Hélène, C. (1991). Short modified antisense oligonucleotides directed against Haras point mutation induce selective cleavage of the mRNA and inhibit T24 cells proliferation. *EMBO J.*, **10**, 1111–1118

99. Minshull, J. and Hunt, T. (1986). The use of single stranded DNA and RNase H to promote quantitative hybrid arrest of translation of mRNA/DNA hybrids in reticulocyte lysate cell-free translations. *Nucleic Acids Res.*, **14**, 6433–6445

100. Cazenave, C., Loreau, N., Thuong, N. T., Toulmé, J. J. and Hélène, C. (1987). Enzymatic amplification of translation inhibition of rabbit β globin mRNA mediated by anti-messenger oligodeoxynucleotides covalently linked to intercalating agents. *Nucleic Acids Res.*, **15**, 4717–4736

101. Gewirtz, A. M., Giovanni, A., Venturelli, D., Valpreda, S., Sims, R. and Calabretta, B. (1989). G1/S transition in normal human T-lymphocytes requires the nuclear protein encoded by c-myb. *Science*, **245**, 180–183

102. Harel-Bellan, A., Durum, S., Muegge, K., Abbas, A. K. and Farrar, W. L. (1988). Specific inhibition of lymphokine biosynthesis and autocrine growth using antisense oligodeoxynucleotides in Th 1 and Th 2 helper T cell clones. *J. Exp. Med.*, **168**, 2309–2318

103. Becker, D., Meier, C. B. and Herlyn, M. (1989). Proliferation of human malignant melanomas is inhibited by antisense oligodeoxynucleotides targeted against basic fibroblast growth factor. *EMBO J.*, **8**, 3685–3691

104. Blake, K. R., Murakami, A., Spitz, S. A., Glave, S. A., Reddy, M. P., Ts'o, P. O. P. and Miller, P.S. (1985). Hybridization arrest of globin synthesis in rabbit reticulocyte lysates and cells by oligodeoxyribonucleoside methylphosphonates. *Biochemistry*, **24**, 6139–6145

105. Miller, P. S., Agris, C.H., Aurelian, L., Blake, K. R., Murakami, A., Reddy, M. P., Spitz, S. A. and Ts'o, P.O.P. (1985). Control of ribonucleic acid function by oligonucleoside methylphosphonates. *Biochimie*, **67**, 769–776

106. Marcus-Sekura, C. J., Woerner, A. M., Shinozuka, K., Zon, G. and Quinnan, G. V. J. R. (1987). Comparative inhibition of chloramphenicol acetyltransferase gene expression by antisense oligonucleotide analogues having alkyl phosphotriester, methylphosphonate and phosphorotiate linkages. *Nucleic Acids Res.*, **15**, 5749–5763

107. Cazenave, C., Stein, C. A., Loreau, N., Thuong, N. T., Neckers, L. M., Subasinghe, C., Hélène, C., Cohen, J. S. and Toulmé, J. J. (1989). Comparative inhibition of rabbit globin mRNA translation by modified antisense oligodeoxynucleotides. *Nucleic Acids Res.*, **17**, 4255–4273

108. Mori, K., Boiziau, C., Cazenave, C., Matsuku, M., Subasinghe, C., Cohen, J. S., Broder, S., Toulmé, J. J. and Stein, C. A. (1989). Phosphoroselenoate oligodeoxynucleotides: synthesis, physico chemical characterization, anti-sense inhibitory properties and anti-HIV activity. *Nucleic Acids Res.*, **17**, 8207–8209

109. Jager, A., Levy, M. J. and Hecht, S. M. (1988). Oligonucleotide N alkylphosphoramidates: Synthesis and binding to polynucleotides. *Biochemistry*, **27**, 7237–7246

110. Drill, W. K. D., Tang, J. Y., Ma, Y. X. and Caruthers, M. H. (1989). Synthesis of oligodeoxynucleoside phosphorodithiates via thioamidites. *J. Am. Chem. Soc.*, **111**, 2321–2322

111. Thuong, N. T., Asseline, U., Roig, V., Takasugi, M. and Hélène, C. (1987). Oligo (alphadeoxynucleotides) covalently linked to intercalating agents: differential binding to ribo and deoxyribopolynucleotides and stability towards nuclease digestion. *Proc. Natl. Acad. Sci. USA*, **84**, 5129–5133

112. Morvan, F., Rayner, B., Imbach, J. L., Thenet, S., Bertrand, J. R., Paoletti, J., Malvy, C. and Paoletti, C. (1987). Alpha-DNA 11. Synthesis of unnatural α-anomeric oligodeoxyribonucleotides containing the four unusual bases and study of their substrate activity for nucleases. *Nucleic Acids Res.*, **15**, 3421–3437

113. Yu, Z., Chen, D., Black, R. J., Blake, K., Tso, P. O. P., Miller, P. and Chang, E. H. (1989). Sequence specific inhibition of in vitro translation of mutated or normal ras p 21. *J. Exp. Pathol.*, **4**, 97–108

114. Chang, E. H., Yu, Z., Shinozuka, J., Zon, G., Wilson, W. D. and Strekowska, A. (1989). Comparative inhibition of ras p21 protein synthesis with phosphorus-modified antisense oligonucleotides. *Anti-cancer Drug Design*, **4**, 221–232

115. Brown, D., Yu, Z., Miller, P., Blake, K., Wei, C., Kung, H. F., Black, R. J., Ts'o, P .O .P. and Chang, E. (1989). Modulation of ras expression by anti-sense non ionic deoxyoligonucleotide analogs. *Oncogene Res.*, **4**, 243–252

116. Reed, J. C., Stein, C. Y., Subasinghe, C., Haldar, S., Croce, C. M., Yum, S. and Cohen, J. (1990). Antisense-mediated inhibition of BCL 2 Protooncogene expression and leukemic cell

growth and survival: comparisons of phosphodiester and phosphorothioate oligo-deoxynucleotides. *Cancer Res.*, **50**, 6565–6570

117. Stein, C. A., Mori, K., Loke, S. L., Subasinghe, S., Shinozuka, K., Cohen, J. A. and Neckers, L. M. (1988). Phosphorothioate and normal oligodeoxynucleotides with 5'-linked acridine: characterization and preliminary kinetics of cellular uptake. *Gene*, **72**, 333–341

118. Loke, S. L., Stein, C. A., Zhang, X. H., Mori, K., Nakanishi, M., Subasinghe, C., Cohen, J. C. and Neckers, L.M. (1989). Characterization of oligonucleotide transport into living cells. *Proc. Natl. Acad. Sci. USA*, **86**, 3474–3478.

119. Yakubov, L. A., Deeva, E. A., Zarytova, V. F., Ivanova, E., Ryte, A. S., Yurchenko, L. V. and Vlassov, V. V. (1989). Mechanism of oligonucleotide uptake by cells: Involvement of specific receptors. *Proc. Natl. Acad. Sci. USA*, **86**, 6454–6458

120. Rabbitts, T. H. and Rabbitts, P. H. (1989). Molecular pathology of chromosomal abnormalities and cancer genes in human tumors. In Glover, D. M. and Hames, B. D. (eds.) *Oncogenes*, pp. 67–102. (New York: Oxford University Press)

121. Rosolen, A., Whitesell, L., Ikegaki, N., Kennett, R. H. and Neckers, L. (1990). Antisense inhibition of single copy N-myc expression results in decreased cell growth without reduction of c-myc protein in a neuroepithelioma cell line. *Cancer Res.*, **50**, 6316–6322

122. Whitesell, L., Rosolen, A., and Neckers, L. M (1991). *In vivo* modulation of N-myc expression by continous perfusion with an antisense oligonucletide.*Antisense Res. Devel.*, **1**, 343–350

123. Leonetti, J. P., Machy, P., Degols, G., Lebleu, B. and Leserman, L. (1990). Antibody-targeted liposomes containing oligo ribonucleotides complementary to viral RNA selectively inhibit viral replication. *Proc. Natl. Acad. Sci. USA*, **87**, 2448–2451

124. Letsinger, R. L, Zhang, G., Sun, D. K., Ikeuchi, T. and Sarin, P. S. (1989). Cholesteryl-conjugated oligonucleoides: Synthesis, properties and activity as inhibitors of replication of human immunodeficiency virus in cell culture. *Proc. Natl. Acad. Sci. USA*, **86**, 6553–6556

125. Knorre, D. G., Vlassov, V. V. and Zarytova, V. F. (1989). Oligonucleotides linked to reactive groups in Cohen, J.S. (ed.) *Oligodeoxynucleotides Antisense Inhibitors of Gene Expression*, pp 173–210. (London: MacMillan Press)

126. Hélène, C. and Toulmé, J. J. (1990). Specific regulation of gene expression by antisense, sense and antigene nucleic acids. *Biochim. Biophys. Acta*, **1049**, 99–125

127. Hélène, C. (1991). The anti-gene strategy: Control of gene expression by triplex-forming oligonucleotides. *Anti-Cancer Drug Design*, **6**, 569–584

128. Maher, L. J. III., Wold, B. and Dervan, P. B. (1989). Inhibition of DNA binding proteins by oligonucleotide-directed triple helix formation. *Science*, **245**, 725–730

129. François, J. C., Saison-Behmoaras, T., Thuong, N. T. and Hélène, C. (1989). Inhibition of restriction endonuclease cleavage via triple helix formation by homopyrimidine oligonucleotides. *Biochemistry*, **28**, 9617–9619

130. Cooney, M., Czernuszewicz, G., Postel, E. H., Flint, S. J. and Hogan, M. E. (1988). Site specific oligonucleotide binding represses transcription of the human c-myc gene in vitro. *Science*, **241**, 456–459

131. Hélène, C., Thuong, N. T., Saison-Behmoaras, T. and François, J. C. (1989). Sequence specific artificial endonucleases. *Trends Biotechnol.*, **7**, 310–315

132. Praseuth, D., Perrouault, L., LeDoan, T., Chassignol, M., Thuong, N. T. and Hélène, C. (1988). Sequence specific binding and photocrosslinking of α and β oligodeoxynucleotides to the major groove of DNA via triple helix formation. *Proc. Natl. Acad. Sci. USA*, **85**, 1349–1353

133. Praseuth, D., Le Doan, T., Chassignol, M., Decout, J. L., Habhoub, N., L'homme, J., Thuong, N. T. and Hélène, C. (1988). Sequence-targeted photosensitized reactions in nucleic acids by oligo-[α]-deoxynucleotides and oligo-[β]-deoxynucleotides covalently linked to proflavin. *Biochemistry*, **27**, 3031–3037

134. Le Doan, T., Perrouault, L., Prazeuth, D., Habhoub, N., Decout, J. L., Thuong, N. T., L'homme, J. and Hélène, C. (1987). Sequence specific recognition, photocrosslinking and cleavage of the DNA double helix by an oligo-[α]-thymidylate covalently linked to an azidoproflavine derivative. *Nucleic Acids Res.*, **15**, 7749–7760

Index